Immunoassay:
Laboratory Analysis
and Clinical Applications

Immunoassay: Laboratory Analysis and Clinical Applications

Edited by

James P. Gosling, Ph.D., H.Dip.Ed.

Statutory Lecturer, Department of Biochemistry, and
Consultant, National Diagnostic Centre, University College
Galway, Ireland

Lawrence V. Basso, M.D., F.A.C.P.

Clinical Associate Professor, Stanford University
School of Medicine, and Division of Endocrinology/Nuclear
Medicine, Palo Alto Medical Foundation, Palo Alto,
California

Butterworth–Heinemann
Boston   London   Singapore   Sydney   Toronto   Wellington

Cover Design by Marcus Gosling

Every effort has been made to ensure that the drug dosage schedules within this text are accurate and conform to standards accepted at time of publication. However, as treatment recommendations vary in the light of continuing research and clinical experience, the reader is advised to verify drug dosage schedules herein with information found on product information sheets. This is especially true in cases of new or infrequently used drugs.

Library of Congress Cataloging-in-Publication Data

Immunoassay : laboratory analysis and clinical applications / [edited by] James P. Gosling and Lawrence V. Basso.
    p. cm.
Includes bibliographical references and index.
ISBN 0-7506-9256-1
1. Immunoassay.   I. Gosling, James P. II. Basso, Lawrence V.
    [DNLM: 1. Immunoassay. QW 570 I326 1994]
QP519.9.I42I436 1994
616.07'56—dc20
DNLM/DLC
for Library of Congress   94-7400
                                           CIP

British Library Cataloguing-in-Publication Data.
A catalogue record for this book is available from the British Library.

Butterworth–Heinemann
313 Washington Street
Newton, MA 02158–1626

10 9 8 7 6 5 4 3 2 1

Printed in the United States of America

CONTENTS

CONTRIBUTING AUTHORS

Wajdi Georges Abdul-Ahad,
B.Pharm., M.Sc. (Clin Bio), Ph.D.
Principal Scientist, Beckman Instruments, Brea, California

Rukhsana Ahsan, Ph.D.
Principal Scientific Officer, Department of Chemical Pathology and WHO CCR for Immunoassays, Hammersmith Hospital, London, UK

Bruno Barenton, Ph.D.
Research Director, INRA Centre de Montpellier, France

Lawrence Basso, M.D., F.A.C.P.
Clinical Associate Professor of Medicine and Radiology (Nuclear Medicine), Stanford University School of Medicine and Divisions of Endocrinology and Nuclear Medicine, Palo Alto Medical Foundation, Palo Alto, California

Arthor Bobrove, M.D.
Clinical Professor of Medicine, Stanford University School of Medicine and Chief, Division of Rheumatology, Palo Alto Medical Foundation, Palo Alto, California

Penelope M. Clarke, Ph.D.
Consultant Clinical Scientist, The Endocrine Department, The Womens Hospital, Birmingham, UK

Sheldon Davidson, M.D.
Associate Clinical Professor, Department of Medicine, UCLA School of Medicine, Los Angeles, California

Mary I Forsling, Ph.D.
Reader in Reproductive Physiology, United Medical and Dental Schools, St. Thomas's Campus, London, UK

Patrick F. Fottrell, Ph.D., D.Sc., M.R.I.A.
Head, Department of Biochemistry and Director, National Diagnostic Research Centre, University College Galway, Ireland

James P. Gosling, Ph.D., H.Dip.Ed.
Statutory Lecturer, Department of Biochemistry and Consultant, National Diagnostic Research Centre, University College Galway, Ireland

Marian Kane, Ph.D., H.Dip.Ed.
Senior Scientist, Immunodiagnostics, National Diagnostic Centre, University College Galway, Ireland

Wieland Kiess, M.D.
Head, Department of Pediatric Endocrinology and Diabetes, Justus Liebig University, Childrens' Hospital, Giessen, Germany

Randolph Linde, M.D.
Clinical Associate Professor of Medicine, Stanford University School of Medicine, and Chief, Division of Endocrinology, Palo Alto Medical Foundation, Palo Alto, California

James H. McBride, Ph.D.
Professor of Chemical Pathology, Department of Pathology, UCLA School of Medicine, Los Angeles, California

Jacob V. Micallef, Ph.D.
Principal Scientific Officer, Department of Chemical Pathology and WHO CCR for Immunoassays, Hammersmith Hospital, London, UK

Michael Power, Ph.D.
College Lecturer, University College Galway, Ireland

Stella Quan, Ph.D.
Associate Director, Diagnostic Division, Chiron Corporation, Berkeley, California

Robert Stebbins, M.D.
Clinical Professor of Medicine, Stanford University School of Medicine, Stanford, California

PREFACE

Without immunoassays the detection or measurement of many clinically important analytes would be much more expensive or even impracticable. Present rates of routine measurements of protein analytes such as the pituitary hormones, apoliproteins or tumor markers, would be impossible.

The early history of the development of immunoassays paralleled the first growth of immunology, but two major inventions have provided much of the impetus: namely, the invention in the late 1950s of limited-reagent, labeled-analyte immunoassays in the laboratories of Rosaleen Yalow and Roger Ekins, and the development in the 1970s of reagent excess immunometric assays by Leif Wide and others. These were truly important scientific advances with far reaching consequences for basic investigations as well as routine applications.

Immunoassay: Laboratory Analysis and Clinical Applications, which was Larry Basso's idea, represents a new departure for single-volume books on immunoassay. While the basic principles and procedures are explained in some detail, this book is primarily concerned with the use and usefulness of immunoassays. It has been designed for both the student of medicine or science with some knowledge of immunology and for the established practitioner of immunoassays. It may prove invaluable to clinical and research scientists and technicians, to clinicians in the relevant specialties, and particularly to commercial specialists developing and validating new or improved immunoassays.

The first four chapters (Introduction to Immunoassay, Reagent Preparation, Immunoassay Development, and Quality Assurance) describe the principal general features of immunoassays and their use. The remaining 14 chapters are concerned with disorders of the endocrine systems (Chapters 5 to 11), blood (Chapter 12), and the immune system (Chapters 13 and 15), with cardiology (Chapter 14), oncology (Chapter 16), infectious diseases (Chapter 17), and pharmacology (Chapter 18). The chapter authors are experts in their fields who have had to work hard to introduce their specialties and to provide comprehensive information on diseases, the roles of immunoassays and diagnostic difficulties, all within strict space limits. These reviews clearly indicate where profound changes with respect to method formats, purity, and selectivity of reagents and the most relevant analytes may occur in the near future.

Both simple and high-performance nonradioisotopic assays are becoming more widespread, multianalyte assays and automated workstations are increasingly important, and reagent excess sandwich assays have almost completely displaced "competitive" assays for some analytes (Chapter 1). Reagent quality is improving, with better standardized calibrants and better characterized antigen preparations (Chapter

2 and throughout text). Some antigens for specific antibody determination are now produced by recombinant DNA methods. In addition, new analytes with greater diagnostic relevance are steadily appearing. For example, insulin-like growth factors (IGFs) for growth disorders, etc. (Chapter 6), renin subforms for the detection of diabetic nephropathy and disorders of the renin-angiotensin-aldosterone axis (Chapter 7), osteocalcin and other markers of bone turnover for the detection and monitoring of osteoporosis (Chapter 10), and cardiac-specific troponin isoforms for the early confirmation of myocardial infarction (Chapter 14).

However, the greatest challenge facing immunoassay methodology is the need to steadily and continuously improve the comparability of the results for the same analyte obtained with assays carried out at different times, in different laboratories, and with different assay kits. The degree to which comparability or standardization is deficient depends on the analyte, but for nearly all analytes substantial improvements are feasible. Improved comparability will greatly enhance the value of studies relating analyte levels to other physiologic or disease parameters, will enable more reliable reference ranges to be established, will improve confidence in clinical laboratory analyses and, because of all of these, will contribute to better wellbeing and health in the community. We hope that this book will support, if only in a small way, this process of improvement.

ACKNOWLEDGMENTS

The editors first of all wish to thank the contributors for participating in this project with enthusiasm and patience in the face of extreme provocation from the editors' knife.

J. P. G. wishes to acknowledge the support of University College Galway (UCG), the National Diagnostic Centre of Bioresearch Ireland, UCG, Galway, and the Station de Physiologie de la Reproduction, INRA Centre de Rescherches de Tours, France, for services and material support during the course of this work. He also wishes to thank Larry Basso for inviting him to participate in preparing this book and Professor Patrick F. Fottrell, Department of Biochemistry, UCG, for advice and encouragement. Finally, but not least, he thanks his partner Elizabeth for the good example that she set and for her cooperation.

L. V. B. wishes to acknowledge the support of the Palo Alto Medical Foundation. He thanks Dr. I. Ross McDougall and Dr. Michael Goris, both of the Division of Nuclear Medicine of Stanford University for asking him to teach a course on immunoassays, thereby providing ongoing stimulation for this project. Finally, a special thank you to his family for support, encouragement, and patience.

The advice and criticism of the many colleagues who read individual, or groups of, chapters is very much appreciated, including Dr. Ernest Egan, Consultant Hematologist, University College Hospital, Galway; Dr. Brendan Fitzpatrick, Consultant Immunologist, University College Hospital, Galway; Dr. Helen Grimes, Chief Biochemist, University College Hospital, Galway; Mr. Anthony O'Connor, Department of Biochemistry, UCG; Dr. Malachy J. McKenna, Consultant Endocrinologist, St. Vincent's Hospital, Dublin; Dr. T. Joseph McKenna, Consultant Endocrinologist, St. Vincent's Hospital, Dublin; Dr. John O'Connor, Consultant Endocrinologist, University College Hospital, Galway; Mr. John Ryan, Chief Technologist, Department of Immunology, University College Hospital, Galway; Dr. John Seth, Senior Lecturer, Department of Clinical Chemistry, University of Edinburgh; Dr. William D. McKee, Consultant in Allergy and Immunology, Palo Alto Medical Foundation and Stanford University; Dr. Randolph B. Linde, Consultant in Endocrinology, Palo Alto Medical Foundation and Stanford University; Dr. Maurice Fox, Consultant in Endocrinology, Palo Alto Medical Foundation and Stanford University; Dr. John F. Scholer, Consultant in Nuclear Medicine and the Clinical Laboratory, Palo Alto Medical Foundation.

CHAPTER 1

Introduction to Immunoassay

James P. Gosling

"Protein binding assay" and "saturation analysis" describe analytic methods dependent on the specific recognition of the analyte by a binding protein. While there are many kinds of high-affinity specific binding proteins in nature (hormone receptors, for example), the special properties of antibodies have made them the most popular choice for such methods. Measurement procedures that use antibodies as specific reagents are termed *immunoassays,* as are assays that use antigens for the determination of specific antibodies.

Because of the extraordinary affinity, specificity and variety of antibody-antigen binding reactions, immunoassays have become essential routine and research tools throughout the biologic sciences, particularly in clinical analysis.

THE ANTIBODY BINDING SITE

Immunoglobulin G

IgG, the class of antibody used predominantly in immunoassays, is a 150,000 mol wt glycoprotein composed of two identical heavy (H, ~ 420 residues) and two identical light (L, ~ 215 residues) polypeptide chains (Fig. 1–1). The diversity of sequences in the variable regions gives rise to the multiplicity of specific IgG antibodies. The remainder of the H chains toward the C-terminals are generally constant within an Ig class and animal species, and the differential functions of each Ig class are determined by structural features in their constant regions (see Table 17–1 for the properties of the Ig classes). L chains in any Ig class can be λ or κ, each having a characteristic, constant sequence toward the C-terminal.

Antibody Diversity

The diversity in the variable region sequences of antibodies, required for the enormous range of binding specificities observed, is generated in B cells by two comple-

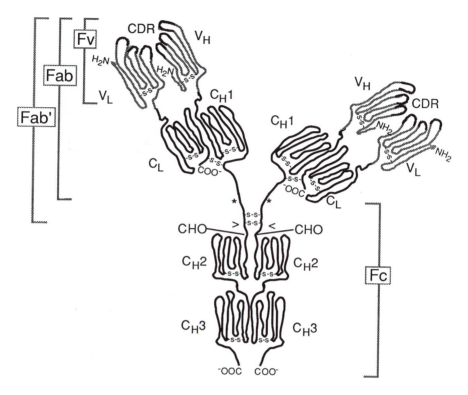

Figure 1.1.   This diagrammatic representation of an IgG molecule is designed to emphasize: (1) that it is made up of six distinct, but structurally analogous globular domains, with the "base" and the "arms" connected by long "tethers" in what has been usually referred to as the hinge region; and (2) its flexibility. It may sometimes be approximately Y- or T-shaped but can assume an extraordinarily large variety of three-dimensional shapes. In addition, the interdomain regions, particularly of the arms, are also flexible (Harris et al., 1992).

The six domains are $2 \times V_L/V_H$, $2 \times C_L/C_H1$, C_H2/C_H2 and C_H3/C_H3, where V indicates variable, C constant, H heavy chain, and L light chain. The V_L/V_H domains, consisting of the approximately 110 residues from the N-terminals of both the H and L chains, constitute the variable regions which contain the two identical binding sites in the intact IgG. The V_L/V_H domains, equivalent to Fv fragments, are shown in gray except for the hypervariable segments making up the complementarity determining regions (CDR) of the binding sites, which are shown in black. The constant domains C_L/C_H1, C_H2/C_H2, and C_H3/C_H3 are also shown in black.

The approximate locations of the sites susceptible to cleavage by papain (*), which is used to prepare Fab and Fc fragments, and to cleavage by pepsin ($<$, $>$), which is used to prepare $F(ab')_2$ and Fab' fragments, are indicated. Compared with Fab, each Fab' has about eight extra residues at the new C-terminal, including at least one free cysteine. The Fv fragment, a ~25,000 mol wt heterodimer of the variable regions of the H and L chains, is the smallest antibody fragment that contains a complete binding site. It is extremely difficult to prepare Fv by proteolytic digestion from most antibodies, but Fv and single-chain Fv, in which the H and L chain sections are joined by an artificial linker peptide, can be prepared by recombinant DNA methods (Huston, et al., 1993).

mentary mechanisms: (1) the shuffling and splicing of multiple variants of genes coding for the segments of the variable regions of the L and H chains and (2) facilitated mutations in the assembled variable region genes which results in the generation of antibodies with progressively improved affinity and specificity of binding. The assembled genes coding for H-chain variable regions are initially joined to genes coding for constant regions of μ chains so that the initial immune response is the secretion of IgM class antibodies. Subsequently, the same section of DNA that coded for the μ-chain variable region recombines with gene segments coding for γ, α, ε, or δ constant regions to give rise to cell lines synthesizing IgG, IgA, IgE, or IgD class antibodies. This is called *class switching* and is an essential aspect of the tailoring of the immune response to meet different kinds of infectious threat.

IgG antibodies occur as subclasses in humans (IgG1, IgG2, IgG3, IgG4), mice (IgG1, IgG2a, IgG2b, IgG3), rats (IgG1, IgG2a, IgG2b, IgG2c) and other species, each IgG subclass molecule containing the corresponding H chain ($\gamma1$, $\gamma2a$ etc.). In a total polyclonal response to immunization the proportions of the specific IgGs belonging to the different subclasses may be influenced by the type of antigen, route of immunization, and the state of health, age, and strain of the animal. The genes coding for the H chain classes and subclasses are thought to have arisen from the gene for a common H chain, which developed through duplication of a primitive gene for the L chain, which arose in turn from duplication of the gene for a 110-residue "proto-immunoglobulin." (Some other aspects of the humoral immune response are described in Chap. 17.)

Investigations of Binding

X-ray crystallographic studies of complexes between antibody fragments and antigens or haptens are contributing greatly to the understanding of the factors that contribute to the affinity and specificity of such binding. Haptens are molecules of limited molecular weight, which are not naturally antigenic, but when conjugated to protein (e.g., bovine serum albumin [BSA], with 20 to 30 hapten molecules per molecule of BSA) yield an immunogen which can be used to generate antibodies that specifically bind free haptens. When an antibody is complexed with its specific hapten, the hapten is generally found to be located in a pocket, cavity or groove at the antibody binding site, surrounded by functional groups of the peptide residues and backbone that are structurally complementary to the adjacent portions of the hapten molecule. In contrast, when an antibody is complexed with the antigenic determinant region (epitope) of its specific protein antigen, the apparent area of close contact is

---

IgG is a glycoprotein because of the carbohydrate (CHO) chains attached via serine residues on the H chains in the C_H2/C_H2 domain. The disulfhydryl bonds making intrachain links in each domain, and in the hinge region, linking L chains to H chains and H chain to H chain are shown as -S-S-. The base of the IgG molecule, consisting of the C_H2/C_H2 and C_H3/C_H3 domains, has a range of essential biologic functions including binding sites for complement and macrophage receptors.

usually very large, being up to 6 nm^2 (600A^2) with about 20 amino acid residues on both reactants apparently participating. Within the large area of contact there may be clefts to accommodate projecting side chains on the antigen, or vice versa. In all antibody-hapten or antibody-antigen complexes the contact is close, with often no room between the two interacting molecules to accommodate water or other small molecules. Such studies, discussed in detail by Day (1990) and Sutton (1993), are of fundamental importance as to how immunoassays are viewed, because they can be used to explore to what extent complete specificity can be regarded as even theoretically feasible. For example, Arevalo, et al. (1993) carried out a comparative analysis of the x-ray structures of five different steroids in complex with the Fab^1 fragment of an antiprogesterone antibody. They found that some of the steroids crossreacted by adopting a different binding orientation of the steroid skeleton that placed the A-Ring in an alternative "pocket" in the antibody binding site. Therefore, the binding of specific hapten and crossreactants is much more haphazard than might have been expected. Alternatively, amino acid residues in antibody binding sites may be characterized by testing the effects on binding of specific chemical modifications (Gudmundsson, et al., (1993).

The interaction of antibody and antigen must also be characterized by means of kinetic studies, in which binding is monitored with respect to time and at different concentrations of antigen or antibody. Such investigations are greatly aided by real-time biospecific interaction analysis (BIA) with the BIAcore instrument (Pharmacia, Uppsala, Sweden) (Malmquist, 1993).

The binding site of an antibody can be further characterized by cross-reactivity studies, by which the ability of each of a range of substances, structurally related to the antigen/hapten, to inhibit the binding of labeled antigen/hapten is investigated. Cross-reaction studies and two-site inhibition binding studies with collections of monoclonal antibodies can be used to "map" the surfaces of large protein antigens (Bidart, 1993) and such investigations are important in the selection of pairs of antibodies for use in immunometric assays.

NOMENCLATURE AND CLASSIFICATION

Naming Immunoassays

The nomenclature of immunoassay systems is confusing to anyone wishing to understand the similarities between different assays as well as the diversity of their designs. In general, most assay names contain *immuno,* the combining form of the adjective 'immune', and another combining word indicating the type of label employed along with the word *assay,* for example, radioimmunoassay (RIA). If receptor is employed rather than antibody the corresponding name is radioreceptor assay. Much of the variety in names comes from the numerous labeling substances that have been exploited. These substances include (with common combining forms in parentheses) radioisotopes (*radio*), enzymes (*enzymo* or *enzyme*), and fluorescent (*fluoro*), chemiluminescent and bioluminescent compounds (*lumino*).

The above names usually refer to limited-reagent, competitive assays; reagent excess assays are commonly distinguished by reversing the order of the combining forms, as an immunoradiometric assay (IRMA), immunofluorometric assay (IFMA), or immunoenzymometric assay (IEMA). The term immunometric assay is used to refer to reagent excess assays in general. However, similar names are sometimes used for competitive assays with labeled antibody. Enzyme-linked immunosorbent assay (ELISA) is used for all kinds of assays with enzymatic labels and cannot be relied upon to indicate a particular assay mechanism. In general, enzyme immunoassay (EIA) is to be preferred for assays equivalent to RIA and IEMA for assays equivalent to IRMA.

Representing Assay Complexes in Text

Most complexes associated with individual assay systems can readily be represented by one-line formulae, and such a system of notation will be used in this text when appropriate. For emphasis the analyte is shown in bold print (e.g., **Ag**, **Ha**, or **Ab** for the general analytes antigen, hapten and antibody, respectively), the hyphen ("-") sign represents associations established before commencement of the assay (e.g., conjugations or the coating of antibody on a solid phase), and the en dash (–) represents associations formed during the course of the assay procedure. Unusual components are accommodated by spelling out their names. For example, the final complex of a solid phase (sp) IEMA for an antigen in which biotin is used as the primary label could be described as sp-Ab–**Ag**–Ab-biotin–avidin-enzyme. Standard abbreviations are used when the class (IgG, IgM) or type of antibody (monoclonal, mAb) or antibody fragment (Fab′, F[ab′]$_2$) or its origin (mouse, M; rabbit, R; goat, G; sheep, S) is relevant.

Antibody Occupancy Principle

Most binding assays, including immunoassays, employing a label can be put into one of two categories, depending on whether at the end of the assay the label is:

1. Associated with antibody-antigen complexes not containing the analyte, for example, in limited-reagent or competitive solid phase fluoroimmunoassay (FIA) the two possible final complexes are sp-Ab–Ag-fluor and sp-Ab–**Ag**
2. Associated with the complexes containing the analyte, for example, in a reagent excess sandwich IEMA the final complex is sp-Ab–**Ag**–Ab-enzyme

In other words, and according to the antibody occupancy principle (Ekins and Chu, 1991), when an immunoassay relies on the observation of binding sites *unoccupied* by analyte, the total number of sites available must be small to minimize error in the (indirect) estimation of *occupied* sites (reagent-limited assays); but when an immunoassay depends on the observation of sites *occupied* by analyte, errors may be minimized by the use of relatively large numbers of sites (reagent-excess assays).

However, when the total number of sites is very small and the volume of analyte is large, the binding of analyte does not significantly change the total concentration of analyte. More importantly, the fractional occupancy of the sites is independent of site concentration but directly dependent on analyte concentration (Fig. 1–2). Assays dependent on this principle have been called ambient analyte immunoassays. Such assays, which are still at an early stage of development and have not yet been applied to routine clinical measurements, may be configured whereby the occupancy of binding sites by analyte is observed directly or indirectly (Ekins and Chu, 1991).

Classifying Immunoassays

Since I informally classified immunoassays by sorting them into six groups (Gosling, 1990), other more systematic approaches (Miyai, 1991; Masseyeff, 1992) have been published. Moreover, in the last 3 years new assay systems have been proposed or

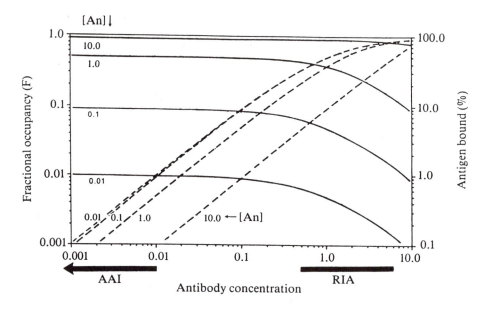

Figure 1.2.   Fractional antibody binding-site occupancy (F) plotted as a function of antibody binding-site concentration for different values of antigen (analyte) concentration (An) (left-hand ordinate, ____). The percentage binding of antigen to antibody, at the same antigen concentrations, is also shown (right-hand ordinate, ------). To make this graph applicable to any antibody, all concentrations are expressed in units of $1/K$, where K is the equilibrium association constant of the antibody in question, so that 1.0 concentration unit of antibody or analyte equals 10^{-10} mol·L^{-1} if the antibody has a K of 10^{10} L·mol^{-1}. For antibody concentrations of less than 0.01 units ($<10^{-12}$ mol·L^{-1} for the above antibody), the percentage binding of antibody is less than 1% and fractional binding-site occupancy is essentially unaffected by very large variations in antibody concentration, being governed solely by antigen concentration. Note also that limited-reagent immunoassays such as RIA are commonly designed with antibody concentrations of from 0.5 to 5 units to give greater than 30% binding of label at antigen concentrations tending to zero. Reproduced with permission from Ekins and Chu (1991).

their potential importance has become more evident. Presently, four main types of immunoassay are evident (Table 1–1), namely precipitation and other assays that generally use nothing that could be called a label, reagent excess assays, limited-reagent assays, and ambient analyte assays.

1. Precipitation Assays

The first immunoassays were precipitation assays developed in the early half of this century as methods for characterizing the interactions of antibodies and antigens. Assays placed in this group include precipitation, nephelometric and turbidimetric immunoassays, gel diffusion assays, immunoelectrophoresis, complement fixation assays, particle or cell agglutination assays, and particle counting immunoassays. In many cases, their endpoints involve the direct detection of insoluble immune complexes ($[Ab–\mathbf{Ag}]_n$ or $[\mathbf{Ab}–Ag]_n$).

Immunoprecipitation Assays. In the classic liquid phase immunoprecipitation assay for antigen or antibody the endpoint is the mass of antibody-antigen complex, determined by weighing or by means of a general protein assay (Tojo, et al., 1988). Al-

Table 1–1 Classification of Immunoassays

Class	*Subclass*	*Examples*
Precipitation	Agglutination	With cells
		With latex particles
	Complement mediated	Complement fixation
	Gel precipitation	Gel diffusion immuno-electrophoresis
	Light interacting	PEG promoted
		Particle enhanced
		Particle counting
		Flow-cytometric
Reagent excess	One-site	Immunostaining
		Western blotting
	Two-site	For antigen
		For antibody
	Selective antibody	For hapten
Reagent limited	Labeled antigen	With separation step
		Separation-free
	Labeled analog	For free analyte
	Labeled antibody	For antigen
		For antibody
		For free analyte
Ambient analyte	Direct	For antigen or antibody
	Indirect	For hapten

PEG, polyethylene glycol.

ternatively, the precipitation may occur in a gel and be readily visible as a precipitin line, as in immunodiffusion and immunoelectrophoretic methods. Another approach is to monitor immune complex formation by nephelometric or turbidimetric techniques (Price and Newman, 1991). Polyethylene glycol is often added to maximize and accelerate precipitin formation and either the "plateau" (representing the maximum degree of complex formation) or, preferably, the rate of complex formation is taken as the endpoint. By means of such assays with specialized automatic nephelometers, or suitable chemical analyzers acting as turbidimeters, a wide range of serum and urinary proteins is determined at concentrations down to 10^{-4} g/L (about 10^{-8} mol/L). Major limitations are their general unsuitability for the quantitation of haptens, their limited analytic ranges, and the requirement for controls and checks to guard against underestimation caused by antigen (or antibody) excess.

Particle-Aided Assays.   Antibody, antigen, or hapten may be coupled to small particles (e.g., latex particles, inorganic colloidal particles, or erythrocytes) to give agglutination, "particle enhanced" or "particle counting" immunoassays. For example, qualitative latex agglutination tests can be carried out on a simple slide without the aid of any instrumentation. Recently a simple fluidic device and ancillary equipment have been developed to allow for the objective determination of the endpoint (Fig. 1–3).

Alternatively, such assays can be performed with the aid of nephelometers or turbidimeters and are now widely employed for the quantitation of specific proteins

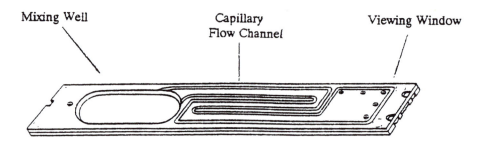

Figure 1.3.   Cambridge Biotech Corporation Recombigen HIV-1/HIV-2 slide immunoassay is a rapid qualitative assay for the detection of antibodies to human immunodeficiency virus type 1 (HIV-1) and/or HIV-2 in human serum or plasma. It is intended as an initial screening test in low-volume testing facilities, in emergencies, and in areas where sophisticated equipment is not available. Two major antigens, $CBre_3$ (from HIV-1) and K_1 (HIV-2), are produced by recombinant DNA technology and coated onto polystyrene latex beads (latex-Ag) to form the basis of a direct latex agglutination assay. The assay is carried out on a special capillary agglutination slide as shown. The slide consists of a well area, for mixing the latex reagent and sample, connected by a capillary flow channel that leads to a viewing window. Samples containing specific antibody (**Ab**) that binds to $CBre_3$ or K_1 cause the antigen-coated latex to agglutinate ($[latex-Ag–\mathbf{Ab}–Ag-latex]_m$) with loss of the milky white appearance of the mixture. Movement of the mixture through the capillary channel enhances specific binding and provides a roughly timed interval before a reading should be taken. The test may also be performed on a special reader unit that gives an objective positive or negative readout result.

and haptens at concentrations down to about $10^{-7}g/L$ (10^{-11} mol/L). Particle counting immunoassays (PACIA) employ special automated instrumentation with the ability to register only particles in a particular size range. Nonspecific interference is minimized by the use of $F(ab')_2$ fragments instead of whole antibodies. There are PACIAs for specific antibodies, for proteins and for haptens, and a PACIA for thyroid stimulating hormone (TSH) with a detection limit of 0.03 mIU/L (about 2×10^{-13} mol/L) has been reported (Wilkins, et al., 1988).

Assays with Complex Biologic Reagents.   Cell agglutination assays resemble latex agglutination assays except that antibody or antigen is immobilized (or is naturally present) on erythrocytes (hemagglutination) or other cells. Complement fixation assays also depend on the use of cells (usually red blood cells) that become lyzed due to the activation of complement, the components of which are supplied by the addition of whole animal serum. While such assays are relatively simple to operate and may require minimal equipment, their principle of operation is not widely applied because their complex biologic reagents are difficult to control and standardize, and are susceptible to degradation during transport and storage. However, they have important roles in blood typing, the diagnosis of hemolytic anemias (see Chap. 12), the identification of bacteria, and testing for the adequacy of the complement system.

2. Reagent-Excess Assays

Assays employing labels in which the principal reagents are used in excess are included in this group. These include immunoblotting and immunohistochemical staining methods as well as two-site sandwich assays such as IRMA, IEMA, IFMA, immunochemiluminometric assay (ICLMA) which have the fundamental advantage that very low detection limits are attainable by maximizing to signal to noise ratio of the label (Ekins and Chu, 1991). However, precautions must be taken that the employment of excess reagents does not lead to high nonspecific binding of label, or degradation of assay specificity (Boscato, et al., 1989). Normally, labeled antibody against the analyte (e.g., Ab-^{125}I) is the principal reagent. To separate bound label (e.g., **Ag**–Ab-^{125}) from free label, any of a range of adsorption or precipitation reagents could be employed, but usually the antigen-label complex is removed by means of excess immobilized antibody which binds to a separate antigenic site on the analyte. This results in the now classic two-site assay complex in which antigen is sandwiched between two antibodies (e.g., sp-Ab–**Ag**–Ab-^{125}I), and plotting the concentration of labeled antibody bound against the concentration of analyte (**Ag**) gives a direct, nonlinear standard curve. Therefore, specificity is determined by the combined selectivity of two antibodies and such assays are observed to be inherently more specific than single-site assays (Seth, et al., 1989). It follows that all candidate analytes for such assays must have two antigenic determinants that can be recognized simultaneously, which excludes simple steroids, small peptides with less than 15 to 20 amino acid residues, and most drugs. The most sensitive of such assays in routine use is capable of detecting less than 1 amole of analyte (Gosling, 1990).

A very large number of variations on the basic two-site sandwich assay for antigen have been described. The most important include the use of alternative labeling

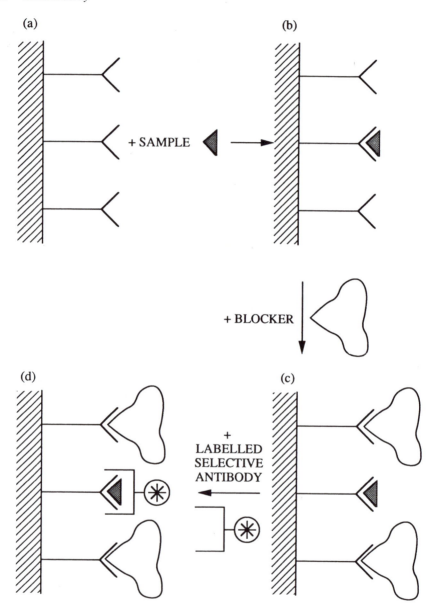

Figure 1.4.   The novel reagent excess assay format for the determination of hapten analytes proposed by Self (1989, 1990). The assay depends on the use of immobilized monoclonal antibody against the analyte (a) to which analyte in the sample can bind (b); next a blocker is added to occupy all free analyte-specific binding sites (c); and finally, labeled antiidiotypic* antibody which can selectively mark the binding sites occupied by analyte is added (d). The blocker envisaged could be a conjugate of hapten and protein, similar to the immunogen used to raise the antianalyte antibody, or an antiidiotypic antibody that can only bind when the binding site of the primary monoclonal antibody is unoccupied by analyte. The labeled antiidio-

substances and indirect labeling, and the use of antibody fragments to decrease non-specific binding. In addition, assay schemes and formulations have been developed which are suitable for a wide variety of applications, from highly sensitive TSH assays to home pregnancy detection kits.

Assays for Haptens.   Because the two-site assays above are unsuitable for analytes with a mol wt less than 200 and because of the inherent limited sensitivity of competitive assays, much effort has been put into the invention of reagent excess assays for haptens. In one such system (Freytag, 1984), analyte is incubated with a calculated *excess* of labeled antibody (usually Fab' or F[ab']₂) and unoccupied labeled antibody is removed by means of excess immobilized analyte before the label associated with analyte is determined. Note that, while the reagents employed here and for labeled-antibody competitive assays may be exactly equivalent, the use of excess label and the determination of the analyte-label complex (**Ha**–Ab-peroxidase, and not immobilized label, sp-Ha–Ab-peroxidase) alter completely the character of the assay. However, it is not apparent that assays of this kind are widely used.

Self (1989, 1990) described a novel alternative assay scheme for the measurement of hapten analytes, in which excess reagents may be used and where the label is associated with the immune complex containing the analyte (Fig. 1–4). This design depends on the use of a blocking reagent to occupy all free analyte–specific binding sites, and on the use of a labeled, suitable antiidiotypic antibody (the selective antibody) to mark the binding sites occupied by analyte (see Fig. 1–4 legend for a definition of antiidiotypic antibody). An equivalent system, but with the "obligatory" use of another antiidiotypic antibody to block the free binding sites, has been described and applied to the determination of estradiol in serum (Barnard, and Kohen, 1980). The major potential advantage of such assays is lower detection limits than with conventional competitive assays. Low nonspecific binding by all reagents would be essential for the achievement of the potentials of these assay schemes, but their major limitation may be the necessity for at least one extra *matched* monoclonal antibody for each assay, which must significantly complicate the process of assay development and validation.

---

typic antibody must be different from the blocker by being capable of binding near occupied binding sites. Both antiidiotypic antibodies are specific for the particular antianalyte monoclonal antibody used. Theoretically, the immobilized monoclonal antibody, the blocker, and the labeled antiidiotypic antibody could all be used in excess to maximize the efficiencies of each step. (This diagram is reproduced with the permission of Professor C. H. Self.)

*An antiidiotypic antibody is an antibody that binds to the variable regions of another (monoclonal) *antibody*. Its site of binding may be anywhere on the variable (idiotypic) regions of the *antibody* and it may or may not block binding of the specific antigen/hapten to the *antibody* or vice versa. Occasionally the binding site of the antiidiotypic antibody closely resembles, in terms of shape and charge distribution, the epitope on the antigen to which the *antibody* binds. Antiidiotypic antibodies are normally monoclonal and are raised by immunizing mice with a specific monoclonal *antibody* and selecting consequent hybridoma cells secreting antibodies that do not bind to other monoclonal antibodies produced by the same strain of mice, and do (or do not) inhibit the binding of antigen/hapten to the original *antibody*.

Assays for Antibodies.   Almost all routine immunoassays for the quantitation of specific antibodies are reagent-excess assays(Kemeny, 1992). Most often, diluted test serum is added to excess antigen immobilized on a solid phase (sp-Ag) and the amount of specific antibody that binds (or is "captured," sp-Ag–**Ab**) may then be quantified by the employment of labeled antibodies that specifically bind to the constant region of the Ig class or classes of interest (e.g., sp-Ag–**IgG1**–Ab-enzyme). To avoid denaturation of surface-adsorbed antigens, biotinylated antigen may be used to capture the specific antibody (**Ab**–Ag-biotin), followed by immobilization of this complex via solid phase protein A (sp-proteinA–**Ab**–Ag-biotin) and detection of solid phase complex with streptavidin–alkaline phosphatase (sp-proteinA–**Ab**–Ag-biotin–streptavidin-enzyme) (Ngai, et al., 1993; see below under Indirect Labeling and under Separation Methods).

Alternatively, and much less frequently, an "antigen capture" approach may be employed. In such assays immobilized anti-Ig class antibodies (sp-Ab) first adsorb relevant immunoglobulins from the sample (sp-Ab–**IgA1**), added antigen is then specifically captured only by the antibodies of interest (sp-Ab–**IgA1**–Ag), and the amount of antigen bound is finally determined by, for example, the use of labeled antibody to antigen (sp-Ab–**IgA1**–Ag–Ab^{125}I). In one such assay F(ab′)$_2$ fragments of antibody against human IgG1 were immobilized and excess antigen with enzyme labeled antibody was used (sp-F[ab′]$_2$–**IgG1**–Ag–Ab-peroxidase; Siddiqi, et al., 1988). In another assay biotinylated antigen and labeled streptavidin were used (sp-Ab–**IgE**–Ag-biotin–streptavidin-enzyme; Olivieri, et al., 1993). Antigen capture assays may be preferable for specific antibodies of the minor Ig classes, as less antigen is needed and antibodies of other classes do not inhibit because they are discarded after the first step. In addition, immune complexes containing intact antigen may be detected with some schemes (Siddiqi, et al., 1988).

Immunoblotting and Immunostaining.   Immunoblotting was recently extensively reviewed by Stott (1989). Immunohistochemical and immunocytochemical staining methods and immunoblotting are generally nonquantitative or semiquantitative and represent the final parts of longer procedures such as histochemical investigations and electrophoretic analysis. The principle of Western blot analysis as applied to the confirmation of a specific infection is explained in Chapter 17. Microscopic immunofluorescence methods are very important in the diagnosis of allergies (Chap. 15), anemias (Chap. 12) and infectious diseases (Chap. 17). In vivo imaging by means of radiolabeled and "electron dense substance"-labeled antibodies is also similar in many respects. For all these procedures, there are many similarities in principle, and in the different strategies and tactics used, with conventional reagent-excess immunoassays and all can be made quantitative, or at least semiquantiative, with the aid of ancillary equipment such as specialized fluorescence microscopes or densitometers.

3. Reagent-Limited Assays

"Competitive" immunoassays are of special relevance because they include the first immunoassays given that name, that is, RIA. They are characterized in general by the use of limited reagent concentrations.

Labeled Antigen Assays. This group includes immunoassays for antigens or haptens equivalent to classic RIA. The labeled analyte is usually formed by tagging the analyte, or a derivative thereof, with radioiodine, a radioiodinated tagging compound, a fluorescent or luminescent compound, or an enzyme. Whereas in classic RIA lower concentrations of label are usually associated with lower detection limits, label is sometimes added late and in great excess to effect an "instantaneous" titration of binding sites unoccupied by analyte. Antibody-bound label and free label are separated to allow one of them, usually the bound fraction, to be determined. Plotting the concentration of label bound to antibody (e.g., Ab–Ag-^{125}I or sp-Ab–Ag-enzyme) against the concentration of analyte (**Ag**) gives inverse, nonlinear standard curves. The detection limits of reagent limited-immunoassays may be improved by the use of high specific activity label, but the smallest amount of analyte detectable is ultimately limited by the affinity of the antibody employed (Ekins and Chu, 1991). However, the most sensitive of these assays can detect less than 1 fmol of analyte (Gosling, 1990).

Labeled Antibody Assays. Labeled antibody reagent-limited assays for antigen or hapten have the advantage that labeled antigens or haptens with undesirable properties (e.g., low solubility in aqueous media) may be avoided. However, immobilized analyte must also be present in a constant, limited amount in each assay vessel. At the end of the assay, plotting the concentration of labeled antibody bound to the immobilized analyte (e.g., sp-Ag–Ab-^{125}I or sp-Ag–Ab-enzyme) against the concentration of analyte (**Ag**) gives an inverse standard curve, as with labeled analyte assays. This approach works well with highly purified monoclonal or affinity-purified polyclonal antibodies, as only then is the nonspecific binding of label not enhanced by contamination with irrelevant antibodies (Diamandis, 1988).

Assays for Specific Antibodies. While most assays for specific antibodies in general use are reagent excess assays, limited-reagent assays can offer certain advantages for some applications (Kemeny, 1992). For example, if only antibodies that bind to a specific region of an antigen (a specific epitope) are to be determined, a monoclonal antibody that binds to the same region is selected and labeled. In the assay, the specific antibodies in the sample (**Ab**) are allowed to compete with a limited concentration of the labeled antibody (Ab-^{125}I) for the antigen immobilized on a solid phase (sp-Ag). The two possible final complexes are sp-Ag–Ab-^{125}I and sp-Ag–**Ab.** Here again, plotting the concentration of labeled antibody bound to the immobilized antigen against the concentration of analyte (**Ab**) gives an inverse standard curve. (See also Measurement of Antibodies in Chapter 17.)

Free Analyte Assays. According to the "free hormone hypothesis," hormones that exist in the circulation as bound and free forms (e.g., thyroxine, most of which is bound by thyroxine-binding globulin and albumin and only 0.03% of which is free) are only biologically active when free; thus the free concentration constitutes a reliable indicator of in vivo hormonal effects even when the concentrations of binding proteins and the total hormone concentration change markedly. Both the free hormone hypothesis itself (Ekins, 1992a) and immunoassay methods for the determination of the concentrations of free thyroxine are controversial (Ekins, 1987; Ekins, 1992b).

While the most accurate methods for the determination of free hormones involve a separation step (e.g., dialysis or ultrafiltration) to allow the isolation and subsequent determination of the free analyte with a conventional competitive assay, the newer "free hormone" immunoassays are more convenient and cheaper to operate. Such assays depend on the introduction into the sample of antibody capable of binding the analyte in such a way that the degree to which this antibody becomes occupied by analyte reflects the original free analyte concentration. Variations on this procedure include one- and two-step protocols and the use of labeled antibody (with immobilized analyte or analog), labeled analyte, or labeled analyte analog with low affinity for serum proteins (Ekins, 1990). Since in one-step assays all reagents are simultaneously present, it is essential that binding of labeled analog by serum hormone-binding proteins be at most insignificant, or else grossly distorted free hormone estimates may be obtained (Ekins, 1990). (See also Chapter 8.)

Separation-Free Assays.   These assays have features in common that result in modulation of signal from the label by the binding reaction, thereby allowing binding to be monitored in the complete reaction mixture, without the necessity for a separation step (Jenkins, 1992). Consequently they are referred to as separation-free or homogeneous immunoassays. (The precipitation and agglutination assays described above also operate without need for a separation step.) An ideal homogeneous assay requires 100% modulation of signal from the label by the binding reaction. In practice this is very difficult to achieve, so that separation-free assays are often much less sensitive than immunoassays with separation steps. They are characterized by simplicity and speed and are widely employed in monitoring blood and urine levels of therapeutic drugs and of drugs of abuse when low detection limits ($<10^{-6}$ mol/L) are not required (see Chap. 18).

The activity of the label is either decreased or increased by the binding reaction. There are two kinds of enzyme-multiplied immunoassay techniques (EMITs): in some the enzyme activity of the label is decreased when the label is bound by the antibody (labels with lysozyme or glucose-6-phosphate dehydrogenase); and in others the activity is increased on binding (labels with malate dehydrogenase) (Jaklitsch, 1985). Apart from enzymes, enzyme mediated separation-free assays may employ as a labeling substance an enzyme prosthetic group, an enzyme inhibitor, an enzyme fragment, or a fluorescent-labeled enzyme substrate (Jenkins, 1992).

Immunochromatographic assays (Houts, 1991) are remarkable separation-free EIA systems in which the concentration of analyte is related to the distance along a chromatographic strip that color develops rather than to the intensity of color development. For combined enzyme donor immunoassay (CEDIA) (Engel and Khanna, 1992), recombinant DNA technology was exploited to produce new strains of *Escherichia coli* that synthesize large inactive fragments of β-D-galactosidase (enzyme acceptors) and small inactive fragments of the same enzyme (enzyme donors) that spontaneously associate to give fully active enzyme.

With fluorescent labels the effect of binding may be monitored by the measurement of one of a wide range of changes in the emitted light; it may be observed as being differentially polarized, quenched, "protected," or activated. Yet another approach to the use of "light emitting" labels in separation-free immunoassay depends on the labeling of both hapten and antibody in such a way that the signal generated by the doubly labeled antibody-hapten complex is modulated in comparison to that of the free reactants. Fluorescence energy transfer immunoassay (FETIA) is the most commonly reported assay using such an approach. See Hemmilä (1991) for a comprehensive review of the applications of fluorescence in immunoassays.

The scintillation proximity assay (SPA) technology marketed by Amershom Int. (Little Chalfont, England) enables separation-free RIA.

4. Ambient Analyte Assays

The ambient analyte immunoassay system (Ekins and Chu, 1991) (see earlier discussion under Antibody Occupancy Principle and below under Multianalyte Microspot Assay) fits into none of the above categories. Its major characteristic is that the primary antibody, immobilized on a microspot, is used at such low concentration that the degree to which it is occupied by analyte (i.e., fractional occupancy) is directly related to the analyte concentration (Fig. 1–2). In the direct assays of this type under development, two fluorescent labels with distinct and separate peak emission wavelengths are used to label the antibody to be immobilized (fluor1-Ab) and the antibody used to complete the sandwich (Ab-fluor2), respectively. On monitoring the final assay complex (sp-[fluor1]Ab]–**Ag**–fluor2), the signal from fluor1 indicates total solid phase antibody, the signal from fluor2 shows occupancy by **Ag** of the immobilized antibody, and the ratio of the two, fluor2/fluor1, is proportional to fractional occupancy.

ANTIBODIES AND OTHER BINDING PROTEINS

The most important binding proteins used in immunoassays and related assays are listed in Table 1–2. The employment of nonimmunoglobulin binding proteins, such as receptors, results in assays dependent on the same basic principles as immunoassays, and although they are not used for most routine assays, they are very useful for some applications.

Other Binding Proteins

Intrinsic factor is the binding protein generally used for the determination of vitamin B_{12} in a variety of reagent-limited assay formats with a variety of labels, including ^{57}Co-B_{12}, acridinium ester-B_{12} (Leonard, et al., 1990), and enzyme-B_{12} (Quinn, et al., 1991). A CEDIA homogeneous system with intrinsic factor as binding protein has also been developed (Khanna, et al., 1989). Purified folate-binding protein from cow's milk is used for the determination of folate in serum and in erythrocytes (Hansen, et al., 1987), and receptor from calf thymus for 1,25-dihydroxyvitamin D is used in assays for that steroid (Oftebro, et al., 1988). (See Chapter 12 where protein binding assays for the measurement of vitamin B_{12} and folate are further discussed.)

Table 1–2   Binding Proteins Used in Immunoassays and Related Assays

Binding Protein	Type or Class	Source
Binding proteins	Avidin	Chicken egg white
	B_{12} intrinsic factor	Porcine gastric mucosa
	Corticosteroid-binding globulin	Equine, etc., serum
	Folate-binding protein	Bovine milk
	Lectin	e.g., *Lotus tetragonolobus*
Immunoglobulins	IgG monoclonal	Mouse, rat, interspecies
	IgG polyclonal	Rabbit, etc.
	IgG F(ab′)₂	Rabbit, mouse, etc.
	IgG Fab′	Rabbit, mouse, etc.
	IgM monoclonal	Mouse
	IgY	Avian serum, egg yolk
Receptors	Acyl-D-alanyl-D-alanine (binds vancomycin-class antibiotics)	Synthetic
	γ-Aminobutyric acid	Rat brain membrane
	1,25-Dihydroxyvitamin D	Calf thymus

Lectin and antibody sandwich immunoassays have been found useful for the determination of different glycosylated forms of proteins (Kinoshita, et al., 1989). Blood binding proteins such as corticosteroid-binding globulin which were widely used for the assay of steroids in the 1960s and 1970s are still occasionally used for cortisol determination (Murphy and Barta, 1987).

Polyclonal Antibodies

Antibodies, usually of the IgG class, offer both convenience and versatility. They are convenient because they are available at relatively enormous titers, because they are stable, and because a wide range of standard procedures and reagents are available which facilitate the development of varied assay procedures and systems. They are versatile because they can be easily raised against nontoxic antigenic substances, and even against most weakly antigenic and nonantigenic compounds (haptens) with a molecular weight of greater than 150 daltons.

Rabbits are still the principal animal used for raising polyclonal antibodies, with sheep and goats being the animals of choice in many commercial enterprises. Other species widely used are guinea pig, donkey, equine, bovine, and porcine. Avian IgY antibodies, which offer the potential of harvesting from the yolks of eggs, are occasionally used. They have the advantages of being produced in large quantities and of exhibiting less interaction with complement, rheumatoid factors, and other interfering factors than is often found with mammalian antibodies (Larsson, et al., 1992).

Antibody Fragments

Immunoglobulins are multifunctional proteins with binding sites on the Fc for complement, phagocyte Fc receptor, staphylococcyl protein A, bacterial Fc receptor, and rheumatoid factor. While many of these properties have been profitably exploited in immunoassays, the presence of the Fc portion of IgG is often unnecessary, and even undesirable, in an antibody to be used as an immunoassay reagent. Eiji Ishikawa and coworkers (Ishikawa, 1987; Ishikawa, et al., 1989) have long advocated the multiple advantages of antibody-enzyme conjugates consisting of Fab[1] linked through a free sulfydryl group, located in what is referred to as the hinge region of intact IgG (see Fig. 1–1). The high specific activity, low nonspecific binding conjugates which they have prepared have enabled the development of assays for antigens and specific antibodies with detection limits down to 0.02 amol per tube. Fv fragments, with no constant region at all, may offer further improvements in reduced nonspecific binding (Huston, et al., 1993).

Monoclonal Antibodies

The versatility of antibodies was greatly extended by the advent of hybridoma technology (see Chap. 2 and a series of papers in Hunter and Corrie, 1983). Monoclonal antibodies offer improved continuity of supply, better defined specificity, and greatly increased opportunities for methodologic advancement. In the last 10 years monoclonal antibodies have become important for the determination by immunometric assay of the most clinically important protein analytes. They are used as matched pairs but more generally with one polyclonal antibody. However, they are still used in less than 20% of immunoassays for hapten analytes. Their popularity may increase further as the number, variety, and quality of commercial antibodies improve, and as the advantages of the simultaneous use of a number of well-characterized monoclonal antibodies become clear (Zenke, et al., 1991). However, monoclonal antibodies must be carefully selected, and their use thoroughly validated, to guard against the nondetection of important isoforms of protein analytes (Pettersson, et al., 1991).

While most monoclonal antibodies are generated by means of mice and murine carcinoma cell lines, rats and rat cell lines may be used (Bazin, et al., 1984). Antibody producing cells from other animals have been used for interspecies fusions with murine carcinoma cells, and some antibodies that have been prepared in this way are of notably high affinity (Groves, et al., 1990).

Combinatorial Library Antibodies

By means of recombinant DNA technology, enormous numbers of different antibodies, but more usually Fab or Fv fragments, can now be generated from combinatorial

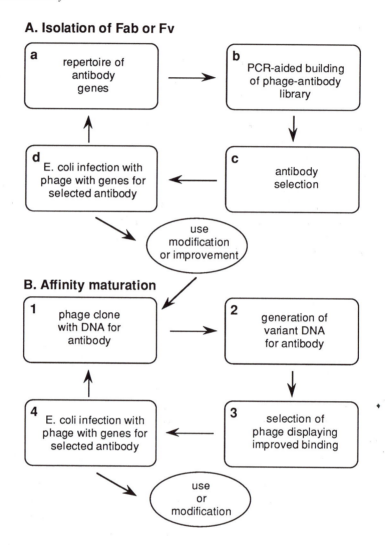

A. Isolation of Fab or Fv

a repertoire of antibody genes

b PCR-aided building of phage-antibody library

d E. coli infection with phage with genes for selected antibody

c antibody selection

use modification or improvement

B. Affinity maturation

1 phage clone with DNA for antibody

2 generation of variant DNA for antibody

4 E. coli infection with phage with genes for selected antibody

3 selection of phage displaying improved binding

use or modification

Figure 1.5.   Combinatorial antibodies and affinity improvement. *A,* Isolation and selection of Fab or Fv antibody fragments. *a.* The repertoire of genes can be derived from lymphocytes in bone marrow, thymus, or the peripheral circulation. IgG mRNA can be used but more diverse repertoires can be generated with IgM mRNA. Alternatively, genes can be derived from a fetal source or can be partially, or completely, artificial. *b.* The gene repertoire is amplified by means of the polymerase chain reaction (PCR) and cloned into bacteriophage or phagemid vectors. Variable region genes for H and L chain genes are amplified separately and spliced with phage coat–protein genes, so that each phage particle displays on its surface the antibody fragment coded for by the genes it is carrying. *c.* Antibody selection is performed by passing the library of phage particles over antigen adsorbed to a solid phase such as sepharose beads held in a column, a coated tube or well, or a membrane. *d.* Phage that are bound can be eluted and used to infect *E. coli* to give stable clones.

cDNA libraries of antibody variable genes (Huse, et al., 1989; Chiswell and McCafferty, 1992), and bacteriophage-based screening systems of increasing efficiency have been progressively developed (Chiswell and McCafferty, 1992; Ditzel, 1993). In this way, starting with mRNA from peripheral blood lymphocytes, specific human antibodies can be obtained (Fig. 1–5). The lymphocytes may be taken at random from a normal person so that no immunization is involved, but it is often advantageous to use an immune individual, in whom the antigen-specific and nonspecific lymphocytes will have been positively and negatively selected, respectively. For example, if an antibody against an HIV antigen is required, the lymphocytes could be taken from a patient who is HIV seropositive or who has acquired immune deficiency syndrome (AIDS) (Ditzel, 1993).

Of greater immediate relevance to the future production of high quality antibodies for use in immunoassays is the development of techniques to improve the affinity and specificity of the antibodies selected from combinatorial libraries (Fig. 1–5). These techniques attempt to mimic, and hope to surpass, the ability of the intact immune system to improve its antibody response by rounds of mutation and selection, that is, affinity maturation (Chiswell and McCafferty, 1992).

In addition, the recombinant DNA approach to the production of antibodies can be used to rescue the genes for an antibody with desirable characteristics from an unstable, or poorly producing, hybridoma cell line (Ditzel, 1993).

LABELS AND THEIR DETERMINATION

The general suitability of a labeling substance depends on its specific activity, solubility, resistance to nonspecific binding, ease of labeling, ease of endpoint determination, associated hazards, and possibilities for convenient assay formulations. Some labeling substances used for immunoassays are listed in Table 1–3.

High specific activity label is essential for assays with low detection limits. The specific activity of a labeled antibody, antigen, or hapten is determined by four main

---

Antibody fragments selected in this way can be used directly, or their genes can be fused with those for Ig constant regions if whole antibodies are required, or they may be subjected to procedures to improve their affinity and specificity.

B, In vitro affinity maturation or selection is a set of manipulations aimed at emulating, and eventually outperforming, the natural processes whereby the antibodies produced during the response to immunization have progressively higher affinities for antigen. *1.* The starting point can be genes for an antibody or fragment selected from a recombinant library, as described above, or from a preexisting hybridoma. *2.* Almost any mutagenesis technique could in principle be used to generate the population of variants to select from. Alternatively, a chain shuffling approach may be taken, whereby either the H or L chain is retained and the partner replaced with a repertoire from another source. *3.* Selection of antibodies displayed by phage is then performed as described above. *4.* Then the selected antibodies are propagated and characterized and the decision is taken to proceed with one selected, or, starting with the best of those generated, to embark on a new round of variant generation and selection (Chiswell and McCafferty, 1992).

Table 1–3   Some Substances Used for Labeling and Methods Used to
Measure Them*

Type	Substance	Assay Method
Enzyme	Acetlycholinesterase	Colorimetric
	Alkaline phosphatase	Amplified colorimetric, colorimetric, electrochemical, enhanced luminometric, time-resolved (TR) fluorimetric, visual assessment
	β-D-Galactosidase	Colorimetric, fluorimetric, luminometric
	Glucose-6-phosphate dehydrogenase	Colorimetric
	Horseradish peroxidase	Colorimetric, fluorimetric, luminometric
	β-Lactamase	Colorimetric
	Malate dehydrogenase	Colorimetric
	Mellitin	Liposome entrapped enzyme, colorimetric
	Urease	Colorimetric
Enzyme related	Cholinesterase inhibitor	Acetylcholinesterase, colorimetric
	FAD prosthetic group	Glucose oxidase, colorimetric
	β-D-Galactosidase fragment	Complementary fragment, colorimetric
Fluorescent	Coumarin derivative	Fluorimetric
	Dysprosium (Dy^{3+})	TR fluorimetric
	Fluorescein	Fluorimetric
	Europium (Eu^{3+})	TR fluorimetric
	Eu^{3+} chelate	TR fluorimetric
	Eu^{3+} chelator	TR fluorimetric
	Phycoerythrin	Fluorimetric
	Samarium (Sm^{3+})	TR fluorimetric
	Terbium (Tb^{3+})	TR fluorimetric
Ligand	Avidin	Biotinylated enzyme
	Biotin derivative	Avidin-acridinium ester, luminometry; avidin-enzyme, colorimetry; avidin-Eu^{3+} chelator, TR fluorimetric; avidin-^{125}I, solid scintillation counting (SSC)
	FITC	anti-FITC-enzyme
Luminescent	Acridinium ester	Luminometry
	Isoluminol derivatives	Luminometry
Microparticle	Colloidal gold	Visual assessment

Table 1–3 (continued)

Type	Substance	Assay Method
	Colored latex	Visual assessment
	Latex, etc.	Nephelometry, particle counting, turbidimetry, visual assessment of agglutination
	Stained bacteria	Visual assessment
Radioisotopic	^{57}Co	SSC
	^{3}H	Liquid scintillation counting
	^{125}I	SSC
	^{125}I-Bolton and Hunter reagent	SSC
Vesicle	Liposome	Entrapped dye, colorimetry; Entrapped enzyme, colorimetry

*Gosling (1990) contains an equivalent table with references.

factors: (1) the fraction available for detection, (2) continuity of detection, (3) efficiency of detection, and (4) substitution ratio. Although only a tiny percentage of a radioisotope such as ^{125}I decays while it is being counted and decayed atoms may not be detected again, radioisotopic decay is very efficiently detected. While haptens are often multiply substituted with tritium (e.g., [1,2,6,7,16,17]-^{3}H-progesterone) (although the substitution efficiency is never 100%), substitution with ^{125}I to give ratios greater than 1 is rarely done in order to minimize radiation and iodination damage. Enzymes (or rather their products) are very inefficiently detected by colorimetry but perform very well in other respects, except that their large size normally restricts the target substitution ratio to about 1. Fluorescent compounds are all available for detection, can be repeatedly excited, and large molecules such as proteins can be multiply substituted. Chemiluminescent molecules can only decay once, and are detected with much lower efficiency than radioisotopes, but they are all potentially available for detection, and multiple substitution is feasible.

Luminescence and Fluorescence

Each category of label may have disadvantages that can be decreased, or abolished, by the use of a different substance and/or by technical developments. For example, the chemiluminescent photoefficiency of isoluminol derivatives is reduced when they are linked to large protein molecules, but the luminescent acridinium esters give a high luminesence quantum yield because of the dissociative nature of the reaction (Weeks and Woodhead, 1984). (Combined luminescence and radioisotope (β or γ) counters that accept samples on suitable microtiter plates are now available.)

In addition, the use of europium^{3+} (Eu^{3+}) and other lanthanide ion-chelates with new equipment for time-resolved fluorescence determination greatly reduces the high background fluorescence often associated with the use of fluorescein and many other fluorescent compounds (Hemmilä, 1991). Time-resolved FIA and IFMA, as immunometric assays with such labels are called, have low detection limits and can also measure analytes over a very wide range of concentrations. Many approaches to the use of lanthanide ion-chelate fluorescence have been employed. Complexed Eu^{3+} may be used as a labeling substance with the Eu^{3+} being eluted and recomplexed with a fluorescence-efficient chelating agent before the fluorescence is estimated (Eu^{3+} labeling) (exemplified by the DELFIAR assays of Pharmacia-Wallac Oy, Turku, Finland), or a fluorescence-efficient chelating agent may be used as a labeling substance and determined in the presence of excess Eu^{3+} (chelator labeling) (exemplified by the early assays of Cyberfluor Inc., Canada). A third approach uses labeling with a Eu^{3+} chelate that is simply determined at the end of the assay (Eu^{3+} chelate labeling), which facilitates the development of homogeneous assays. Alternatively, an auxiliary chelator functionally blocked by phosphorylation (5-fluorosalicyl phosphate) can be used as substrate for alkaline phosphatase label. In the resulting enzyme-labeled assays the 5-fluorosalicylic acid (FSA) product can form a highly fluorescent ternary complex of the form, FSA-Tb^{3+}-EDTA, which is efficiently determined by time-resolved fluorimetry (Cyberfluor Inc.) (Christopoulos and Diamandis, 1992).

Lanthanide cryptates are a group of highly stable macrocyclic, cage-type chelates that have been "tipped" as potentially important alternates to the lanthanide chelates presently used. However, the actual cryptates initially tried in immunoassays were difficult to prepare and prone to nonspecific binding to proteins and surfaces (Hemmilä, 1991).

Radioisotopes

In recent years the use of radioisotopes has declined significantly, but about 70% of commercial assays still use isotopic labels. Radioisotopes are totally impervious to normal environmental changes and this may partly account for the widespread opinion that RIA and IRMA methods are inherently stable with low between-assay variability and hence their continued popularity in large-scale clinical analytic service laboratories. Because of the relative convenience of gamma counting (especially with multiheaded, computer-assisted modern counters), tritiated labels are now rarely used and ^{125}I is the predominant choice, even where high specific activity is unnecessary.

Enzymes

Enzymes are the most popular nonisotopic labeling substances, with horseradish peroxidase being the most popular enzyme (Gosling, 1990). A feature of the employment of enzymes in labels is the wide variety of assay methods available to determine the activities of the most popular of them (Table 1–3).

Indirect Labeling

Quite often the label determined at the end of an immunoassay procedure is not the primary label. This trend can be said to have started with the employment of a labeled "second" antibody in solid phase antigen immunoassays. For example, if the analyte binds to immobilized sheep antibody and unlabeled rabbit antibody is used to complete the sandwich (sp-SAb–**Ag**–RAb), the concentration of the bound rabbit antibody may be determined with a labeled goat antibody raised against whole rabbit IgG or its Fc fragment (sp-SAb–**Ag**–RAb–GAb-^{125}I). Here the constant region of the rabbit IgG can logically be said to be the primary label. Alternatively, labeled protein A can be used as a general purpose reagent for the quantification of immobilized Fc.

Combined Primary and Secondary Labeling

The use of biotin conjugated to antibody (or antigen/hapten) as primary label, with labeled avidin or streptavidin as a secondary label (Guesdon, et al., 1979), is a logical, universally applicable extension of the above approach. Biotin and avidin are chosen because of the high affinity of the binding reaction and the quadravalency of avidin or streptavidin. However, streptavidin is often preferred as it has a lower pI (5.5 to 6.5) and is not glycosylated, both of which properties help to decrease nonspecific binding. The concentration of biotinylated antibody is determined with iodinated avidin or avidin conjugated to an enzyme, a luminescent compound, or a Eu^{3+} chelate.

Fluorescein isothiocyanate (FITC) is also used as a primary label, as opposed to a fluorimetric labeling substance, in which case the concentration of FITC primary label is determined by means of enzyme-labeled monoclonal antibodies to FITC (Harmer, et al., 1989).

Label Complexes

A recurring approach to maximizing the final signal obtained in an immunoassay is to attempt to attach multiple molecules of the final labeling substance for each immune complex or component to be detected (Avrameas, 1992). This may be achieved with biotin as the primary label and multiply labeled streptavidin. If a biotinylated antigen or antibody is multiply substituted with biotin the degree of amplification may be further enhanced. The use of an "avidin bridge" as suggested by Guesdon, et al. (1979) may provide another level of multiplication because of the quadrivalency of avidin. However, attempts to amplify the signal obtained by assembling large label-containing complexes are inherently limited by steric effects and by a pronounced tendency for the nonspecific binding of label to increase in parallel.

Alternatively, the use of liposomes containing dye (O'Connell, et al., 1985) or enzyme (Canova-Davis, 1986) as primary labeling substances leads to amplification because the lysis of each vesicle releases many molecules of the trapped indicator. Such assays are usually separation-free.

Hazardous Reagents

The most hazardous procedure associated with radioimmunoassays is radioiodination but, unlike toxic chemicals (carcinogens, teratogens, etc.), contamination with the hazardous substance involved (^{125}I) is readily detected by means of inexpensive monitoring equipment. Care should be taken with all known or potentially hazardous substances, whether radiochemical or not (Gosling, 1980).

SEPARATION METHODS

Most immunoassays, particularly those designed to operate in the nmol/L range or lower, involve a distinct separation step or steps. Although absorption (e.g., with ac-

Table 1–4   Some Separation Methods used in Immunoassays

Type	Reagent/Solid Phase
"Liquid phase" absorption	Anion resin
	Dextran "coated" charcoal
	Diatomaceous earths, e.g., florisil
"Liquid phase" precipitation	ammonium sulfate
	polyethylene glycol
	"Second" antibody
	"Second" antibody with PEG
Solid phase adsorption	Glass fiber membrane
	Glass fiber membrane-latex
	Large bead
	Microtiter plate
	Nylon membrane
	Tube
Solid phase indirect adsorption	Biotin-antibody, solid phase-avidin
	FITC-antibody, solid phase-anti-FITC
	Microtiter plate-"second" antibody
Solid phase precipitation	Magnetizable bead-antibody
	"Microbeads"-antibody
	"Microbeads"-"second" antibody
	Staphylocossus aureus-protein A

tivated charcoal) and precipitation ("second" antibody or polyethylene glycol, etc.) separation procedures are still used, the employment of solid phase antibodies or antigens/haptens has become predominant because of their convenience and efficiency, and a wide range of solid phases are commonly used (Table 1–4) (Gosling, 1992).

Indirect binding via "second" antibody is sometimes employed in competitive assays because often less specific antibody is required, variability may be reduced, and the properties of the "first" antibody may be protected.

Immobilization via Ligand "Anchors"

It is widely held that many immune complexes form more efficiently in solution and that detection limits may be lowered by allowing such complexes to form in solution before being trapped on a solid surface (Ishikawa, et al., 1989). In one such assay procedure the nonlabeled antibody in a two-site sandwich complex is biotinylated, with the biotin functioning to anchor the complex to immobilized avidin when the solid phase is added (sp-avidin–biotin-Ab-**Ag**-Ab-^{125}I) (Zahradnick, et al., 1989). Alternatively, FITC can be used as an anchor ligand when combined with solid phase anti-FITC antibody as capture protein (sp-Ab–FITC-Ab-**Ag**-Ab-^{125}I) (Kang, et al., 1986). FITC's advantages over the use of biotin and streptavidin include low nonspecific binding and the coloration of FITC-labeled antibodies which aids in their preparation and characterization.

AUTOMATION AND MULTIPLE ANALYSIS

Automatic Immunoassay Workstations

The adaptation of immunoturbidimetric and separation-free assays to allow their use on chemistry analyzers has constituted a quiet revolution by which a very wide range of higher-concentration blood proteins, therapeutic drugs, and certain hormones can now be routinely determined automatically. However, most hormones, tumor markers, and many other analytes determined by immunoassay must be assayed at such low concentrations that such methods are inappropriate.

At present there is intense commercial competition in the development and marketing of specialized immunoassay workstations of two main types: sophisticated liquid-handling systems allowing the use of lower-cost bulk reagents, and lower capital cost systems based around relatively expensive, analyte-specific plastic trays or cassettes containing most reagents (Litman, 1991).

An alternative system for classifying such systems is on the basis of "access," or when and how new samples may be added or new tests requested (Gorman, et al., 1991). Thus analyzers may be regarded as "batch assay" if they can run samples through a single test or a prefixed panel of tests; as "random-batch" if they can run multiple samples through multiple tests, scheduling them to optimize instrument performance; and as "random-access" if they can offer complete flexibility. This means that additional tests may be requested in any order or test sequence, with the ability to give a new sample priority over all the waiting samples.

To enable such features, standard immunoassay formats are often extensively reformulated with solid phase reagents, facilitating automated draining and washing. For example, microparticles in a vessel with a porous bottom, magnetizable particles and insertable/removable magnets, or a spinning disk over which reagents flow, may be used.

However, automation inevitably leads to decreased involvement by highly skilled clinical scientists and, since a single company normally supplies both the instrument and the matching reagents, there is usually much less opportunity for a user to obtain alternative reagents. These are important disadvantages. As the number of such automated systems increases, it will become clear whether they yield results which are more or less accurate than the manual assays they are replacing.

Multianalyte assays

There are obvious practical advantages to the simultaneous determination of a number of analytes in single samples, especially if the results are routinely required at the same time in order to make certain diagnoses or decisions. The screening of blood donations is an important example. Many dual-analyte immunoassays have been developed and advocated (Gosling, 1990), including assays with two radioisotopes (^{57}Co and ^{125}I), two enzymes (horseradish peroxidase and alkaline phosphatase [Porstmann, et al., 1993]), two rare earth metal ions (Eu^{3+} and terbium^{3+} [Tb^{3+}]), or two differently colored kinds of latex particles. A quadruple-label time-resolved fluorimetric system for the neonatal screening of TSH, 17α-hydroxyprogesterone, immunoreactive trypsin, and creatine kinase MM isoenzyme in dried blood spots has been described (Xu, et al., 1992). The four labels contained ions of the four lanthanide metals Eu^{3+}, Tb^{3+}, samarium (Sm^{3+}) and dysprosium (Dy^{3+}), which were allocated to the analytes so as to match higher specific activity labels with assays requiring lower detection limits.

An alternative approach is to use only one kind of labeling substance but to have spatially distinct groups of specific binding sites; this has the advantage that the number of analytes determined is limited only by the number of groups of sites. Kakabakos and colleagues (1991) described a method based on the coating of distinct areas of polystyrene with analyte-specific antibodies and applied it to the simultaneous determination of luteinizing hormone (LH), follicle-stimulating hormone (FSH), choriogonadotropin (CG), and prolactin in serum. A qualitative immunoassay test pack for the simultaneous qualitative detection of seven drugs of abuse (phencyclidine, benzodiazepine, cocaine, amphetamine, tetrahydrocannabinol, barbiturate, and opiate has also been described (Buechler, et al., 1992). Nine bands on a nylon membrane held in a special plastic device are coated with specific antibodies against analyte (seven bands), a positive control reagent or a negative control reagent, and conjugates of colloidal gold to each drug are used as labels. Another multianalyte immunoassay with many more spatially distinct groups of binding sites has been in widespread use for a number of years. The multiallergo sorbent test (MAST) system is a reagent excess, antibody capture assay with solid phase antigen and labeled anti-human lgE antibody (Brown, et al., 1984). MAST employs 38 individual allergen-coated cellulose threads mounted in a special pipette-like test chamber to measure pmol amounts of allergen-specific IgE against up to 35 different allergen classes.

Multianalyte Microspot Assay

Roger Ekins (one of the original inventors of immunoassays) and his coworkers have been developing a multianalyte microspot immunoassay (Ekins and Chu, 1991) (see earlier discussion, Antibody Occupancy Principle and Ambient Analyte Assays). This is based on multiple miniature solid-phase regions on a relatively large, flat surface, dual fluorescence-labeling of antibodies, and confocal fluorescence microscopic detection system. This proposed system, which would use spatially distinct groups of binding sites, may lead to the emergence of a range of automated multianalyte immunoassay workstations, not just for determining simultaneously a wide range of analytes, but perhaps even for measuring individually each clinically significant isoform of more complex analytes. However, as there would be a requirement of one labeled specific antibody for each analyte determined, and all binding sites apparently must be exposed to all labels, special care will be needed to minimize nonspecific binding.

REFERENCES

Arevalo JH, Taussig MJ, Wilson IA. Molecular basis of cross reactivity and the limits of antibody-antigen complementarity. London: Nature, 1993; 365:859–863.

Avrameas S. Amplification systems in immunoenzymatic techniques. J Immunol Methods 1992;150:23–32.

Barnard G, Kohen F. Ideometric assay: a non-competitive immunoassay for haptens typified by the measurement of serum estradiol. Clin Chem 1990;36:1945.

Bazin H, Xhurdebise L-M, Burtonboy G, et al. Rat monoclonal antibodies. I. Rapid purification from in vitro culture supernatants. J Immunol Methods 1984;66:261–269.

Bidart J-M. Functional mapping of proteins with monoclonal antibodies. In: Gosling JP, Reen DJ, eds. Immunotechnology. London: Portland Press, 1993:77–90.

Boscato LM, Egan GM, Stuart MC. Specificity of two-site immunoassays. J Immunol Methods 1989;117:221–229.

Brown CR, Higgins KW, Frazer K, et al. Simultaneous determination of total Ig and allergen-specific IgE in serum by the MAST chemiluminescent assay system. Clin Chem 1984;31:1500–1505.

Buechler KF, Moi S, Noar B, et al. Simultaneous detection of seven drugs of abuse by the Triage™ panel for drugs of abuse. Clin Chem 1992;38:1678–1684.

Canova-Davis E, Redemann CT, Vollmer YP, Kung VT. Use of a reversed-phase evaporation vesicle formulation for a homogeneous liposome immunoassay. Clin Chem 1986;32:1687–1691.

Chiswell DJ, McCafferty J. Phage antibodies: will new 'coliclonal' antibodies replace monoclonal antibodies? Tibtech 1992;10:80–84.

Christopoulos TK, Diamandis EP. Enzymatically amplified time-resolve fluorescence immunoassay with terbium chelates. Anal Chem 1992;64:342–351.

Day ED. Advanced Immunochemistry, Chap. 4. New York: Wiley-Liss, 1990.

Diamandis EP. Immunoassays with time-resolved fluorescence spectroscopy: principles and applications. Clin Biochem 1988;21:139–150.

Ditzel H. Combinatorial libraries: an approach for generating human antibodies. In: Gosling JP, Reen DJ, eds. Immunotechnology. London: Portland Press, 1993;27–38.

Ekins R (answered by Midgley JEM, Moon CR, Wilkins TA). Validity of analog free thyroxin immunoassays. Clin Chem 1987;33:2137–2152.

Ekins RP. Measurement of free hormones in blood. Endocrinol Rev 1990; 11:5–46.

Ekins RP. The free hormone hypothesis and measurement of free hormones. Clin Chem 1992a;38:1289–1293.

Ekins RP (with answers from Christophedes N, Sheehan C; Midgely JEM, Wilkins TA). One-step, labeled-antibody assay for measuring free thyroxine. 1. Assay development and validation. Clin Chem 1992b;38:2355–2358.

Ekins RP, Chu FW. Multianalyte microspot immunoassay—microanalytical "compact disk" of the future. Clin Chem 1991;37:1955–1967.

Engel WD, Khanna PL. CEDIA in vitro diagnostics with a novel homogeneous immunoassay technique: current status and future prospects. J Immunol Methods 1992;150: 99–102.

Freytag JW, Lau HP, Wadsley JJ. Affininity-column-mediated immunoenzymometric assay: influence of affinity-column ligand and valency of antibody-enzyme conjugates. Clin Chem 1984;30:1494–1498.

Gorman E, Hochberg A, Knodel E, Leflar C, Wang C-C. An overview of automation. In: Price CP, Newman DJ, eds. Principles and Practice of Immunoassay. London: Macmillan, 1991;219–245.

Gosling JP. The hazards of enzyme immunoassay as compared to radioimmunoassay. In: Malvano R, ed. Immunoenzymatic assay techniques. The Hague: Martinus Nijhoff, 1980;259–272.

Gosling, JP. A decade of development in immunoassay methodology. Clin Chem 1990;36:1408–1427.

Gosling, JP. Solid phase concepts and design. In: Masseyeff RF, Albert WH, Staines NA, eds. Methods of Immunological Analysis, vol. 1. Weinheim, Germany: VCH Verlags Gesellschaft, 1992, MB, 1993, in press.

Groves DJ, Sauer MJ, Rayment P, Foulkes JA, Morris BA. The preparation of an ovine monoclonal antibody to progesterone. J Endocrinol 1990;126:217–222.

Gudmundsson B-ME, Young NM, Oomen RP. Characterization of residues in antibody binding sites by chemical modification of surface-adsorbed protein combined with enzyme immunoassay. J Immunol Methods 1993;158:215–227.

Guesdon J-L, Ternynck T, Avrameas S. The use of avidin-biotin interaction in immunoenzymatic techniques. J Histochem Cytochem 1979;27:1131–1139.

Hansen SI, Holm J, Nexø E. Immobilized purified folate-binding protein: binding characteristics and use of quantifying folate in erythrocytes. Clin Chem 1987;33:1360–1363.

Harmer IJ, Samuel D. The FITC–anti-FITC system is a sensitive alternative to biotin-streptavidin in ELISA. J Immunol Methods 1989;122:115–121.

Harris LJ, Larson SB, Hasel KW, Day J, Greenwood A, McPherson A. The three-dimensional structure of an intact monoclonal antibody for canine lymphoma. London: Nature, 1992; 360:369–72.

Hemmilä IA. 1991. Applications of Fluorescence in Immunoassay. New York: Wiley Interscience, 1991.

Houts T. Immunochromatography. In: Price CP, Newman DJ, eds. Principles and Practice of Immunoassay. New York: Stockton Press, 1991; 563–583.

Hunter WM, Corrie JET, eds. Immunoassays for Clinical Chemistry. Edinburgh: Churchill Livingstone, 1983.

Huse WD, Sastry L, Iverson SA, et al. Generation of a large combinatorial library of the immunoglobulin repertoire in phage lambda. Nature 1989;246:1275–1281.

Huston JS, Keck P, Tai M-S, et al. Single-chain immunotechnology of Fv analogues and fusion proteins. In: Gosling JP, Reen DJ, eds. Immunotechnology. London: Portland Press, 1993:47–60.

Ishikawa E. Development and clinical application of sensitive enzyme immunoassay for macromolecular antigens—a review. Clin Biochem 1987;20:375–385.

Ishikawa E, Hashida S, Tanaka K, Kohno T. Methodological advances in enzymology: development and application of ultrasensitive enzyme immunoassays for antigens and antibodies. Clin Chim Acta 1989;185:223–230.

Jaklitsch A. Separation-free enzyme immunoassay for haptens. In: Ngo TT, Lenhoff, eds. Enzyme-mediated Immunoassay. New York: Plenum Press, 1985;33–55.

Jenkins SH. Homogeneous enzyme immunoassay. J Immunol Methods 1992:150:91–97.

Kakabakos SE, Christopoulos, Diamandis EP. Multianalyte immunoassay based on spatially distinct fluorescent areas quantified by laser-excited solid-phase time-resolved fluorometry. Clin Chem 1992;38:338–342.

Kang, J, Kaladas, P, Chang, C, et al. A highly sensitive immunoenzymometric assay involving "common-capture" particles and membrane filtration. Clin Chem 1986;32:1682–1686.

Kemeny DM. Titration of antibodies. J Immunol Methods 1992;150:57–76.

Khanna PL, Dworschack RT, Manning WB, Harris JD. A new homogenous enzyme immunoassay using recombinant enzyme fragments. Clin Chim Acta 1989;185:231–240.

Kinoshita N, Suzuki S, Matsuda Y, Taniguchi N, α-Fetoprotein antibody-lectin enzyme immunoassay to characterize sugar chains for the study of liver diseases. Clin Chim Acta 1989;179:143–152.

Larsson A, Wejåker P-E, Forsberg P-O, Lindahl T. Chicken antibodies: a tool to avoid interference by complement activation in ELISA. J Immunol Methods 1992;156:79–83.

Leonard H, Blake M, Chang S, McLaughlin L. An automated chemiluminescent receptor assay for vitamin B12. Clin Chem 1990;36:1105.

Litman DJ. Immunoassay automation—progress and perspectives. Clin Chem 1991;37:1097.

Malmquist M. Real-time BIA for the direct measurement of antibody-antigen interaction. In: Gosling JP, Reen DJ, eds. Immunotechnology. London: Portland Press, 1993:61–76.

Masseyeff RF. Classification of immunomethods. In: Masseyeff RF, Albert WH, Staines NA, eds. Methods of Immunological Analysis, vol 1. Weinheim, Germany: VCH Verlags Gesellschaft, 1993:116–133.

Miyai K. Classification of immunoassay. In: Price CP, Newman DJ, eds. Principles and Practice of Immunoassay. New York: Stockton Press, 1991:246–264.

Murphy BEP, Barta A. One-tube radiotransinassay for determination of cortisol at ambient temperature. Clin Chem 1987;33:1137–1140.

Ngai PKM, Ackermann F, Wendt H, Savoca R, Bosshard HR. Protein A antibody-capture ELISA (PACE): an ELISA format to avoid denaturation of surface-adsorbed antigens. J Immunol Methods 1993;158:267–276.

O'Connell JP, Campbell RL, Fleming BM, Mercolino TJ, Johnson MD, McLaurin DA. A highly sensitive immunoassay system involving antibody-coated tubes and liposome-entrapped dye. Clin Chem 1985;31:1424–1426.

Oftebro H, Falch JA, Holmberg I, Haug E. Validation of a radioreceptor assay for 1,25-dihyroxyvitamin D using selected ion monitoring GC-MS. Clin Chim Acta 1988; 176:157–168.

Olivieri V, Beccarini I, Gallucci G, Romano T, Santoro F. Capture assay for specific IgE: an improve quantitative method. J Immunol Methods 1993;157:65–72.

Pettersson K, Ding Y-Q, Huhtaniemi I. Monoclonal antibody-based discrepancies between two-site immunometric tests for lutropin. Clin Chem 1991;37:1745–1848.

Porstmann T, Nugel E, Henklein P, et al. Two-colour combination enzyme-linked immunosorbent assay for the simultaneous detection of HBV and HIV infection. J Immunol Methods 1993;158:95–106.

Price CP, Newman DJ, Light scattering immunoassay. In: Price CP, Newman DJ, eds. Principles and Practice of Immunoassay. New York: Stockton Press, 1991; 446–481.

Quinn B, Edwards N, Longhurst S, Chan DW. Evaluation of an automated non-isotopic immunoassay for measurement of serum vitamin B12. Clin Chem 1991;37:978.

Self CH. Method, use and components. World Intellectual Property Organization International Publ No. 89/05453, 1989.

Self CH. Hapten determination method; its components, its uses and kits including it. Chemical Abstracts 1990;112:51813.

Seth J, Hanning I, Bacon RRA, Hunter WM. Progress and problems in immunoassays for serum pituitary gonadotrophins: evidence from the UK external quality assessment schemes, (EQAS) 1980–1988. Clin Chim Acta 1989;186:67–82.

Siddiqi MA, Abdullah S. An 'antigen capture' ELISA for secretory immunoglobulin A antibodies to hepatitis B surface antigen in human saliva. J Immunol Methods 1988;114:207–211.

Stott DI. Immunoblotting and dot blotting. J Immunol Methods 1989;119:153–187.

Sutton BJ. Molecular basis of antigen-antibody reactions. In: Masseyeff RF, Albert WH, Staines NA, eds. Methods of Immunological Analysis, vol 1. Wienheim, Germany: Verlags Gesellschaft, 1993:66–79.

Tojo M, Shibata N, Osanai T, Mikami T, Suzuki M, Suzuki S. Quantitative precipitin reaction and enzyme-linked immunosorbent assay of mannans of *Candida albicans* NIH A-207 and NIH B-792 strains compared. Clin Chem 1988;34:2423–2425.

Weeks I, Woodhead JS. Chemiluminesence Immunoassay. J Clin Immunoassay 1984;7:82–89.

Wilkins, TA, Brouwers, G, Mareschal, JC, Limet, J, Masson PL. Immunoassay by particle counting, in: Collins, WP (ed), Complementary Immunoassays. Chichester: John Wiley & Sons Ltd., 1988:227–240.

Xu Y-Y, Pettersson K, Blomberg K, Hemmilä, Mikola H, Lövgren T. Simultaneous quadruple-label fluorimetric immunoassay of thyroid stimulating hormone, 17a-hydroxyprogesterone, immunoreactive trypsin, and creatine kinase MM isoenzyme in dried blood spots. Clin Chem 1992;38:2038–2043.

Zahradnik R, Brennan G, Hutchison JS, Odell WD. Immunoradiometric assay of corticotropin with use of avidinbiotin separation. Clin Chem 1989;35:804–807.

Zenke G, Strittmatter U, Tees R, Andersen E, Fagg B, Kocher H, Schreier MH. (1991) A cocktail of three monoclonal antibodies significantly increases the sensitivity of an enzyme immunoassay for human granulocyte-macrophage colony-stimulating factor. J Immunoassay 12:185–206.

CHAPTER 2

Reagent Preparation

Wajdi G. Abdul-Ahad and
James P. Gosling

Whether assays are developed for use "in house" or for commercial exploitation, individual reagents, such as label or antibody, are often purchased from specialist suppliers. This has many advantages with respect to costs and convenience but reagent preparation by the assay developer gives the ability to achieve exceptionally high quality and more opportunities for innovation. In this chapter the common types of immunoassay reagents and their preparation are reviewed.

ANTIBODIES

The techniques already current for the preparation, manipulation, and derivation of antibodies are very powerful and are, in large part, responsible for the immense popularity of antibodies as binding proteins in immunoassays and related techniques. Although invaluable for some specific applications, the alternatives, such as receptors, blood binding proteins, and lectins (see Table 1–2), have individual sets of properties and they each require particular conditions for their manipulation. Therefore, in this chapter relevant discussions are confined to antibodies. The new methods for the preparation and improvement of combinatorial library antibodies, which may become important in the future, are discussed in Chapter 1.

Polyclonal Antibodies

Although many immunoassays for protein analytes, and an increasing number of immunoassays for hapten analytes, employ monoclonal antibodies, polyclonal antibodies have many strong advocates and will remain important in immunoassays for the foreseeable future, particularly as "second" antibodies for indirect labeling or for immobilization.

Choice of Animal Species

The major species used are the rabbit, sheep, goat, guinea pig, and donkey, with the larger animals being more popular for commercial scale production and for "second" antibodies. Animals for immunization should be young, but mature, well nurtured, disease-free, and unstressed. Particular strains or breeds of individual species may offer certain advantages with respect to the antigenicity of some antigens or to the affinity or specificity of the antibodies obtained. This area of expertise is poorly documented and almost anecdotal. Opinions are occasionally strongly expressed: "With TSH goats give higher affinity antibody then sheep" and "The best antibodies to human insulin are produced almost exclusively in guinea pigs." Avian species such as chickens or turkeys have long been advocated as suitable for the production of antibodies against "difficult" mammalian antigens.

Immunization Procedures

There is no generally agreed procedure for immunization to produce antibodies, although there are some important guidelines (Hurn and Chandler, 1980; Burrin and Newman, 1991). The nature of the immunogen and the type of animal may be very important, and the other parameters which are varied include the dose of immunogen, the route of immunization, the adjuvant, and the immunization schedule. A suitable primary dose for a rabbit would be about 100 μg (200 to 500 μg for a goat or sheep) and low doses are regarded as essential for the production of high affinity antibodies. Booster doses may be 10% to 50% of the primary dose. While the route varies, administration is always by injection. Multiple-site intradermal injections at 30 to 50 sites on the back and neck are often recommended for the primary treatment, although the route may be subcutaneous and the number of sites as low as 4. The most popular adjuvants are Freund's complete and incomplete adjuvants, but liposomes are now being advocated as an alternative (Alving, 1991). Normally the titer of serum samples taken at regular intervals increases steadily after the primary injections to reach a maximum at 4 to 6 weeks and then declines. Initial boosting, after an interval of up to several months, normally gives much higher titers within 10–14 days of injection, at which time harvesting is recommended.

Monoclonal Antibodies

Monoclonal antibodies are single idiotype antibodies produced by immortal, monoclonal, hybridoma cell lines which are formed by the fusion of antibody-secreting spleen (or plasma) cells and myeloma cell lines. The great majority of monoclonal antibodies are generated with spleen cells from immunized mice and murine myeloma cell lines, and, because of space limitations, the following discussions are confined to murine homohybridoma antibodies. While an outline is given in Figure 2–1, the detailed information necessary for carrying out these procedures is available in specialist manuals (Campbell, 1984; Goding, 1986; Harlow and Lane, 1988)

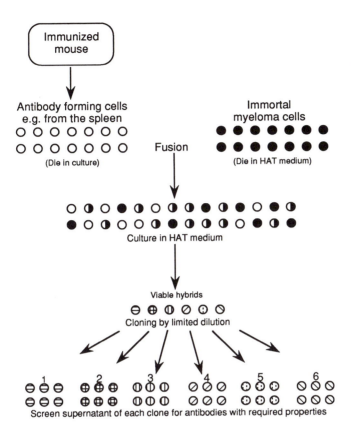

Figure 2–1. Procedure for preparing a monoclonal antibody. The mice are mainly of the BALB/c strain, as most of the available myeloma cell lines are of BALB/c origin and the resulting hybridomas grow well as ascites in BALB/c mice. Immunization is usually with 10 to 100 μg protein in 250 μL of emulsion with Freund's complete adjuvant per mouse, injected intradermally or subcutaneously. Boosting is with similar amounts of incomplete adjuvant. Bleeds are tested so that spleen cells from mice giving the greatest response can be used for fusions.

The myeloma cells to be fused with the antibody producing cells have a genetic defect (normally an inability to survive in growth medium containing hypoxanthine, aminopterin and thymidine [HAT medium]) that is absent in genuine hybrids, thus allowing their selection. The myeloma cells used should also have a good reputation as fusion partners and, when hybridized, as producers of antibody. Polyethylene glycol is the most popular fusing agent; other techniques used involve Sendai virus or electroporation. Successful fusion is uncommon and must be followed by rapid loss of excess chromosomes, so that many fused cells never become established as stable lines. In turn, many of these do not secrete antibody, and even if they do, many will not secrete antibody specific for the antigen of interest. Still less will secrete antibody with the minimum degree of affinity and specificity necessary to be selected by a well-designed screening system. Hence the need for efficient procedures to give a high rate of formation of viable hybrids, and the need to clone and screen thousands of hybridoma clones. Cloning is the process of dilution and culture of small aliquots of culture medium designed to ensure that individual cultures contain only cells derived from a single parent cell. The screening procedure should be very sensitive to identify positive cultures as soon as possible in their growth cycle, and very selective to avoid wasted effort with lines producing inadequate antibody.

The quality of monoclonal antibodies is very largely determined by the screening procedure used to select clones for further investigation, and therefore it should reflect as closely as possible the situation in which the desired antibody will be used, while allowing for the elimination, as early as possible, of a high percentage of clones producing antibodies with inadequate specificity or affinity; perhaps by a series of tests carried out in parallel. Portions of selected clones are frozen according to a defined procedure, stored at −70°C and tested for viability and continued ability to secrete antibody.

Most screening procedures are standard, solid phase, antibody capture, reagent excess, enzyme labeled assays for specific antibodies carried out on microtiter plates or as dot blot procedures (sp-Ag–**Ab**–Ab-enzyme) (see Chap. 1). However, special precautions may be necessary when screening for antibodies against small peptides (Smith, et al., 1993) or to detect antigen-conformation sensitive antibodies (Lolov, et al., 1993).

Production

There are two main ways to produce monoclonal antibodies in significant quantities. BALB/c-compatible hybridomas can be established in the peritoneal cavity of BALB/c mice as tumors that secrete ascites fluid. After 7 to 10 days this fluid accumulates with the specific antibody at 1 to 10 mg/mL and contaminated with 10% of nonspecific antibody. Eventually 5 to 15 mL of ascites containing 40 to 100 mg of antibody can be withdrawn. Repeated removal of fluid can increase greatly the yield per mouse, but this is widely regarded as contrary to basic animal welfare principles. Although in vivo antibody production in ascites fluid requires no complicated equipment, welfare considerations, as well as the fact that the antibody produced in this way is impure, means that this method of production is not used for large-scale production.

In vitro hybridoma culture is applicable to all hybridoma cell types and can be carried out at scales up to that necessary for the production of antibodies for immunotherapy, when kg quantities per batch may be required. Production in homogeneous suspension in flat culture flasks is sufficient for most antibody production for immunoassays. "Hollow fiber," "stirred tank," or "air lift" culture techniques are used for larger scale production.

Purifying Antibodies and Preparing Fragments

Purification

While for some applications antiserum, ascites fluid, or culture medium (which may contain 10% fetal bovine serum) can be used without prior fractionation, it is necessary to purify antibodies when conjugation or immobilization is intended. Purification is also necessary as a preliminary to the preparation of fragments such as Fab'. For polyclonal antibodies purification of the whole IgG fraction may often be adequate, but since specific antibody represents at best only 10% of the IgG, affinity extraction with immobilized antigen may be desirable to give a sufficient density of antibody on a solid phase or to obtain conjugate with a high enough specific activity.

Recommended procedures for obtaining pure or nearly pure antibody include (1) caprylic acid fractionation followed by ammonium sulfate fractionation, (2) fractionation with ammonium sulfate plus DEAE ion exchange chromatography, (3) affinity chromatography with immobilized protein A or protein G, or (4) affinity chromatography with immobilized antigen/hapten, or anti-Ig class antibody (Harlow and Lane, 1988). The precipitation and ion exchange methods are cheap and suitable for large volumes but do not give the highest purity, while the affinity methods, although often single-step, are expensive. Chromatography on staphylococcal protein A is the easiest and most useful method but it is not suitable for antibodies of all classes (e.g., human IgG$_3$) or from all species (e.g., sheep, goat, or rat). Streptococcal protein G is suitable for most IgG subclasses not bound by protein A. Brooks, et al. (1992) described a simplified method for the purification of mouse IgG from hybridoma culture supernatant, with polyethylene glycol 6000 and ammonium sulfate precipitation steps.

Fragmentation

The use of Fab' fragment of specific antibody for the preparation of label conjugates for immunoenzymometric assays (IEMA) has long been advocated by Eiji Ishikawa, who has described procedures for their preparation and purification (Ishikawa, let al., 1983). The preparation of Fab' from mouse monoclonal IgG requires some modifications (Parham, 1986); who also reviewed the preparation for Fab and of Fc from mouse IgM, IgA, IgD, and IgE, and from rat monoclonal antibodies. Akita and Nakai (1993) describe the production and purification of Fab' from chicken egg yolk IgY. Briefly, to prepare Fab', purified IgG is incubated with pepsin and the resultant F(ab')$_2$ is purified from the digest by molecular sieve chromatography on Sephadex G-200, G-150, or Ultrogel AcA 44. Rea and Ultee (1993) propose the addition of ammonium sulfate to the pepsin digestion mixture to improve the specificity of cleavage. Fab' is then formed by reduction with dithiotreitol or 2-mercaptoethylamine in the presence of EDTA. In addition, all solutions should be degassed to prevent reoxidation. Finally, reagents are removed on a desalting column and the Fab' is best used immediately if a conjugate with an enzyme, etc., is required. If not required, the free sulfhydryl can be blocked with *N*-ethylmaleimide and monoiodoacetate.

Characterization of Antibodies

The affinity and specificity of an antibody may be estimated at two to three stages, often initially with a radioactive tracer, then with one or more labels similar to that proposed for use in the assay. For two-site assays with two different antibodies, the antibodies must be evaluated as pairs, perhaps as part of an extensive mapping of the epitopes of the antigen. Specificity may be investigated in detail by means of a range of compounds closely related structurally and biologically to the analyte, but is implicitly being tested during most validation experiments with real samples (see Chaps. 1 and 3 for complementary information and references).

Affinity

Affinity, normally characterized by the equilibrium association constant (K_a; $L \cdot mol^{-1}$, $K_a = k_1/k_2$, where k_1 is the association rate constant [s^{-1}] and k_2 is the dissociation rate constant [$L/mol \cdot s$]) or by the equilibrium dissociation constant (K_d; $mol \cdot L^{-1}$, $K_d = k_2/k_1$), is a characteristic of a single binding site. Antibodies that are bi-, quadra-, or decivalent bind more strongly to antigens with multiple epitopes and can form dense aggregates with soluble antigens. Such complex binding affinity is described by the term *avidity,* which is not precisely defined kinetically. In addition, polyclonal antibodies consist of a number of subpopulations of antibodies, each subpopulation binding with a certain affinity and specificity. Therefore, an affinity constant determined for a polyclonal antibody represents an average of the affinities of the individual subpopulations and is dependent on their relative affinities and concentrations. The methods used to study the affinity and kinetics of antibody-antigen reactions are comprehensively reviewed by Steward (1986).

Specificity

The specificity of an antibody is defined by cross-reactivity studies, but it is important to be aware that these have some important limitations. Many possible cross-reactants may be unavailable in pure form, compounds structurally unrelated to the analyte (and therefore not likely to be included in a formal cross-reactivity study) may cross-react, and if the standard curves for analyte and the cross-reactant are not parallel no single numerical value can adequately represent the cross-reactivity.

For many protein analytes the range of potential cross-reactants that are available in pure form is very limited and a similar situation exists for many drugs. However, a series of highly purified structural components and relatives of immediate interest are available for some protein hormones (e.g., glycoprotein hormones), and a very wide range of steroids may be purchased commercially; it is for analytes like these that cross-reactivity studies are most useful.

As stated above, polyclonal antibodies are heterogeneous, with subpopulations binding analyte and cross-reactants with certain affinities, and an estimate of cross-reactivity represents a balance that is dependent on the relative concentrations of all the substances present that can bind. Therefore, as the concentration of analyte simultaneously present increases, the degree to which a crossreacting substance binds to an antibody may decrease or increase. Here the line between the study of the binding specificity of an antibody and the evaluation of the specificity of an immunoassay becomes evident. For preliminary binding specificity studies the widely used method of Abraham (1969) may be used. According to this method, "standard" curves are constructed with standard and with each potential interferent, and a percentage cross-reactivity is the dose of analyte causing 50% displacement of label divided by the dose of interferent causing 50% displacement, multiplied by 100.

The importance of any potential cross-reactant is greatly dependent on its maximum concentration relative to the lowest, clinically relevant analyte concentration in patient samples. For example, and particularly relevant to antibodies to steroids, 1% cross-reactivity from dehydroepiandrosterone sulfate or cholesterol (for which concentrations of 9 μmol/L or 6000 μmol/L, respectively, would be normal) would contribute 90 or 60,000 nmol/L, respectively, of apparent analyte in an assay.

LABELS

Labeled Proteins

Radioiodination

Although the labeling of proteins by the insertion of ^{125}I into tyrosine, histidine, or tryptophan residues is older than radioimmunoassay (RIA), the requirement for iodinated, but otherwise unaltered, proteins for RIA stimulated the development of a wide range of procedures for their preparation. The oxidative formation of active iodine, such as H_2OI^+, may be promoted electrochemically (little used) or by means of chemical oxidants (e.g., chloramine-T, or iodogen). With the lactoperoxidase method the H_2O_2-dependent oxidation of iodide is enzymatically catalyzed. "Enzymobeads" (Bio-Rad, Richmond, CA) containing immobilized glucose oxidase and lactoperoxidase were designed to minimize exposure to oxidant. The oxidase, along with glucose and dissolved oxygen, serves to continuously generate H_2O_2 for use by the peroxidase, and the beads facilitate removal of the enzymes at the end of the reaction. Recent or comprehensive reviews of iodination methods include Edwards (1991) and Butt (1984).

Tagging Protein Molecules

The range of tagging reagents has expanded greatly and promises to continue to do so. Table 2–1 lists some of the available reagents which vary both with respect to the nature of the labeling substance and the groups on the protein, etc., with which they react. The protein to be labeled may be biotinylated, radioiodinated, or chemiluminescence or fluorescence labeled by attachment of appropriate tags via amino or sulfhydryl groups. Alternatively, a wide range of common antibodies, antigens, and reagents (avidin, streptavidin, protein A, etc.) are commercially available already tagged.

Protein-Protein Conjugation

Antibody- or antigen-enzyme are the most common examples of protein-protein conjugates, but proteins and peptides are also conjugated to carrier proteins to increase their antigenicity. With the multiple antigen peptide (MAP) system, carrier protein is replaced by a small immunogenically inert core of lysine residues for anchoring multiple copies of a peptide (Briand, et al., 1992). Immunization with peptides is also done to generate antibodies against cognate large proteins, but has a low success rate

Table 2–1   Tagging Reagents for the Preparation of Labeled Proteins, etc.*

Label	Label Compound	Reagent Name	Notes	Groups Substituted
Fluor	Coumarin	7-Hydroxy-coumarin-3-carboxylic acid-succinimide ester		Amino
	Fluorescein	5(6)-Carboxyfluorescein-*N*-hydroxysuccinimide ester		Amino
		5-Iodoacetamido-fluorescein		Sulfhydryl
	Rhodamine	5(6)-Carboxy-rhodamine 101–*N*-hydroxysuccinimide ester		Amino
Fluor, TR	Eu^{3+}	N^1-(p-Isothiocyanatobenzyl)-diethylene-triamine-N^1, N^2, N^3-tetraacetic acid-Eu^{3+} chelate	Eu^{3+}-chelate	Amino
Ligand	Biotin	D-Biotinoyl-1,8-diamino-3,6-dioxaoctane	(Biotin-DADOO)	Aldehyde
		N-Hydroxysuccinimidobiotin	NHS-biotin	Amino
		Succinimidyl 6-(biotinamido) hexanoate	Long chain	Amino
		D-Biotinoyl-ϵ-aminocaproic acid–*N*-Hydroxysuccinimide ester	Long chain	
		(1-Biotinamido-4-[4'-(maleimidomethyl) cyclohexane-carboxamido] butane	Biotin-BMCC	Sulfhydryl
		3-(*N*-maleimido-propionyl) biocytin	MPB	sulfhydryl
Luminescent compound	Acridinium Esten	4-(2-Succinimidyloxy-carbonylethyl)phenyl-10-methylacridinium-9-carboxylate		Amino
Radioisotope	^{125}I	*N*-Succinimidyl 3-(4-hydroxy-5-[^{125}I]iodophenyl) propionate	Bolton and Hunter reagent	Amino

*These are available from various suppliers including Pierce, Rockford, Ill; Boehringer Mannheim, Mannheim, Germany; and Pharmacia-Wallac Oy, Turku, Finland.

(Friede, et al., 1993) To prepare conjugates with enzyme, the method of conjugation should be particularly mild so as to retain the immuno- and enzymatic activities and to give stable conjugates. When monoclonal antibodies were carefully prepurified and optimum antibody to enzyme ratios were achieved, the resulting antibody-horseradish peroxidase conjugates improved IEMA sensitivities by up to 6-fold (Madersbacher, et al., 1992).

Glutaraldehyde Methods

Glutaraldehyde, a homobifunctional reagent, is very simple to use for linking together amino groups of lysine residues in different proteins, but homodimers and aggregates may also be produced, particularly in what are called one-step procedures. In two-step procedures one of the proteins (the enzyme, for example) is first allowed to react with glutaraldehyde, the excess reagent is removed, and only then is the second protein (IgG, for example) added and the conjugate allowed to form (Avrameas, et al., 1978). The coupling efficiency is greater, and higher activity is retained, than with one-step methods, although the recovery of enzyme activity may be very low (<10%).

Periodate Oxidation of Glycoproteins

The oxidation of glycoproteins with sodium periodate, horseradish peroxidase for example, gives cleavage of vicinal glycols of the carbohydrate residues to generate dialdehydes, which can react with free amino groups on other protein molecules to form Schiff base linkages. These linkages may then be stabilized by reduction with sodium borohydride. The method has been optimized by Tijssen and Kurstak (1984) who reported 90% coupling efficiency and 90% retention of perioxidase activity. Glucose oxidase is another glycoprotein that can be conjugated in this way.

Heterobifunctional Reagent Methods

Such methods employ reagents that can react with two different functional groups, one on each of the two proteins to be conjugated. The functional groups most often used are amino groups, such as lysine ϵ-amino groups, and sulfhydryl groups, as found on cysteine residues. The reactive moieties found in the reagents are most often succinimides, which react with amino groups, and maleimides or halogenated functions, which react with sulfhydryl groups, all under mild conditions (Table 2–2).

While the great majority of proteins and most peptides have free amino groups, free sulfhydryl groups are relatively rare in intact proteins and peptides. Important exceptions are Fab' and β-*D*-galactosidase from *Escherichia coli*. The reaction sequence for the conjugation of an Fab' to an enzyme with a heterobifunctional coupling reagent is shown in Figure 2–2. Fab'-enzyme conjugates normally retain full immunologic activity because of the favorable geometry of the linkage and can retain full enzymic activity because of the mildness of the reaction conditions (Abdul-Ahad and Gosling, 1987). Careful control of the molar ratios of reactants ensures a high yield of enzyme-Fab' heterodimers with no unwanted aggregation.

Free sulfhydryl groups may be generated by reductive cleavage of native cysteine residues with reagents such as dithiotreitol or mercaptoethylamine, or may be introduced chemically. One of a number of available reagents (Table 2–2) may be used, sometimes with a second step to remove the protective group and expose the sulfhydryl. An important limitation to this approach is the difficulty of ensuring a high degree of substitution but at a low or fixed level (often a 1:1 ratio is desired).

Table 2–2   Reagents for Protein-Protein Coupling, and for Inserting sulfhydryl groups into proteins*

Acronym	Name	Group 1 Reacts with	Group 2 Reacts with
ABDP	N-(4-Aminobenzoyl-N'-(pyridyl-dithioproprionyl)-hydrazine	–SH	–OH (tyrosine)
	Glutaraldehyde	–NH$_2$	–NH$_2$
HSAB	N-Hydroxysuccinimidyl-4-azidobenzoate	–NH$_2$	Unspecific
MBS	m-Maleimidobenzoyl-N-hydroxy-succinimide ester	–NH$_2$	–SH
SMCC	Succinimidyl 4-(N-maleimido-methyl) cyclohexane-1-carboxylate	–NH$_2$	–SH
SATA	N-Hydroxysuccinimide S-acetylthioacetic acid (inserts protected –SH)	–NH$_2$	
SPDP	N-Succinimyl 3-(2-pyridyldithio) propionate (inserts protected –SH)	–NH$_2$	
	2-Iminothiolane (Traut's reagent) (inserts –SH)	–NH$_2$	

*These are available from various suppliers including Pierce, Rockford, Ill; Boehringer Mannheim, Mannheim, Germany; and Pharmacia, Uppsala, Sweden.

Conjugates with Haptens

Immunogens

The chemistry of linking small nonpeptide molecules to a protein (see below under Enzyme Labeled Haptens) for use as an immunogen, or to an enzyme for use as a label, is exactly the same, although the desired substitution ratio is usually much higher in the case of immunogens. The site of attachment on the hapten should be selected on the principle that the antibodies raised will be most specific for those portions of the hapten furthest removed from that site, although this rule of thumb needs to be taken in conjunction with information in regard to the structures of the most important potential cross-reactants. For example, early immunoassays for cortisol used antibodies raised against immunogens with cortisol-21-hemisuccinate and many of these cross-reacted up to about 100% with 21-deoxycortisol, 11-deoxycortisol, and other metabolites. Cortisol is largely distinguished from its metabolic relatives by groups on or near the carbon 20-21 side chain and cortisol linked through the carbon-3 position could be expected to expose these more effectively. Immunogens with cortisol-3-(O-carboxymethyl)-oxime greatly improved the specificity with respect to most metabolites but there is still very strong interference from prednisolone, which differs from cortisol in having an extra double bond in the A ring (Gosling, et al., 1993).

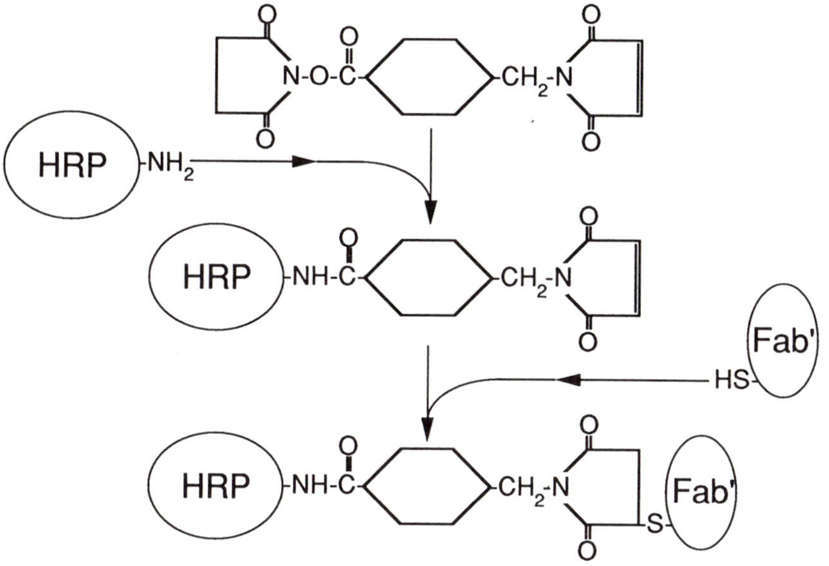

Figure 2–2.   The conjugation of Fab′ to horseradish peroxidase with *N*-succinimidyl 4-*N*-maleimidomethyl) cyclohexane-1-carboxylate (SMCC). The cyclohexane bridge is claimed to give stability to the maleimide group. A sulfonated derivative of SMCC with improved water solubility is also available (Pierce, Rockford, Ill). *m*-Maleimidobenzoyl-*N*-hydroxysuccinimide ester (MBS) has the same reactive groups but a benzoyl bridge.

   In the first step SMCC is reacted with a protein with free amino groups, but no free sulfhydryl group, in this case horseradish peroxidase (HRP). The consequent maleimide-substituted HRP is then reacted with the sulfhydryl-containing protein, in this case Fab′. Both reactions proceed efficiently under mild conditions which facilitates retention of enzyme and antigen-binding activities.

   The retention of the native integrity of the "hapten-substituted" protein in an immunogen may not be essential. The proteins most often used are bovine and human serum albumin, ovalbumin, thyroglobulin, and keyhole limpet hemocyanin (KLH), and preferences have been expressed for those with large numbers of exposed lysine residues and/or those which are from species phylogenetically distantly related to the animal species being immunized. Common carrier proteins, KLH, bovine serum albumin (BSA), and ovalbumin are available commercially with maleimide groups already inserted, for the preparation of immunogens with peptides or haptens containing innate or previously inserted sulfhydryl groups (Pierce, Rockford, ILL).

Enzyme Labeled Haptens

The procedure for coupling is dependent on the functional groups available on the molecules. Although the most popular procedures link haptens to free α- or ε-amino (lysine) or sulfhydryl (cysteine) groups, others including phenolic (tyrosine), imidazole (histidine), or carboxyl (glutamic or aspartic acid) groups can be the linkage site on the enzyme (or other protein). On the hapten a carboxyl or an amino group is most commonly used and, if neither of these is already present (or if such a group is present but necessary for the functional integrity of the hapten molecule), one may be added by derivation. In addition, a spacer group 4 to 6 carbon or oxygen atoms long between the hapten and the enzyme is usually necessary to allow adequate immunologic recognition. A wide variety of common steroids (Steraloids, Wilton, NH; Sigma Chemical Company, St. Louis, MO) and other haptens derived by the addition of potential bridging groups are available commercially. A range of haptens, including estriol, estradiol-17β, digoxin, theophylline, triiodothyronine and thyroxine, with bridging groups and active functions already attached are available from Boehringer Mannheim, Germany (Immunologicals for the Diagnostic Industry Catalogue).

In an immunoassay for hapten, the type of spacer group and its site of attachment to the hapten molecule may be the same in the labeling substance-hapten conjugate as in the hapten-protein immunogen used to raise the antibody (homology) or they may be different (heterology). Heterology may concern the bridging group and/or the site of attachment, or even the hapten itself (Colburn, 1975). Site or bridge heterology decreases the affinity of the antibody for the enzyme-hapten conjugate and it used to be widely claimed that heterology is a necessary precondition for an EIA with a low detection limit. But most hapten EIAs are homologous, and some of them are highly sensitive. On the other hand gross heterology may result in reduced specificity. A labeled-antigen immunoassay for a protein is described as heterologous if the antigen/protein in the label is from a different species and/or has a different amino acid sequence from the protein used to generate the antibody.

The optimum hapten to enzyme ratio in conjugate for an EIA should be investigated each time by preparing a range of test conjugates starting with different ratios of reactant molarities. Most often an incorporation ratio of 1:1 is suitable and a higher ratio results in a decrease in sensitivity (Hosada, et al., 1985). Determination of the ratio for hapten-horseradish peroxidase conjugates can be by spectral differences if such exist (as they do for steroids such as progesterone), but radioactive hapten may be used as a quantifiable tracer, or an immunoassay may be used to estimate the accessible haptens. The recovery of enzyme activity should be at, or near 100%, and there should be negligible nonspecific binding; conjugates not meeting these criteria should normally be rejected for use in high performance assays.

The most common coupling procedures for haptens and proteins are the carbodiimide, the mixed anhydride, and the active ester procedures.

Mixed Anhydride Procedure.   Here the carboxyl group of the hapten is first converted to an acid anhydride which is then allowed to react with a protein amino group. We recommend the procedure as described by Munro and Stabenfeldt (1984), by which the hapten reacts with isobutyl chloroformate in the presence of *n*-ethylmorpholine for 2 minutes at $-20°C$, and is then transferred to react with the protein at the desired molar ratio of hapten to enzyme. It is important to maintain the pH of the protein near its isoelectric point; for example, with conjugates of horseradish peroxidase a pH of 8.0 should be maintained for efficient incorporation of hapten.

Carbodiimide Procedure.   This process consists of the condensation at pH 5.5 between an amino group on a protein and a carboxyl group on a hapten, previously activated with carbodiimide to form an *o*-acylisourea intermediate. It is suitable for the synthesis of immunogen but enzymes may be inactivated and the quality of enzyme conjugates is inconsistent.

Active Ester Procedure.   In this instance carbodiimide is used to enable the formation of an active *N*-succinimidyl ester from the carboxyl-containing hapten and *N*-hydroxysuccinimide (Hosada, et al., 1985) (Fig. 2–3). The active ester can then be used directly or, more effectively, isolated in solid form. A range of such activated derivatives of steroid and thyroid hormones is available commercially from Boehringer Mannheim (Mannheim, Germany).

Tagging Hapten Analytes

Conjugation of a labeling reagent to a hapten-bridge derivative is carried out much as is the tagging of proteins, if the groups to be connected are the same; otherwise chemical synthetic expertise may be required.

SOLID PHASE REAGENTS

Most commonly, the reagent immobilized is a protein; for example, an antibody in two-site assays or in labeled-antigen competitive assays, or an antigen in assays for specific antibody. For labeled-antibody competitive assays, hapten is immobilized. The hapten may be coupled directly and covalently to the solid phase material (e.g., Verschoor, et al., 1990; Yonezawa, et al., 1993), or indirectly by conjugating the hapten to a protein and then immobilizing the protein (e.g., Rajkowski, et al., 1989).

Indirect Immobilization

Indirect binding of antibody or antigen to a solid phase usually means that a second antibody (Howard, et al., 1989), protein A (Sisson and Castor, 1990) or streptavidin (Davies et al., 1994) is first immobilized (normally noncovalently) and then the first antibody (or antigen, etc.) is allowed to specifically adsorb to the bound antibody, etc. Such procedures have the advantages that less first antibody is used, variability may be reduced, and some antibodies perform much better when indirectly bound (Davies, et al., 1994). In addition, the second antibody may bind to a region of the protein to be immobilized "distal" to the site of interest for the next step of the assay (e.g., antibody raised against Fc of IgG), giving improved efficiency by promoting suitable orientation on the solid matrix.

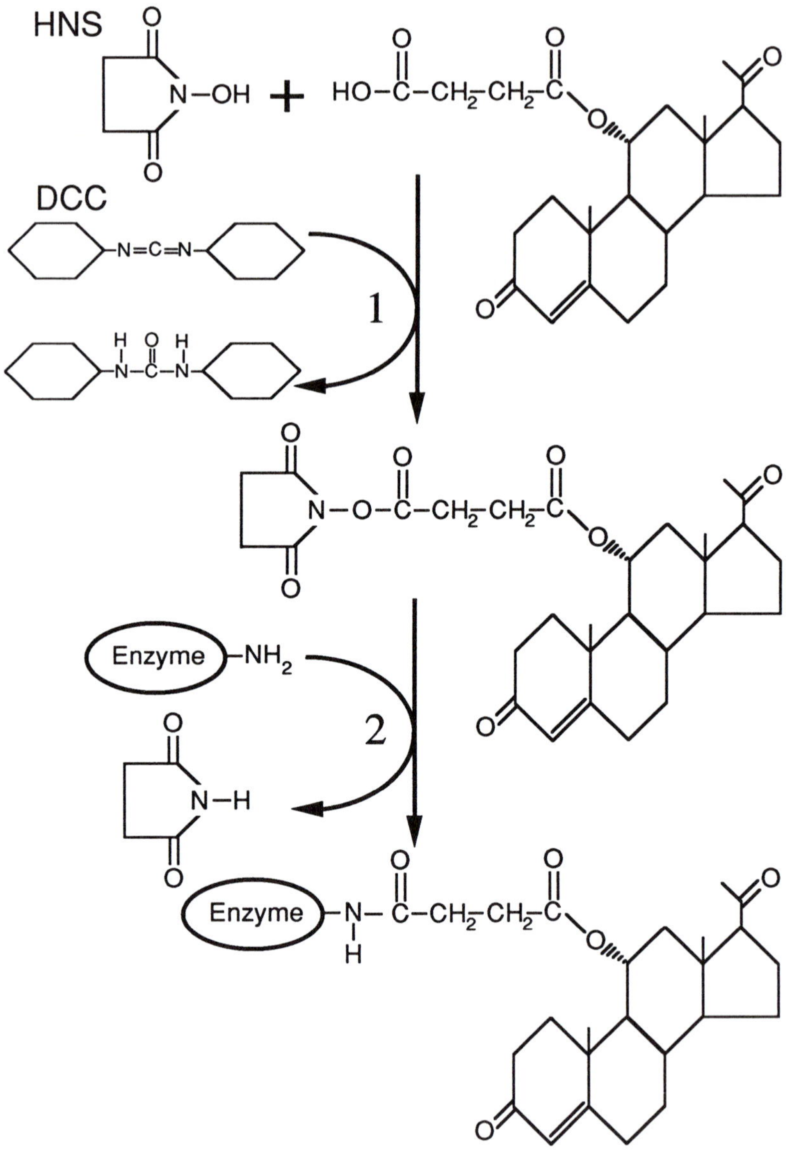

Figure 2–3.   Active ester procedure for the conjugation of steroid hapten to an enzyme or protein. This procedure is carried out in two steps, the first to generate the active ester derivative of the carboxyl-containing hapten, which can then be used directly or stored until needed, and the second for the reaction of the activated hapten with the protein.

  1. 11α-Hydroxyprogesterone hemisuccinate, the steroid to be conjugated, is reacted with *N*-hydroxy succinimide (NHS) in the presence of dicyclohexylcarbodiimide (DCC) in dioxane at room temperature (14° to 20°C) for at least 2 hours, with stirring. As the carbodiimide is transformed to *N,N′* dicyclohexyl urea, the NHS active-ester of the 11α-

Noncovalent Binding

Noncovalent binding of proteins to solid support such as plastics, glass, etc., is a natural and spontaneous process that is often a source of difficulty when μg amounts of protein are being handled. It arises mainly from hydrophobic interactions between surface and subsurface hydrophobic amino acid residues in the protein and hydrophobic regions on the solid surface, and is facilitated by the large molecular weights of proteins. The tightness of binding is not necessarily weaker than when binding is covalent (Rasmussen, 1988). Gamma irradiation of polystyrene induces charged groups on the polystyrene and promotes the binding of some proteins such as IgG, possibly by helping to overcome the effect of intermediate-distance repulsive interactions.

The great advantage of noncovalent methods for coating solid phase materials is their simplicity. Generally, the protein to be adsorbed is put into neutral or mildly alkaline, low concentration buffer and exposed to the solid phase for 30 minutes to 16 hours, before being thoroughly washed to remove loosely bound material. Conditions suitable for adsorption to microtiter plates, tubes (Tijssen, 1985; Rasmussen, 1988) and glass (Tijssen, 1985) are discussed and described in manuals and books concerned with practical aspects of immunoassays. Coating in the presence of precipitating reagents ("forced adsorption") (Hechemy and Anacker, 1983) and partial denaturation of coating antibody (Conradie, et al., 1983) have also been reported as promoting adsorption.

Many developers of solid phase immunoassay methods carry out an extra immobilization step whereby the solid phase already coated with specific antibody or antigen is incubated with inert protein such as BSA or gelatin in buffer in order to minimize nonspecific binding of label. However, in most normal circumstances such "post coating" is not necessary (Mohammed and Esen, 1989) and other approaches to reducing nonspecific binding are more important. The constitution of assay and wash buffers should discourage nonspecific binding, for example, assay buffers may contain detergent with or without inert protein. In addition, only labels that have a low tendency to bind nonspecifically should be used. Thorough washing at every step is also essential. For immunoblot assays an unsuitable blocking reagent may aggravate the sample-dependent high background and, if one proves to be necessary, the blocking protein should be carefully chosen and tested (Craig, et al., 1993).

---

hydroxyprogesterone hemisuccinate is formed. The NHS ester is then isolated after dilution with water and extraction with ethylacetate, and can be stored until needed. This procedure also removes residual carbodiimide, which could deactivate the protein during step 2, and facilitates the adjustment of the molar ratio of hapten to enzyme for step 2.

2. Here the active ester and enzyme (or carrier protein if an immunogen is being synthesized are mixed together in 10 mmol/L phosphate buffer, pH 7.0, and allowed to react at 4°C overnight, before the conjugate is separated from the reactants by means of dialysis (with removal of precipitate by centrifugation) and gel filtration chromatography with Sephadex G-25. This procedure is similar to that described in Tijssen (1985), who reviews many of the alternative approaches.

Covalent Coupling

By its nature the covalent immobilization of proteins on solid phase materials involves the use of materials and proteins with suitable reactive groups and/or coupling reagents. Immobilization onto polysaccharide or polyacrylamide particles, which are not naturally adsorptive, is generally covalent (e.g., Zaidi, et al., 1988). For materials that are naturally adsorptive, covalent coupling has been employed in an attempt to increase the apparent tightness of binding (Place and Schroeder, 1982) or to give more control over the binding process. Materials already substituted with reactive groups such as amines, carboxyls, etc. (Zahradnik, et al., 1989; Kakabakos, et al., 1990; Yonezawa, et al., 1993) may be purchased. Alternatively, reactive groups are inserted (Tijssen, 1985), or a reactive coating is applied in a preliminary step (Hobbs, 1988).

BUFFERS AND AUXILIARY REAGENTS

Buffers

The nature of the buffer used in an immunoassay can significantly influence the assay performance as many antigen-antibody interactions are ionic strength- and pH-dependent, usually unpredictably (Kajubi, et al., 1981). Phosphate buffered isotonic saline, 10 mmol NaH_2PO_4/Na_2HPO_4, 150 nmol NaCl/L, with 0.1% bovine serum albumin (Cohn Fraction V powder) or with 0.1% to 0.5% Tween 20 surfactant, is a popular assay buffer; the protein or surfactant serves to minimize nonspecific interactions. Coating buffer to promote noncovalent adsorption is often 50 mmol/L $NaHCO_3/Na_2CO_3$, pH 9.5. The solution used to thoroughly wash solid phase reagents and hence, to remove nonspecifically bound substances, is often 150 mmol NaCl, 0.5% Tween 20 per liter. In solid phase immunoassays carried out in small vessels such as microtiter wells, procedures to promote mixing (Boraker, et al., 1992; Zhong, et al., 1993) and efficient washing (Beumer, et al., 1992) can have significant advantages.

Auxiliary Reagents

The most important auxiliary reagents include displacing reagents for releasing hapten from serum binding proteins in non-extraction assays, separation reagents for liquid phase assays, enzyme assay mixture for enzyme immunoassays, and enhancement solution for fluorescence endpoint determination in time-resolved fluorimetric immunoassays. To discuss these in detail is beyond the scope of this book.

REFERENCES

Abdul-Ahad WG, Gosling JP. An enzyme-linked immunosorbent assay (ELISA) for bovine LH capable of monitoring fluctuations in baseline concentrations. J Reprod Fertil 1987;80:653–661.

Abraham GE. Solid-phase radioimmunoassay of estradiol-17β. J Clin Endocrinol Metab 1969;29:866–870.

Akita EM, Nakai S. Production and purification of Fab' fragments from chicken egg yolk immunoglobulin Y (IgY). J Immunol Methods 1993;162:155–164.

Alving CR. Liposomes as carriers of antigens and adjuvants. J Immunol Methods 1991;140:1–13.

Avrameas S, Ternynck T, Guesdon JL. Coupling of enzymes to antibodies and antigens. Scand J Immunol 1978;8(suppl 7):7–20.

Beumer T, Stoffelen E, Smits J, Carpay W. Microplate washing: process description and improvements. J Immunol Methods 1992;154:77–87.

Boraker DK, Bugbee SJ, Reed BA. Acoustic probe-based ELISA. J Immunol Methods 1992;155:91–94.

Briand J-P, Barin C, Van Regenmortel MHV, Muller S. Application and limitations of the multiple antigen peptide (MAP) system in the production and evaluation of anti-peptide and anti-protein antibodies. J Immunol Methods 1992;156:255–265.

Brooks DA, Bradford TM, Hopwood JJ. An improved method for the purification of IgG monoclonal antibodies from culture supernatants. J Immunol Methods 1992;155:129–132.

Burrin J, Newman D. Production and assessment of antibodies. In: Price CP, Newman DJ, eds. Principles and Practice of Immunoassay. New York: Stockton Press, 1991;19–52.

Butt WR. Problems of iodination. In: Butt WR ed. Practical Immunoassay: The State of the Art. New York: Marcel Dekker, 1984;19–36.

Campbell AM. Monoclonal Antibody Technology. Amsterdam: Elsevier, 1984.

Colburn WA. Radioimmunoassay for cortisol using antibodies against prednisolone conjugated at the 3-position. J Clin Endocrinol Metab 1975;41:868–875.

Conradie JD, Govender M, Visser L. ELISA solid phase: partial denaturation of coating antibody yields a more efficient solid phase. J Immunol Methods 1983;59:289–299.

Craig WY, Poulin SE, Collins MF, Ledue TB, Richie RF. Background staining in immunoblot assays. J Immunol Methods 1993;158:67–76.

Davies J, Dawkes AC, Haymes AG, et al. A scanning tunnelling microscopy comparison of passive antibody adsorption and biotinylated antibody linkage to streptavidin on microtiter wells. J Immunol Methods 1994;167:263–269.

Edwards R. Radiolabelled immunoassay. In: Price CP, Newman DJ, eds. Principles and Practice of Immunoassay. New York: Stockton Press, 1991;265–294.

Friede M, Muller S, Briand JP, Schuber F, Van Regenmortel M. HV. Generation of antibodies cross-reactive to proteins by peptide immunization. In: Gosling JP, Reen DJ, eds. Immunotechnology. London: Portland Press, 1993:1–12.

Goding JW. Monoclonal Antibodies: Principles and Practice. London: Academic Press, 1986.

Gosling JP, Middle J, Siekmann L, Read G. Improvement of the comparability of results from immunoprocedures for the measurement of hapten analyte concentrations: cortisol. Scand J Clin Invest 1993;53(suppl 216):3–41.

Harlow E, Lane D. Antibodies: A Laboratory Manual. New York: Cold Spring Harbor Laboratory, 1988.

Hechemy KE, Anacker RL. Coating of polymeric surfaces for immunoassay by a forced adsorption technique. J Immunoassay 1983;4:147–157.

Hobbs RN. Solid-phase immunoassay of serum antibodies to peptides. Covalent antigen binding to adsorbed phenylalanine-lysine copolymers. J Immunol Methods 1988;117:257–266.

Hosada H, Takasaki W, Arihara S, Nambara T. Enzyme labeling of steroids by N-succinimidyl ester method. Preparation of alkaline phosphate-labeled antigen for use in enzyme immunoassay. Chem Pharm Bull (Tokyo) 1985;33:5393–5398.

Howard K, Kane M, Madden A, Gosling JP, Fottrell PF. Direct solid-phase enzymoimmunoassay of testosterone in saliva. Clin Chem 1989;35:2044–2047.

Hurn BAL, Chandler SM. Production of reagent antibodies. Methods Enzymol 1980;70: 104–141.

Ishikawa E, Imagawa M, Hashida S, Yoshitake S, Hamaguchi Y, Ueno T. Enzyme-labelling of antibodies and their fragments for enzyme immunoassay and immunohistochemical staining. J Immunoassay 1983;4:209–327.

Kajubi SK, Yang R-K, Li H-R, Yalow RS. Differential effects of non-specific factors in several radioimmunoassay systems. Ligand Quarterly 1981;4:63–66.

Kakabakos SE, Livaniou E, Evengelatos GP, Ithakissios DS. Immobilization of immunoglobulins onto surface-treated and untreated polystyrene beads for radioimmunoassays. Clin Chem 1990;36:492–496.

Lolov S, Tyutyulkova S, Marinova I, Kehayov I, Kyurkchiev S. Conformation-sensitive immunoassay: optimization, validation and evaluation. J Immunol Methods 1993;157:19–23.

Madersbacher S, Wolf H, Gerth R, Berger P. Increased ELISA sensitivity using a modified for conjugating horseradish peroxidase to monoclonal antibodies. J Immunol Methods 1992;152:9–13.

Mohammad K, Esen A. A blocking agent and a blocking step are not needed in ELISA, immunostaining dot-blots and Western blots. J Immunol Methods 1989;117:141–145.

Munro C, Stabenfeldt G. Development of a microtitre plate enzyme immunoassay for the determination of progesterone. J Endocrinol 1984;101:41–49.

Parham P. Preparation and purification of active fragments from mouse monoclonal antibodies. In: Weir DM ed. Handbook of Experimental Immunology, vol 1. Oxford: Blackwell Scientific Publications, 1986;14.1–14.23.

Place JD, Schroeder HR. The fixation of anti-HB$_s$Ag on plastic surfaces. J Immunol Methods 1982;48:251–260.

Rajkowski KM, Hanquez C, Bouzoumou A, Cittanova N. A competitive microtitre plate enzyme immunoassay for plasma testosterone using polyclonal anti-testosterone immunoglobulins. Clin Chim Acta 1989;183:197–206.

Rasmussen SE. Solid phases and chemistries. In: Collins WP, ed. Complementary Immunoassays. Chichester, England: John Wiley & Sons, 1988;43–55.

Rea DW, Ultee ME. A novel method for controlling the pepsin digestion of antibodies. J Immunol Methods 1993;157:165–173.

Sisson TH, Castor CW. An improved method of immobilizing IgG antibodies on protein A-agarose. J Immunol Methods 1990;127:215–220.

Smith SC, McIntosh N, James K. Pitfalls in the use of ELISA to screen for monoclonal antibodies raised against small peptides. J Immunol Methods 1993;158:151–160.

Steward MW. Overview: introduction to methods used to study the affinity and kinetics of antibody-antigen reactions. In: Weir DM ed. Handbook of Experimental Immunology, vol 1. Oxford: Blackwell Scientific Publications, 1986;25.1–25.30.

Tijssen P. Practice and Theory of Enzyme Immunoassays. Amsterdam: Elsevier, 1985;297–328.

Tijssen P, Kurstak E. Highly efficient and simple methods for the preparation of peroxidase and active peroxidase-antibody conjugates for enzyme immunoassays. Anal Biochem 1984;136:451–457.

Verschoor JA, Vermeulen NMJ, Visser L. Haptenated nylon-coated polystyrene plates as a solid phase for ELISA. J Immunol Methods 1990;127:43–49.

Yonezawa S, Kambegawa A, Tokudome S. Covalent coupling of a steroid to microwell plates for use in a competitive enzyme-linked immunosorbent assay. J Immunol Methods 1993;166:55–61.

Zahradnik B, Brennan G, Hutchison JS, Odell WD. Immunoradiometric assay of corticotropin with use of avidin-biotin separation. Clin Chem 1989;35:804–807.

Zaidi M, Girgis SI, MacIntyre I. Development and performance of a highly sensitive carboxyl-terminal-specific radioimmunoassay of calcitonin gene-related peptide. Clin Chem 1988;34:655–660.

Zhong L–Z, Gong Y–F, Fong Y, Zhang Y–S, Gu F–S. Use of microwaves in immunoenzyme techniques. Clin Chem 1993;39:2021.

CHAPTER 3

Immunoassay Development

Jacob Micallef and
Rukhsana Ahsan

Modern immunoassay systems exist in many different forms with diverse ancillary technologies. However, several basic elements are common to most assay development, including selection of suitable reagents, optimization of assay conditions, and analytic and clinical validation.

Immunoassays are usually developed to a specification which includes items relating to analytic and clinical performance, stability of reagents, resistance to operator errors, and cost of manufacture. Aspects such as the instrumentation, label, and separation system to be used may also be fixed by practical considerations or by a requirement for methodologic uniformity.

Reagent selection includes identification of suitable antibodies, label, calibrant, calibrant matrix, buffers, solid phases, and ancillary components such as enzyme substrates. In addition, the forms the various components are to take (e.g., solution, suspension, frozen, powdered, tablet, or lyophilized) must be determined. Reagent selection, optimization, and validation are not sequential steps and their roles are overlapping. Selection of reagents, for example, intrinsically requires some optimization of the process in which they are being evaluated. In practice assay development tends to be a cyclic process as decisions taken at early stages (e.g., reagent selection or incubation conditions) are provisional and may be changed because of results obtained later.

In this chapter assay development is illustrated by examples of immunoassays for hormones developed in our laboratory for the Special Programme of Research in Human Reproduction of the World Health Organization. These assays are used in laboratories in developing countries and have specifications that differ in some respects from those of most commercial manufacturers. In addition to assay validity and operational simplicity, we are particularly concerned that the reagents are stable at temperatures exceeding 40°C for several weeks and that the assays can be used with robust instrumentation requiring little or no servicing.

In this chapter the development and optimization of the three most common types of immunoassays, a two-site assay for antigen, an assay for hapten, and an assay for specific antibody are described, and then, because the main parameters of validation are not method dependent, analytic and clinical validation is covered separately.

DEVELOPMENT OF A TWO-SITE IMMUNOASSAY

The essential requirements of a sandwich assay (see Chap. 1 for a general description) are a matched pair of antibodies with high combined affinity and specificity, a solid phase support for the immunoextractant antibody, a labeling substance that remains highly detectable when covalently linked to antibody and does not reduce antibody affinity, and an analyte preparation to be used as calibrant. A sandwich assay should produce a large, highly reproducible signal in the presence of analyte, and an extremely low signal in its absence. It is the relative sizes and reproducibility of these specific and nonspecific signals that determine the sensitivity and precision of the assay.

Selection of Reagents

Selection of Antibody Pairs

The first stage in the development of a sandwich assay is to identify pairs of antibodies that bind simultaneously to spatially separate epitopes on the antigen. Samples of as many as possible available monoclonal and polyclonal antibodies to the antigen should be collected. All of the antibodies are immobilized on solid phase as potential immunoextractants and also labeled as potential marker antibodies. Every combination of immobilized and labeled antibodies is incubated with antigen to test for sandwich formation. Pairs of antibodies found to give a high signal when exposed to antigen are then further tested for combined specificity. Where possible, antibody pairs with established characteristics should be used, as their identification is a time-consuming procedure. (See also Chap. 1.)

Antibodies used for coating to a solid phase must be purified in order to obtain high specific antibody loading (see also Chap. 2). This allows the use of a minimum surface area of solid phase in the assay, producing low nonspecific binding of label as well as economic benefits. The antibody to be labeled must be highly pure in order to achieve maximum signal/noise response from the assay. In our laboratory antisera are purified by affinity chromatography on protein A or protein G, or by diethylaminoethyl (DEAE) ion exchange chromatography to isolate the IgG fraction. We use monclonal or polyclonal antibodies to produce immunoextractants (particulate solid phase antibody), although we prefer monoclonals as they are available almost indefinitely. Normally we use a purified monoclonal antibody in the label. Where practical, polyclonal antibodies to be labeled should be purified by affinity chromatography to isolate specific IgG (Edwards, et al., 1991).

Substances with structural similarities to the analyte, or present as impurities in the immunogen, may interfere in sandwich assays by binding to either or both of the solid phase and labeled antibodies. This phenomenon is referred to as cross-reactivity and any such substances may contribute to the apparent analyte concentration. Specificity data for individual antibodies in reagent-limited experiments may not relate to their combined specificity in a reagent excess system (Boscato, et al., 1989). Initial specificity tests may be performed in a similar manner to the simultaneous binding experiments. The selected antibody pairs are incubated together with various concentrations of possible interfering substances. Pairs of antibodies found to produce no significant signal with any potential cross-reactant at 10 to 100 times their likely concentrations in physiological fluids are used in further assay development. However, specificity data for two-site assays obtained from such experiments must be treated with caution, as they can produce misleading results (Chapman, 1992).

Solid Phase and Labeling Substance

A variety of solid supports are available for the preparation of immunoextractants. The properties of a good solid support are high antibody loading capacity and low nonspecific binding. Commonly used solid phase materials are described in Chapter 1, and immobilization methods are reviewed in Chapter 2.

A range of particulate supports with magnetic cores surrounded by cellulose, latex, or polystyrene are available commercially (e.g., Piechaczyk, et al., 1989), and their protein binding characteristics vary with the nature of the surface layer. We use magnetic particles as solid support for assays to be distributed to developing countries because they can easily be prepared in large batch sizes, are resistant to degradation at high temperature, and form the basis of a convenient and efficient separation method (Ahsan, et al., 1991).

Substances commonly used to label antibodies for use in sandwich assays include radioisotopes, chemiluminescent molecules, fluorophores, and enzymes. We use alkaline phosphatase as marker for assays to be distributed to developing countries. Antibody-alkaline phosphatase conjugates are resistant to degradation at high temperature and enzyme determination is simple and rapid to perform with inexpensive robust instrumentation (Ahsan, et al., 1991).

Standards and Calibrants

For most protein analytes there is a recognized primary standard, often an "International Reference Preparation" (Bangham, 1976). In theory any stable analyte preparation may be used as the assay calibrant, but this must itself be calibrated against the primary standard for potency and parallelism in the assay system in which it is expected to be used.

It must be noted that some protein analytes exist in multiple isoforms, although this does not always present an analytic problem (Jeffcoate, 1992). The glycoprotein hormones LH, FSH, and TSH are good examples, and their molecular heterogeneity can be demonstrated by electrophoresis, electrofocusing, or chromatofocusing (Snyder, et al., 1989). In such cases a standard preparation of "pure" hormone may react differently in different assay systems according to the relative affinities of the antibodies for their different isoforms and their relative concentrations in the preparation. This causes nonparallelism between standards and may make attempts at standardization of assays for these hormones analytically invalid (Jeffcoate, 1992). In addition, interindividual variation in isoforms can lead to different results for the same serum when assayed in different two-site assays. The origin of this heterogeneity has been attributed to post-translational differences in protein glycosylation (Wide, 1985), but may have a genetic origin (Pettersson, et al., 1991).

The calibrant matrix should ideally be identical to the fluid in the samples to be tested, as the assay response may vary in different media. In the case of human samples this is difficult to achieve and calibrant matrices are often animal serum or protein-loaded buffer.

Individual patient samples may contain endogenous factors that interfere in the chemistry of the assay. The most commonly recognized example is the presence in human serum samples of heterophilic anti-IgG antibodies (Chapman, 1992). These antibodies can cause false negative results by binding, and rendering inactive, the antibodies in the assay, or they can cause false positive results by crosslinking the marker and capture antibodies. The prevention of this interference is important, as the prevalence of human antimurine IgG antibodies may be as high as 40% (Nahm and Hoffmann, 1990), and the number of two-site assays utilizing murine monoclonal antibodies is increasing rapidly. The effect can usually be countered by the addition of up to 3% mouse serum or nonimmune IgG to the assay buffer. Other potential sources of endogenous interference include rheumatoid factors, antianalyte autoantibodies, complement, and factors interacting with antibody-enzyme conjugates (Weber, et al., 1990).

Optimization

When the component reagents have been selected the assay design must be adjusted to optimize the analytic performance of the assay over the range of clinical interest. The dose range, sensitivity, precision, and specificity of the assay must be tailored to meet the clinical diagnostic requirements, while ensuring analytic validity.

Titration of Reagents

The dose range of a two-site assay is limited at the low end by the signal/noise ratio and reproducibility of the assay response. This is determined by the combined affinity of the two antibodies, the detectability of labeled antibody, and the nonspecific signal produced in the absence of analyte. The assay response increases with increasing amounts of immunoextractant and labeled antibodies, but eventually a limit may be reached beyond which increasing background offsets the benefits of increasing signal magnitude. The upper limit of the dose range may be determined by the amounts of antibodies used or by the method used to determine the endpoint. Both the solid phase and labeled antibodies must be titrated to ensure sufficient amounts of both to operate in excess in the presence of the highest analyte concentrations to be measured, while maximizing precision at critical diagnostic levels.

With coated plastic surfaces, such as microtiter wells, the concentration of IgG in the coating solution is changed to vary the coating density, but particulate immunoextractants coated to a fixed density can also be serially diluted for testing, In both cases the various concentrations of immobilized antibody are reacted with excess labeled antibody in the presence of zero analyte and at the highest concentration of analyte specified to be measured. Results for the titration of a magnetizable solid-phase polyclonal antibody used in a two-site enzyme-labeled assay for prolactin are shown in Figure 3–1. The specific signal for the highest standard reaches a maximum value with increasing antibody concentration (i.e., excess reagent conditions prevail). Further increases serve only to increase the nonspecific or zero signal and, hence, decrease the signal/noise ratio. The labeled antibody must be similarly tested at serial dilutions using excess immunoextractant.

Incubation Conditions

To achieve maximum signal sizes and to minimize drift in results, it is usual to incubate for sufficient time to allow all reactions to achieve or approach equilibrium. The time required varies from a few minutes for a modern particulate immunoextraction step at 37°C, to several hours for some other assay systems at 4°C. The rate of reaction may be different for the samples and standard and may also vary with the concentration of analyte. Typically, low analyte concentrations require longer times to reach equilibrium than high concentrations.

Determination of the rate of equilibrium is carried out by incubating a few patient samples and standards of different concentrations for varying lengths of time and plotting the resultant signals against time. The incubation time and temperature

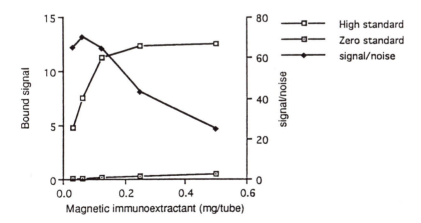

Figure 3–1. Titration of protein G–purified polyclonal antiprolactin IgG coated on magnetic particles for use as an immunoextractant detected by excess enzyme-labeled monoclonal antibody in a two-site sandwich assay.

chosen should be sufficient so that the signals for samples and standards for all concentrations approach stable maxima.

There are two basic assay procedures for two-site immunoassays. The first has a single step and involves the simultaneous reaction of the immunoextractant and labeled antibody with the analyte. This is convenient but has the disadvantage that very high antigen concentrations lead to a "hook effect," whereby increasing concentrations of antigen cause a paradoxic fall in signal (Nomura, et al., 1982). The signal decreases because at high analyte concentrations there tends to be sufficient analyte to saturate both the labeled and immunoextractant antibodies, thereby preventing sandwich formation. The importance of this effect varies with different analytes but it may lead to misdiagnoses.

The alternate procedure involves two separate reaction incubations. The first incubation is to allow reaction of the immunoextractant with the analyte, after which the assay mixture is discarded and the solid phase is washed. The second incubation is for the reaction of the immobilized analyte with the labeled antibody. The complete solid phase sandwich is then washed and the bound labeled-antibody measured. This protocol is less convenient but no hook effect occurs, as any analyte not extracted in the first step is physically removed by washing.

DEVELOPMENT OF A LIMITED-REAGENT ASSAY

Small molecular weight analytes, such as thyroid and steroid hormones and many drugs, cannot be detected by two-site assays, because sandwich formation is only possible for antigens large enough to bind two molecules of immunoglobulin independently without steric hindrance. Consequently, they are measured by limited-reagent assays, for which there are no limitations on the nature of analyte, provided a specific antibody can be obtained.

The requirements of a labeled-analyte, reagent-limited assay are a high-affinity specific antibody, a marker that remains highly detectable when covalently linked to the hapten (or a chemical derivative of it), a calibrant preparation, and usually a method for separation of the free and antibody-bound analyte. An alternative design for limited-reagent assays involves analyte immobilized on a solid phase and detection of bound labeled-antibody (e.g., Bodmer, et al., 1989). (See also Chap. 1.)

Selection of Reagents

Selection of Antibody and Labeled Hapten

Antibodies used in reagent limited-assays may be monoclonal or polyclonal. The main factors in selection of reagents include antibody affinity, specificity, and bridge binding effects (Tiefenauer, et al., 1989).

The antibody selected must be capable of binding analyte at the concentrations of clinical interest, which are usually in the 10^{-6} to 10^{-9} mol/L range, but may be as low as 10^{-12} mol/L. For a particular antibody, analytic performance is optimal at analyte concentrations near the inverse of its affinity. Therefore, antibody affinities of 10^{10} L/mol are adequate for most analytes, but affinities of up to 10^{12} L/mol are required for some analytes. Antibody affinity can be estimated from Scatchard plots (Soos and Siddle, 1982; see also Chaps. 1 and 2).

Antibodies can be tested for binding to labeled hapten by incubating them together at various dilutions. Labels substituted with tritium atoms are usually chemically identical to the endogenous analyte, but antibody affinity for labeled haptens (hapten-bridge-marker) may be much greater than that for endogenous analyte due to bridge binding effects. Therefore, antibodies should be tested with the labeled hapten intended for use in the assay. When present, bridge binding effects may be reduced by the use of heterologous hapten conjugates in the immunogen and label (Tiefenauer, et al., 1989). In fact, the majority of commercial hapten immunoassays are homologous, employing immunogen and label with identical bridges and sites of attachment.

Separation Systems

An efficient assay separation step is critical for maximizing assay precision. The most reproducible and efficient separation is given by solid phase systems. The most commonly used separation agent is solid phase anti-IgG, although in some assays the primary antibody is itself immobilized. The range of supports is similar to that for two-site assays.

Other separation methods include liquid phase precipitation of antibody-bound labeled-analyte with anti-IgG antiserum, and charcoal adsorption of free labeled-hapten. These methods are less reproducible and efficient, and are rarely encountered in commercially produced immunoassays (see also Chap. 1).

Standards and Calibrants

Hapten analytes can normally be obtained in pure form and absolute standardization by mass is usually possible. There are no internationally recognized primary standards for analytes, although preparations of certified quality for some hapten analytes are available from the National Institute for Science and Technology (NIST), Washington DC. In any case, a master calibrant set should be prepared against which routine calibrants can be checked to avoid batch to batch variation.

The standard matrix should ideally be identical to the fluid in the samples, but animal serum or buffer is often used in place of human fluids. Assays for human serum analytes, such as thyroid or steroid hormones which use blocking agents (Ratcliffe, et al., 1982), as well as for free thyroid hormones (Ekins, 1982), may require human serum as standard matrix because the interaction of the analyte with serum binding proteins is central to the chemistry of the assay.

Displacement of Analyte from Binding Proteins

Some hapten analytes, including many steroids, thyroid hormones and some drugs, are largely bound to binding proteins in serum. Some assay methods measured such analytes after extraction from serum with an organic solvent.

Direct assay of these analytes without solvent extraction is possible with the use of blocking analogs. These analogs must be selected, either individually or in combination, for binding to serum proteins. Concentrations must be sufficient to displace the analyte from binding proteins, while not binding to the antibody. Typical examples include the displacement of triiodothyronine (T_3) and thyroxine (T_4) from thyroid binding globulin (TBG), albumin, and prealbumin by 8-anilino-1-naphthalene sulfonic acid (ANS) and the displacement of progesterone from corticosteroid binding globulin (CBG) and albumin by danazol or cortisol (Ratcliffe, et al., 1982).

Alternatively, the binding proteins in the samples may be irreversibly denatured by heating (e.g., at 56°C after dilution with alkaline buffer).

Optimization

When a suitable antibody, labeled hapten, calibrant preparation and blocker analog (if applicable) have been selected, the assay design must be optimized for precision at analyte concentrations corresponding to clinical decision limits. A number of authors have described approaches to the systematic derivation of conditions for maximal sensitivity of reagent-limited immunoassays (e.g., Ekins, 1991; Ezan, et al., 1991).

Selection of Reagent Concentrations.   The concentration range over which acceptable precision may be obtained is narrower for reagent limited-assays than for two-site reagent excess assays. The range of acceptable precision, and hence the limiting sensitivity of limited-reagent assays, can be shifted, within limits, to higher or lower concentrations of analyte by changes in the concentrations of antibody and labeled hapten used. Figure 3–2 shows the effect of changes of antibody concentration on the precision profile with other factors held constant. An analogous effect can be obtained for changes in labeled hapten concentration.

Selection of approximate antibody and labeled-analyte concentrations is performed by making serial dilutions of both, and testing the combinations of each antibody dilution with every labeled hapten dilution in the presence of zero analyte and analyte concentrations corresponding to the anticipated highest and lowest standards. The initial "optimum" reagent concentrations are those giving the greatest, and most reproducible, changes in signal with increasing analyte concentration. The concentrations finally selected are those giving the best precision in the clinical diagnostic ranges required. Many workers simplify this process by initially selecting a convenient label concentration (usually between 10^4 to 10^5 counts per minute for radioimmunoassay [RIA]) to get a suitable maximum signal size. They then determine the optimum antibody dilution at this prefixed labeled-analyte concentration. Results of an antibody dilution experiment for a T_3 RIA are shown in Figure 3–3.

Optimal times and temperatures of incubation are determined in a similar fashion to that described for two-site assays, bearing in mind that antibody affinity may be temperature dependent.

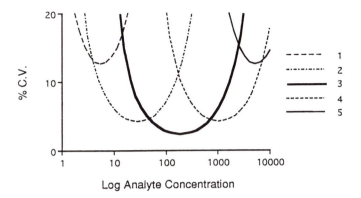

Figure 3–2. Effect of antibody concentration on precision profile. Curve 3 represents a notional within-batch precision profile for a reagent-limited assay optimized for a certain dose range. Curve 2 represents a shift in the range of best precision to lower concentrations due to a decrease in antibody concentration. Curve 4 represents a similar shift to higher concentrations due to an increase in antibody concentration. Curves 1 and 5 illustrate how at extremes of antibody concentration there will also be a marked deterioration of precision.

DEVELOPMENT OF AN ASSAY FOR SPECIFIC ANTIBODY

Immunoassays for specific antibody can be of reagent-limited or two-site sandwich design (see Chaps. 1, 15, and 17). The most common design is a two-site sandwich assay where the solid phase is coated with purified antigen (e.g., rubella or hepatitis sur-

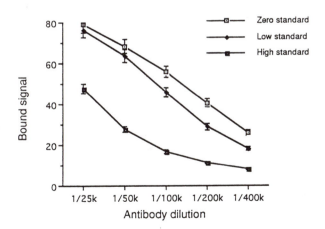

Figure 3–3. Antibody dilution and displacement curves for T_3 RIA using a polyclonal anti-T_3 antibody with ^{125}I-T_3 tracer and anti-IgG coated to magnetic particles. The error bars represent ±SD.

face antigen which may be of "recombinant" origin or consist of inactivated pathogen). Specific antibodies from the test sample that are captured by the solid phase are then detected by reaction with a labeled, anti-human immunoglobulin antibody.

When the detection of the presence of specific IgG antibodies is of no diagnostic value, class specificity may be required as, for example, in the diagnosis of recent viral infection by assay of viral-antigen-specific IgM antibodies, and an antigen capture assay design may be used (see Chap. 1; Kemeny, 1992).

Commercial assays frequently use microtiter plates, as these are well suited to large sample throughput and automation, but other solid phases are also used. The anti-human class or subclass antibody used may be common to any number of assays, but must be of high affinity for maximal assay sensitivity. Enzyme labels are frequently used.

Optimization of an Antibody Capture Assay

Assays for specific antibody are normally qualitative, and therefore are optimized to minimize false positive and false negative results, as well as for a low detection limit. The solid phase and marker antibody and antigen concentrations are titrated with dilutions of known, strongly positive and weakly positive sera. Sufficient of both must be used to ensure that reagent excess conditions prevail for strongly positive samples, while keeping nonspecific binding and the imprecision of low assay response levels as low as possible. This maximizes the signal/noise ratio and the sensitivity of the assay for weakly positive samples.

Incubation times and temperatures should be sufficient to ensure that immunochemical reactions approach equilibrium. Reaction rates can be determined by incubating a few patient samples for varying lengths of time and plotting the resultant signals against time. Reaction is slower for low concentrations of specific antibody, and reaction kinetics should be determined using weakly positive samples as well as samples producing a stronger assay response.

ANALYTIC VALIDATION

All assays developed for use in clinical chemistry should be validated in accordance with the guidelines published by the International Federation of Clinical Chemistry (IFCC, 1980; 1983; 1984a; 1984b). The most commonly used parameters of assay validation are assay specificity, sensitivity, within-batch and between-batch precision at concentrations reflecting clinical decision limits, tests of identity of patient analyte and assay calibrant, and tests for analytic recovery. Finally, patient results must be compared with those obtained by other independent methods of assay. Validation experiments are only reliable when carried out under the same assay conditions as used in the final, fully developed assay.

Specificity

Even if all available likely cross-reactants are shown not to produce a response in an assay, specificity is not unequivocally established. This is because potential cross-reactants may not be available in pure form or may be unknown. However, cross-reactivity studies are essential and should be as comprehensive as possible.

The nature of likely cross-reactants varies with the nature of the analyte. TSH, for example, is a glycoprotein produced in the pituitary consisting of α and β subunits. The β subunit is not unique to TSH but common to TSH, LH, FSH, and hCG. Likely cross-reactions for TSH, therefore, include LH, FSH, hCG and the unassociated α and β subunits, as well as other pituitary hormones (e.g., prolactin and growth hormone) which are possible contaminants of the pituitary extract material commonly used in immunogen. Likely cross-reactants for a new drug, or a steroid analyte would include all structurally related molecules (including any binding protein-blocker analog used for assays without an extraction step) and metabolites.

To characterize the specificity of an assay system, dose response curves are constructed in the presence of the analyte and potential cross-reactants tested at concentrations greater than likely pathophysiologic concentrations. These tests should be performed using the final assay design with the intended sample matrix. The results of such an experiment for an enzyme-labeled two-site sandwich FSH assay with separate magnetic solid phase immunoextraction and labeled antibody incubations are shown in Figure 3–4.

The importance of testing the effects of the interaction of cross-reactants with analytes is even more important with two-site immunometric assays. This is because a cross-reactant that binds to only one of the two antibodies will prompt little or no

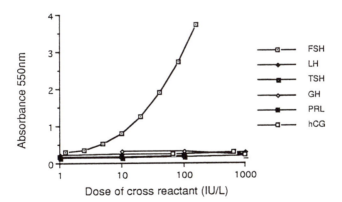

Figure 3–4. Specificity of a two-site sandwich assay for FSH employing one monoclonal anti- FSH antibody coated to magnetic particles and another monoclonal antibody conjugated with enzyme.

assay response when presented alone as a pure standard, but may significantly reduce analyte binding if simultaneously present in sufficiently high concentrations, causing false low results. Even when binding of cross-reactant by both antibodies occurs, some cross-reactions may be concealed by the high dose hook effect, if this is present. The assessment of the recovery of pure hormone standard (preferably an international Reference Preparation that is of high purity) from patient samples containing pathophysiologic levels of potential cross-reacting substances is recommended as the most reliable indicator of cross-reaction problems (Chapman, 1992).

Cross-reactivity can be expressed in a variety of ways (Miller and Valdes, 1992) including the apparent concentration of analyte resulting from the assay response due to an arbitrary concentration of cross-reactant, and the percentage ratio of the concentrations of analyte and cross-reactant that produces a 50% displacement of tracer in a limited-reagent assay (see also Chap. 2). Miller and Valdes (1992) also proposed a new protocol for evaluating and expressing cross-reactivity data involving the construction of interferographs for analytically important cross-reactants.

Precision and Sensitivity

Overall assay reproducibility is best derived from patient sample data or from the analysis of control samples that resemble patient samples as closely as possible. Most simply, it can be expressed as the coefficient of variation of patient sample duplicate results (within-sample, within-batch precision), but this varies markedly with analyte concentration. Therefore, sufficient duplicate data should be collected and sorted by concentration into a number of groups, the between-replicate coefficient of variation calculated for each group, and the resultant information represented graphically as a plot of coefficient of variation against analyte concentration. Such plots are known as precision profiles and can be constructed for other levels of reproducibility such as within-sample, between-batch precision. An acceptable level of imprecision for assay results is dependent on the clinical application and on intraindividual biologic variation (Ricós and Arbós, 1990). Prevision requirements are usually more rigorous at, or near, clinical decision limits (see also Chap. 4).

Clinical requirements for assay sensitivity vary widely, and for many analytes maximizing assay sensitivity is not necessary. Other analytes ideally require detection limits below levels achievable with current technology. The operational definition of the sensitivity of assay is the smallest detectable dose at which the assay response is significantly different from zero. This is estimated empirically as 2 or 3 times the standard deviation in the measurement of zero dose (Ezan, et al., 1991), but a factor of 3 should be universally adopted.

Tests for Analytic Recovery

To test for analytic recovery, graded doses of calibrant are added to patient samples and allowed to equilibrate with the matrix. The samples should be as varied and as numerous as is practical and the amounts of calibrant added should cover the intended dose range of the assay. When the samples are analyzed the observed results should equal the endogenous concentrations plus the amounts of calibrant added.

Recovery experiment data is analyzed by plotting for each sample the amount of material detected on the abscissa against the amount introduced on the ordinate and fitting the points to a straight line by regression analysis. For 100% recovery the slope should be unity and the intercept equal to the endogenous level. More simply, the individual percentage recoveries for each concentration of calibrant added to each sample may be calculated and tabulated.

Analytic recoveries consistently greater or less than 100% (within experimental error) often result from disparity between the calibrant and patient sample matrices, but may have other causes, for example, susceptibility of the assay to cross-reactants in patient samples.

Tests for Identity of Analyte and Calibrant

In the validation of any assay, it is essential to demonstrate that the calibrant and unknown materials produce parallel assay response curves. Although parallelism of dose response curves does not prove identity of materials, lack of parallelism proves nonidentity. The usual test for parallelism is linearity of results of patient samples with dilution.

To set up a linearity test, patient samples are progressively diluted in sample or calibrant matrix, and analyzed to calculate the apparent amount of material present. The samples should be as varied and as numerous as possible, and the dilutions should be arithmetic not serial (e.g., 1/1, 4/5, 3/5, 2/5, 1/5 and not 1/1, 1/2, 1/4, 1/8, and so on) and include dilutions lower than normally analyzed. Any substances present in patient samples that affect the assay response, but are not identical to the calibrant, may give patient and standard dose response curves that are nonparallel. Several methods have been developed for testing of parallelism (Rodbard, et al., 1977). The simplest is to plot assay result (expressed as pg or nmol per tube or well) against the effective volume of sample analyzed (μL) and the points obtained should fall on a straight line of negligible intercept. The observation, in even only one sample, of a significant deviation from linearity at higher volumes (lower dilutions) would clearly indicate that the sample volumes or dilutions routinely determined should be limited to those safely within the linear region. The use of serial dilutions and the plotting of results as a series of "parallel" "standard curves" can hide even pronounced effects (Power and Fottrell, 1991).

Comparisons with Independent Methods

Immunoassays should produce patient results similar to those of other reliable immunoassays as well as independent methods of assay. Samples from a variety of clinical conditions are analyzed by both methods and the results compared. A statistically significant number of varied patient and normal samples (30 at least) must be used. Plotting the data on a scattergram with identical axes, along with the (bisecting) line of perfect agreement, allows a good assessment to be made of the degree of agreement between the two methods. Simple regression analysis is very widely used to estimate the measure of correlation, but this has been strongly criticized by Bland and Altman (1986) because the correlation coefficient obtained is nearly always very large, even in the face of poor agreement. Disagreement, and whether or not it is concentration dependent, is better assessed by plots of difference in the two assay results against the mean result (Bland and Altman, 1986; Pollock, et al., 1992).

Where possible, comparison should be made with an established reference method, for example isotope dilution–gas chromatography mass spectrometry (ID-GCMS) for hapten analytes (Tunn, et al., 1990; Gosling, et al., 1993). For protein analytes, a well validated and well established clinical test should be used, if possible one that has given accurate and precise results in external quality assessment schemes.

CLINICAL VALIDATION

When an immunoassay is developed for a specified clinical purpose the effectiveness of the assay in achieving clinical objectives must be assessed.

With respect to clinical validation, the percentage of patients known to have the disease who test positive is called the "sensitivity" of a test. Similarly, the percentage of patients known to be free of the disease who test negative is called the "specificity" of the test. (Please note that clinical specificity and sensitivity are quite different from analytic specificity and sensitivity.) The overall efficiency of the test is the proportion of all patients for whom the test correctly predicts the presence or absence of the disease. For qualitative tests the proportion of false positive results can usually be minimized at the expense of an increase in false negative results, and vice versa, by changing the diagnostic cutoff limits. Assessment of the clinical validity of an assay is made by mathematical evaluation of these parameters in light of clinical requirements and by comparison with other tests for the diagnosis of the same disorder.

High clinical sensitivity is essential in, for example, screening tests for HIV or hepatitis infection in blood or organ donation. Such tests may inevitably produce some false positive results but this may be acceptable if all the samples designed positive can be further investigated by means of more specific tests. On the other hand, high clinical specificity is especially important when treatment of the disease diagnosed is potentially dangerous, for example chemotherapy or radiotherapy. False negative results may be identified by other means, but the possibility of a healthy person being subjected to treatment is minimized.

For quantitative assays the same principles apply but numeric results can indicate the probability of disease being absent or present. Normal and diagnostic ranges must be established by the analysis of a large number of patient samples with verified normal or pathologic conditions. Patient samples verified as free of disease should include as wide a variety of types as possible. Occasional or abnormal states that may affect the interpretation of results include pregnancy, confinement to bed, hyperthyroidism, liver disease, and treatments with any of a wide variety of drugs. Diagnostic ranges are calculated by standard epidemiologic methods (Armitage and Berry, 1987) and may vary between populations because of genetic, dietary, or environmental factors or within population groups because of additional factors such as age, sex, body weight, lifestyle, occupation, and previous clinical history. Inadequate and inappropriate reference ranges constitute a very serious deficiency in some areas of clinical immunoanalysis (Seth, et al., 1991).

For many analytes well-defined changes in their normal levels occur naturally or can be induced, and these should be measured to corroborate clinical validity. Such changes may be due to diurnal rhythms (e.g., cortisol), menstrual rhythms (e.g., progesterone), pregnancy (e.g., hCG), or be induced by administration of drugs or hormones (e.g., corticotropin-releasing hormone and corticotropin).

EVALUATION OF COMMERCIAL ASSAYS

In-house immunoassays are normally validated in the laboratory that developed and runs them routinely, but their use is diminishing in favor of commercially produced and increasingly automated kits (Wheeler, 1992). The number of kits on the market is steadily expanding and an *Immunoassay Kit Directory* is now being regularly published (Seth, 1991).

The suitability of a commercial assay for a particular clinical purpose cannot be assumed, and the first step in its evaluation is the compilation of as much available data as possible. The manufacturer's product information must be read carefully to establish that the assay is designed for the user's intended purpose. Product information usually includes some data on analytic and clinical validity. Certain analytes present problems of calibration and it is important to ascertain the nature of the calibrant and, where applicable, the validity of its calibration against internationally recognized reference preparations. A literature search may yield information describing other users' experience with the assay and further data may be obtained by personal contact. Additional valuable information can be obtained from national or commercial external quality assessment schemes, including the number of users for any particular method, bias relative to other methods of assay, between-batch variability of bias, between-laboratory precision, and analytic recovery (Middle, 1992). Even when the names of manufacturers are not included in reports, external quality control scheme organizers may be willing to give advice on choosing a method.

Full evaluation of a commercial assay includes independent analytic and clinical validation, as described earlier, to confirm the manufacturer's product information data. The manufacturer's assay instructions must be followed rigorously. In addition, the reproducibility of results from at least four assay kits, ideally from more than one production batch, should be assessed. This is done by repeated assay of at least six samples with analyte concentrations of clinical interest up to 10 times with each kit. An assessment of the shelf life of complete kits (as well as individual critical reagents) should also be performed by storage at elevated temperatures so that degradation is rapid and can be detected in a relatively short time (Kirkwood, 1977). From data collected in such accelerated degradation studies, the shelf lives of reagents under more normal conditions can be predicted with software based on the Arrhenius and Eyring equations (Tydeman and Kirkwood, 1984).

It is worth noting that proper evaluation of commercial free-hormone assays should involve tests to show genuine measurement of the free fraction, in addition to the above noted criteria (Ekins, 1982). These tests should include independent confirmation that the antibody affinity is adequate for free hormone concentrations and estimates of assay response to increases in the free concentration induced by addition of agents that partially displace the bound fraction. For free T_4, the lack of dependence of assay result on sample dilution should also be demonstrated.

The full evaluation of commercial assays is a time-consuming undertaking, rarely performed in routine pathology laboratories. Most laboratories establish the analytic and clinical validity of commercial assays by a review of product information and published data followed by a brief practical assessment of assay precision and bias. Selection of a particular commercial kit is usually based on cost, reputation, and available instrumentation as well as assay performance. However, the performance of an assay in external quality assessment schemes should *always* be examined critically and taken into consideration.

REFERENCES

Ahsan R, Cekan S, Hayes MM, Latif A, Micallef JV, Sufi SB. Multicentre trial of isotopic and non-isotopic assays of reproductive hormones: a comparison of assay performance and reagent stability. In: Developments in radioimmunoassay and related procedures. Vienna: IAEA, 1991;529–538.

Armitage P, Berry G. Statistical Methods in Medical Research, ed 2. Oxford: Blackwell Scientific Publications, 1987.

Bangham DR. Standardisation in peptide hormone immunoassays: principle and practice. Clin Chem 1976;22:957–963.

Bland JM, Altman DG. Statistical methods for assessing agreement between two methods of clinical measurement. Lancet 1986;i:307–310.

Bodmer DM, Tiefenauer LX, Andres RY. Antigen versus antibody-immobilised ELISA procedures based on a biotyinyl-estradiol conjugate. J Steroid Biochem 1989;33: 1161–1166.

Boscato LM, Egan GM, Stuart MC. Specificity of two-site immunoassays. J Immunol Methods 1989;117:221–229.

Chapman RS. Interference in immunoassay. Communications in Laboratories Medicine 1992;1:49–56.

Edwards R, Little JA, Zaman MR, Knott JA, Newman DJ. Affinity chromatography of polyclonal antibodies: a practical alternative to monoclonal antibodies. In: Developments in Radioimmunoassay and Related Procedures. Vienna: IAEA, 1991;205–212.

Ekins R. The biological significance and measurement of 'free' hormones in blood. Recent Adv Endocrin Metab 1982;2:287–327.

Ekins R. Immunoassay design and optimisation. In: Price CP, Newman DJ eds. Principles and Practice of Immunoassay. New York: Stockton Press, 1991;96–153.

Ezan E, Tiberghien C, Dray F. Practical method for optimizing radioimmunoassay detection and precision limits. Clin Chem 1991;37:226–230.

Gosling JP, Middle J, Siekmann L, Read G. Improvement of the comparability of results from immunoprocedures for the measurement of hapten analyte concentrations: cortisol. Scand J Clin Lab Invest 1993;53 (suppl 216):3–41.

IFCC. Approved recommendations (1978) on QC in clinical chemistry. Part 2. Assessment of analytical methods for routine use. J Clin Chem Biochem 1980;18:78–88.

IFCC. Revised recommendations (1983) on evaluation of diagnostic kits. Part 2. Guidelines for the evaluation of clinical chemistry kits. J Clin Chem Biochem 1983;21: 899–902.

IFCC. IFCC/WHO principles and recommendations on evaluation of diagnostic reagent sets used in health laboratories with limited resources. Part 3. Selection and evaluation using reference materials, general considerations. J Clin Chem Biochem 1984a;22: 573–582.

IFCC. IFCC/WHO principles and recommendations on evaluation of diagnostic reagent sets used in health laboratories with limited resources. Part 4. Evaluation of performance using reference materials of analytes commonly determined in blood serum or plasma. J Clin Chem Biochem 1984b;22:817–826.

Jeffcoate SL. Heterogeneity of peptide hormones: analytical and clinical significance. Communications in Laboratory Medicine 1992;1:6–15.

Kemeny DM. Titration of antibodies. J Immunol Methods 1992;150:57–76.

Kirkwood TBL. Predicting the stability of biological standards and products. Biometrics 1977;33:736–742.

Middle JG. The state of the art of steroid hormone assays: a UK NEQAS perspective. Communications in Laboratory Medicine 1992;1:84–113.

Miller JJ, Valdes R Jr. Methods for calculating crossreactivity in immunoassays. J Clin Immunoassay 1992;15:97–107.

Nahm MH, Hoffmann JW. Heteroantibody: phantom of the immunoassay. Clin Chem 1990;36:829.

Nomura M, Imai M, Usuda S, Nakamura T, Miyakawa Y, Mayumi M. A pitfall in two-site sandwich 'one-step' immunoassay with monoclonal antibodies for the determination of human alpha-fetoprotein. J Immunol Methods 1982;56:13–17.

Pettersson K, Ding, YQ, Huhtaniemi I. Monoclonal antibody-based discrepancies between two-site immunometric tests for lutropin. Clin Chem 1991;37:1745–1748.

Piechaczyk M, Baldet L, Pau B, Bastide JM. Novel immunoradiometric assay of thyroglobulin in serum with use of monoclonal antibodies selected for lack of cross-reactivity with autoantibodies. Clin Chem 1989;35:422–424.

Pollock MA, Jefferson SG, Kane JW, Lomax K, MacKinnon G, Winnard CB. Method comparison—a different approach. Ann Clin Biochem 1992;29:556–560.

Power MJ, Fottrell PF. Osteocalcin: diagnostic methods and clinical applications. Crit Rev Clin Lab Sci 1991;28:287–335.

Ratcliffe WA, Corrie JET, Dalziel AH, Macpherson JS. Direct ^{125}I-radioligand assays for serum progesterone compared with assays involving extraction of serum. Clin Chem 1982;28:1314–1318.

Ricós C, Arbós MA. Quality goals for hormone testing. Ann Clin Biochem 1990;27:353–358.

Rodbard D, Munson PJ, DeLean A. Improved curve fitting, parallelism testing, characterisation of sensitivity and specificity, validation and optimisation for radioligand assays. In: Radioimmunoassay and Related Procedures in Medicine. Vienna: Symposium proceedings of the International Atomic Energy Agency 1977;469–503.

Seth J, ed. The Immunoassay Kit Directory, Series A: Clinical Chemistry. Dordrecht: Kluwer Academic Publishers, 1991.

Seth J, Sturgeon CM, Al-Sadie R, Hanning I, Ellis AR. External quality assessment of immunoassays of peptide hormones and tumour markers: principles and practice. Ann Ist Super Sanità 1991;27:443–452.

Snyder PJ, Bashey HM, Montecinos A, Odell WD, Spitalnik SL. Secretion of multiple forms of human luteinizing hormone by cultured fetal human pituitary cells. J Clin Endocrinol Metab 1989;68:1033–1038.

Soos M, Siddle K. Characterization of monoclonal antibodies directed against human thyroid stimulating hormone. J Immunol Methods 1982;51:57–68.

Tiefenauer LX, Bodmer DM, Frei W, Andres RY. Prevention of bridge binding in immunoassays: a general estradiol tracer structure. J Steroid Biochem 1989;32:251–257.

Tunn S, Pappert G, Willnow P, Kreig M. Multicentre evaluation of an enzyme-immunoassay for cortisol determination. J Clin Chem Clin Biochem 1990;28:929–935.

Tydeman M, Kirkwood TBL. Design and analysis of accelerated degradation tests for the stability of biological standards. III. Principles of design. J Biol Standards 1984; 12: 215–224.

Weber TH, Kapyaho KI, Tanner P. Endogenous interference in immunoassays in clinical chemistry: A review. Scand J Clin Invest 1990;50(suppl 201):77–82.

Wheeler MJ. Automated immunoassay analysers: an overview. Communications in Laboratory Medicine 1992;1:1–5.

Wide L. Median charge and charge heterogeneity of human pituitary FSH, LH and TSH. II. Relationship to sex and age. Acta Endocrinol 1985;109:190–197.

CHAPTER 4

Quality Assurance

James P. Gosling and
Lawrence V. Basso

The trueness of the concentrations measured by an assay is dependent on correct calibration, resistance to interference, ruggedness of the assay procedure, and the suitability of the data interpolation algorithm. For immunoassays, the determination of true concentrations is beset by particular problems related to the use of complex biologic materials as reagents, calibration standards, and quality control materials. These difficulties are compounded when it is desired to measure extremely low concentrations of analytes that are structurally complex and heterogeneous. Consequently, the comparability of the results of measurements carried out in different places and over long periods of time may be much less than is required for consistently accurate diagnoses (Bergmeyer, 1991). Improving the present situation, and even the maintenance of current levels of quality, is dependent on thorough assay validation, properly executed procedures, correct calibration, accurate interpolation of data, internal quality control, and external quality assessment. The last four are the concerns of the present chapter.

CALIBRATION

Although each has a somewhat different meaning, the terms comparability, standardization, and calibration are often used interchangeably when referring to the abilities of assays to measure true concentrations. While comparability implies agreement but not necessarily trueness, true measurements automatically entail comparability. Standardization implies a concern that all measurement procedures should be related to internationally recognized standard preparations. Calibration is mainly concerned with the analyte-containing preparations that are compared with the unknown samples to enable calculation of a final result; without correct calibration standardization and comparability are unattainable.

Low Molecular Weight Analytes

Many lower molecular weight analytes have chemically defined structures, are homogeneous, are available in pure form, and, when necessary, can be measured by reference procedures which return true values and are resistant to interference. In spite of these advantages, immunoassays for many low molecular weight analytes give results that are inadequately comparable. Some poorly standardized assays, such as assays for follicular phase estradiol or testosterone in women (Middle, 1992), are for analytes that must be measured at very low concentrations, while others, such as assays for cyclosporine (Lensmeyer, et al., 1990), are for analytes that exist in isoforms variably detectable by current assays. Since it is impossible to standardize different immunoassays which variably measure mixtures of analytes of variable composition (Ekins, 1991), the first requirement for a standardized immunoassay is specificity for a defined analyte.

Analytes with assays that exhibit relatively good comparability of results, such as (total) thyroxine, have distinctive molecular structures or are present in high concentration. However, assays for cortisol, measured at concentrations almost always greater than 10 nmol/L in serum, exhibit deficient comparability and were chosen on behalf of the Bergmeyer Conference Organizing Committee as the subject of a report designed to foster improved comparability of immunoassays for hapten analytes in general (Gosling, et al., 1993).

One recommendation of the Bergmeyer conference report is that master calibrators for use in the production of the calibrators included in commercial kits should be certified with a reference assay such as isotope-dilution gas chromatography mass spectrometry (ID-GCMS) (Thienpont, et al., 1991), so that the concentrations of analyte present in routine calibrators can be traced back to concentrations determined by a reference assay. It was also recommended that occasional checks with a reference assay be made on kit calibrators to ensure that they contain the concentration of analyte indicated on the label. The objective of these recommendations is to ensure that abnormally high readings resulting from the use of antibodies with poor specificity are not compensated for by calibrants with increased concentrations of analyte.

Complex Analytes

Protein analytes cannot be readily defined chemically, because they are subject to proteolytic "nicking," or loss of amino acid residues at either terminal of each constituent polypeptide chain; loss from glycoproteins of sugar residues; and nonenzymatic glycosylation. In addition, many proteins occur in multiple isoforms (due to differences in amino acid sequence or degree of glycosylation) or as genetically determined isoforms which may be present in, dominant in, or absent from the blood of any one individual (Pettersson, 1992). Consequently, the comparability of the results obtained with different immunoassays for some complex protein analytes is often very poor (e.g., thyrotropin, Rei and Drake, 1991; carcinoembryonic antigen and chorionic gonadotropin, Sturgeon, et al., 1992).

With immunoassays for some analytes the use of common calibrants, in place of the calibrants normally used, results in a marked improvement in comparability, demonstrating that a significant portion of between-method variability may be due to differences in the calibration materials used (Rei and Drake, 1991; Whicher, 1991). In addition, it was clearly demonstrated many years ago that, while the accuracy of a nonspecific assay system is clearly affected by the presence of cross-reacting material in patient samples, even greater inaccuracies occur when the cross-reacting material is also present in the calibrator (Seth, 1991). For example, highly specific immuno-metric assays for FSH with calibrants based on the relatively crude International Reference Preparation (IRP) 78/549 for FSH tend to give lower patient results than do less specific competitive immunoassays, because the samples have less cross-reacting impurities than the calibrants (Seth, et al., 1992). Use of the more pure International Standard (IS) 83/575 for FSH is to be preferred.

Stenman, et al., (1993) in their report to the Fourth Bergmeyer Conference on Immunoassay Standardization made a comprehensive series of recommendations aimed at improving the standardization of immunoassays for chorionic gonadotropin, and these are very relevant to protein analytes in general.

Nevertheless, while it is quite obvious that immunoassay results can be more comparable, and that regulators, manufacturers and users must all constantly work at improving comparability, the clinical usefulness of present reagents and methods must be maintained by daily attention to good laboratory practices.

DATA PROCESSING

The method used for processing the data from immunoassays can significantly influence the results obtained. Manual plotting of standard curves and interpolation of unknown results is time-consuming, and liable to subjectivity and random error, but it ensures constant intimacy between operators and their results and limits the blame that can be ascribed to the immunoassay processing machine. However, computerized data logging, curve fitting, interpolation, and patient data handling are essential for the efficient analysis of large numbers of samples.

David Rodbard and his coworkers (Rodbard and Lewald, 1970; Rodbard, et al., 1977; Dudley et al., 1985) have played a very important role in recognizing and solving the major problem areas of computerized immunoassay data processing, but the lessons learned so long ago are still not always applied. A good data processing method uses a suitable, weighted mathematical model with calculation and analysis of the residuals for each data point, involves appropriate truncation to identify samples with levels falling below or above the useful range of the assay, and allows the determination of confidence limits for each result (Raggatt, 1991).

There is insufficient space in the present volume to allow a full discussion of this subject, but its importance is attested to by the occasionally observed, and recently confirmed, finding that identical data issued to different laboratories using the same commercial assay yield widely scattered results (J. Middle, UK NEQAS for steroid hormones in preparation). Wide variation was even observed when the curve-fitting algorithm was apparently the same. This leads to the inevitable conclusion that the exact interpolation method is an essential part of an assay procedure and must not be changed without very careful consideration. In addition, the suppliers must be able to assure compatibility if different software packages with apparently identical curve-fitting algorithms are to be regarded as interchangeable.

INTERNAL QUALITY CONTROL

In accord with modern management practice, quality control and assurance must be regarded as a collaborative exercise with the active and committed participation of all personnel concerned, from the most neophyte to the most qualified. Low or zero rejection rates require corrective actions to be taken before actual problems arise, which is impossible without the full participation of those most closely involved. Good assay precision is dependent on the precision of pipettes, diluters, and readout devices such as colorimeters or radioactivity counters and these should be subject to regular validation checks and preventive maintenance. Good operator technique is also essential. Drifting or changes in bias may be caused by reagent deterioration or batch changes, volumetric miscalibration, or errors in the preparation of standards. The rejection of results should always be by joint decision and should never be seen as imposed from above. Regular "quality circle" discussions can serve to evaluate longer term performance, interpret jointly internal and external quality control results, examine the merits of present and alternative kit suppliers, and provide a forum for the continued education of all concerned.

Samples for Quality Control

The samples used for quality control purposes must resemble as closely as possible the patient samples and, if possible, should be identical. While identity is impossible to achieve for some purposes, important control statistics can be derived from patient results or the repeat analysis of small groups of patient samples available in adequate amounts. However, for most purposes special quality control pools, which are available in sufficient quantity and are of sufficient stability to allow even daily repeat analyses over many months, are essential. Such quality control samples may be supplied by the kit manufacturer, purchased commercially, or prepared by the user in the laboratory. "In house" quality control samples, if prepared with attention to detail, forward planning and adequate safety precautions, can offer significant advantages with respect to similarity to patient unknown samples (they may be frozen rather than freeze dried), and economy (Seth, 1991). Some quality control materials available commercially or from regulatory agencies may have a target concentration assigned by a reference method (e.g., freeze-dried materials for cortisol and progesterone produced for the Community Bureau of Reference-BCR, Commission of the European Community, 200 rue de la Loi, B-1049, Brussels, Belgium) (Thienpont, et al., 1991).

Generating and Interpreting Quality Control Statistics

The results from the analysis of quality control samples and patient samples may be tabulated to calculate statistics which act as indicators of the performance of an assay, both relative to the performance of the same assay in the past and relative to other assays. There are two major aspects of performance that are of concern: the first is described by the absolute terms trueness and accuracy, and by the relative term bias; and the second is described as imprecision, precision, or variation. Trueness and bias are represented by percentages of the true or relative analyte concentration, respectively. Imprecision is described by means of statistics related to the standard deviation (SD), and total imprecision may be partitioned in order to allow evaluation of its causes. All levels of precision are dose dependent.

Within-Sample, Within-Batch Precision

This is the most fundamental level of precision and is most simply assessed by assaying, all in one batch, 10 to 20 replicates of 5 to 10 samples containing a range of analyte concentrations evenly distributed along the dose response curve. After calculating the mean, SD, and Coefficient of Variation (CV) for each set of replicates, a graph relating precision to analyte concentration is plotted, which is referred to as the within-sample, within-batch precision profile.

Alternatively, duplicate data from accumulated patient sample results may be used, thus saving reagent and labor costs and reflecting more closely actual routine precision (Fig. 4–1). Performing analyses on duplicate, as opposed to single, aliquots of patient samples improves, in itself, within-sample, within-batch precision by a factor of $\sqrt{2}$ or 1.414.

Between-Sample, Within-Batch Precision

This is related to within-batch drift and can be estimated by means of inserting standard curves at the beginning and at the end of the batch, placing internal quality control pools at intervals within the batch, or by repeat determinations of patient samples at intervals within the batch. Note that drift can also cause within-sample imprecision, especially if the addition of reagents to replicates is not sequential; this can occur when replicates on a microtiter plate are side-by-side but reagents are added column-by-column, or vice versa. Drift is most often caused by temperature variations across racks or microtiter plates during incubations, inadequate incubation times, and inefficient mixing after addition of reagent. It is often not linear and should not be corrected for.

Within-Sample, Between-Batch Precision

This statistic is normally estimated with internal quality control pools placed in each batch to be analyzed, then the SD and CV for each pool are calculated from the collected results over the required number of batches; each result is the average of duplicate determinations if patient samples are assayed in duplicate. Normally, there

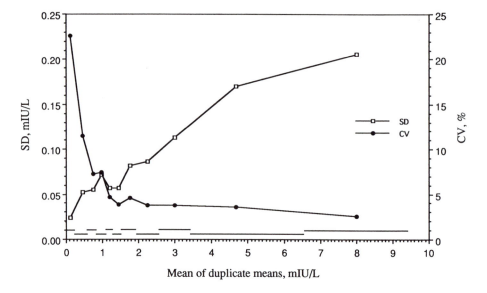

Figure 4–1.   Within-sample, within-batch imprecision profile for a thyroid-stimulating hormone (TSH) immunometric assay estimated from 515 duplicate measurements (Raggatt, 1989).

In the absence of specialized software, this is the best done with the aid of a standard spreadsheet program. Select at least a few hundred pairs of duplicate patient data at random and enter them in two columns. In the third to sixth columns calculate each duplicate mean, difference (d), SD ($d/\sqrt{2}$), and variance (SD^2) and sort the six column set in order of increasing mean. After surveying the range and distribution of the means, select 5 to 10 subranges with an adequate (≥ 50) number (N) of data in each. This may be done on the basis of fixed analyte concentration intervals (e.g., 0.31 to 0.5, 0.51 to 0.7 mIU/L, and so on, but then the number of data per interval will vary widely. Alternatively, fixed numbers of data points can be included in each interval, with the interval limits varying in consequence. Obviously, to obtain reliable statistics for concentration ranges into which few measured levels fall, very large total numbers of data will have to be analyzed. For each interval, count the number of points and calculate the mean duplicate-mean, mean duplicate-SD and CV, where:

$$\text{Mean} = \Sigma \text{ duplicate mean}/N,$$
$$\text{SD} = \sqrt{(\Sigma \text{ duplicate variance}/(N-1))}, \text{ and}$$
$$\text{CV} = \text{SD} \times 100/\text{mean}.$$

As shown in the above graph, plot SD and CV against mean over the range of sample concentrations. Here each interval (shown by the horizontal lines at the bottom) contained data from 50 duplicate measurements, except where the TSH concentration was below the average lower detection limit for the assay (< 0.25 mIU/L), where N was 32; and for the top range (6.61 to 9.41 mIU/L), where N was only 20. Data for the 13 samples with the highest measured TSH concentrations were omitted because they covered too wide a range to be meaningful.

should be three such pools with concentrations representing the low, medium, and high concentrations encountered in routine samples and spanning all diagnostically relevant concentrations. Occasionally, an assay has a dual diagnostic purpose and batches of samples involving different reference interval concentrations are analyzed; for example, the measurement of estradiol during the follicular phase for the diagnosis of infertility, or to monitor follicular development in women in an in vitro fertilization program. In such cases, because the concentration ranges of interest are so different, different sets of control samples with appropriate concentrations should be used.

Quality Control Charts

The immediate charting of quality control statistics assists in their evaluation and encourages rapid action when this is required. The most useful and common form of presentation of such statistics is the Shewhart chart (Fig. 4–2) (Westgard, et al., 1981). The batch number or, if there is never more than one batch per day, the working day is plotted on the *x*-axis and the analyte concentration on the *y*-axis. Horizontal lines are drawn to indicate the positions of the target mean concentrations and the concentrations representing three or four standard deviations above and below the mean. Alternatively, charts graduated on the *y*-axis in terms of SD units may be used to give neater plots, although at the expense of more preliminary calculations. A set of such charts, including one for each control, represents the between-batch variability of one assay and should be displayed together. At the beginning, the target means and SD values should be estimated from data obtained by the analysis of about 15 batches (Seth, 1991).

Also included in the set of Shewhart graphs (but not necessarily taken into consideration when decisions to accept data are being made) may be plots of within-sample, within-batch precision over a specified range of concentrations, a within-batch average of all normal samples and plots of statistics describing the standard curve (e.g., slope). However, it is important to limit the statistics plotted to the most representative and important; plots of less important statistics distract attention from the more important ones. A new batch of assay kits, and any other change of reagent, should be clearly indicated on the combined chart, as should changes of quality control pools.

Criteria for Acceptance of the Results of an Assay Batch

A set of clear rules for the objective acceptance or rejection of the results from an assay batch or run must be established and followed. These rules should take account of diagnostic requirements and the consequences of positive or negative misdiagnoses, generally accepted norms for the relevant analyte, and professional experience. A second person other than the assayist (normally the laboratory supervisor) should be routinely involved in decisions to accept or reject data, as the absence of such a check has been reported to be strongly associated with poor assay performance (Seth and Hanning, 1988).

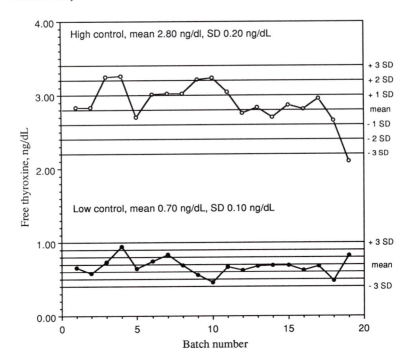

Figure 4–2.   Example applications of the multirule Shewhart procedure for a free thyroxine (T₄) immunoassay with two control pools. One batch was analyzed per day and the data for the high and low standard are plotted against batch number. The horizontal lines indicate the previously determined mean and ± 1, 2, and 3 SD limits for each control. Here are some comments for days on which all is not as would be desired:

Day 3: The high control is greater than + 2 SD but the low control is within ± 1 SD. Warning.

Day 4: Both high and low controls are greater than + 2 SD. Reject batch. Systematic error?

Day 9: High control greater than + 2 SD and low control less than − 1 SD constituting a warning but, in addition, the high control has now been greater than 1 SD for 4 days. Reject batch. Systematic error?

Day 10: High control greater than + 2 SD and low control less than − 2 SD. Reject batch. Random error? Would also have been rejected on the grounds that the high control has now been greater than 1 SD for 5 days. Continuing systematic error?

Day 11: High control has now been greater than 1 SD for 6 days. Reject batch. Continuing systematic error?

Day 18: Low control less than − 2 SD and high control within ± 1 SD constituting a warning, but, in addition, the low control has now been less than the mean for 10 days. Reject batch. Systematic error?

Day 19: The high control is greater than − 3 SD but the low control is greater than 1 SD, so their concentrations differ by greater than 4 SD. Reject batch. Random errors?

The rules based on the use of Shewhart charts presented by Westgard, et al. (1981) have been widely applied and adapted to individual circumstances. These rules vary depending on the number of control poor measurements taken into consideration (see Table 4 in Westgard, et al., 1981). The control samples may be assigned randomly to positions in a run or placed in specific locations that bracket patient samples. The progressive interpretation of data for two controls over a series of 19 batches is discussed in Figure 4–2, and the rules used are summarized in Figure 4–3.

Westgard, et al., (1981) and Seth (1991) discussed circumstances in which a batch might be accepted, at least in part, despite failure to meet an internal quality control rule. These include occasions when the problem is obviously due to the control material itself, when two samples were evidently interchanged, when the out-of-control control sample is of a concentration around which few or none of the patient samples lie, or when the error detected is small in relation to an urgent clinical requirement. When appropriate, patient samples with concentrations near the out-of-control control would be selectively repeated.

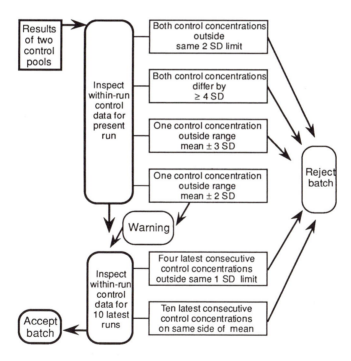

Figure 4–3.   Decision algorithm for use with Shewhart charts with two controls (Westgard, et al., 1981; Seth, 1991). Note that the particular test failed by the batch may suggest the reason for the failure, and therefore when a batch must be rejected the control data should be carefully reviewed (Seth, 1991).

EXTERNAL QUALITY ASSESSMENT

Most clinical chemistry laboratories participate in external quality assessment schemes and are able, retrospectively, to compare their performance with that of others for each analytic method and method group. Participating laboratories are also made aware of what constitutes achievable good performance and of the relative biases associated with results obtained with different commercially available methods

Sample Material Distributed

Ideally the sample materials distributed should closely resemble patient samples in physical state, age and composition, subjection to minimal treatment, and the use of endogenous analyte(s). Preservative must be carefully selected (Thijssen, 1992) and used sparingly. Some schemes with relatively few but larger participating laboratories distribute frozen samples containing only added preservative and endogenous analytes (Middle, 1992), but for schemes with thousands of small laboratories this could pose insuperable difficulties. In these cases the samples are often spiked with a cocktail of analytes and freeze dried before distribution. The distribution, together or separately, of pairs of samples, identical except that one contains an additional known amount of analyte, allows estimation of the abilities of different methods to efficiently measure added standard (Middle, 1990; Thijssen, 1992).

Distributions of external quality assessment materials should be frequent enough to supply regular information to scheme members, and reports of the results of each distribution should be returned early enough for the information to be more than of historical interest. Distributions are monthly with the reports of each batch sent with the next lot of samples in some schemes (Seth, 1991; Middle 1992), and bimonthly (Thijssen, 1992), or every 3 or 6 months in others (Vicari, 1991).

Target Values

Much of the value of external quality assessment schemes is related to estimating the bias of commercial kits and of assays as run in individual laboratories. However, bias can only be calculated relative to a target value that is taken to be the correct value. There are four main ways in which target values are estimated (Seth, 1991):

1. *Reference method value.* Agreed reference methods that measure the true concentration and are resistant to interference from normal sample constituents are expensive to perform and do not exist for many analytes, particularly protein analytes. However, they are routinely used in the German schemes for some steroids and are recommended wherever possible (Gosling, et al., 1993).
2. *Mean of all laboratory results.* This is the method most commonly used, although it has very important limitations, particularly when there is marked dom-

ination by the "market leading" method *and* there is evidence that the dominant method itself is significantly biased or wrongly calibrated (e.g., human placental lactogen in the United Kingdom) (Seth, et al., 1990). The mean of all laboratory results should not be used when a reference method that gives true values is available or else manufacturers may unnecessarily be pressurized by commercial considerations to calibrate their assays relative to a market leader rather than relative to true concentrations. Valuable evidence as to which methods display accuracy or bias may be obtained with samples that allow calculation of the recovery of added standard (Seth, 1991).

3. *Mean of expert laboratory group.* This method may appear to be preferable to obtaining the mean of all laboratory results, but there is some evidence that laboratories initially accepted as expert often perform no better than average.

4. *Mean of method group.* This is usually used in conjunction with other ways, as it is always of interest to individual laboratories how they perform relative to others using the same reagents and procedure.

Method Performance

External quality assessment schemes are the source of much valuable information on the comparative performance of commercial immunoassay methods under routine conditions and such information should be sought by anyone choosing a method for a new analyte or considering a change of method (see also Chap. 3). For example, EQAS data indicate that reagent excess immunometric assays are more specific and give better between-laboratory agreement than competitive radioimmunoassays or, in other words, they are more rugged. Distribution of external quality assessment samples with known possible interferents is sometimes done and this can identify methods that are especially susceptible to interference from heterophilic antibodies or human antimouse antibodies (Seth, et al., 1991). Without the use of such special samples, the effects of even common interfering substances are not easily detectable by either internal or external assessment methods; however, the consequences for patient care can be serious.

The reliability of estimates of cumulative laboratory performance derived from external quality assessment data depends on the number of samples taken into account. Even with a monthly distribution of samples and data accumulated over 6 months this can be no more than 20 to 30. Therefore, while an indication of satisfactory performance may be reliable within the limitations outlined above, gross estimates of precision and bias indicating poor performance should be carefully examined for concentration-dependent and other effects before any action is taken (Seth, 1991).

In conclusion, internal and external quality assessment results are both essential elements in the pursuit of quality, efficiency and productivity, but to maximize their value they must be considered together. In general, internal quality assessment data are best for the assessment of precision, whereas accuracy is most reliably confirmed by external quality assessment data.

This chapter has been primarily concerned with quality assurance in the context of a professionally organized clinical laboratory. However, the accuracy and precision of results are also highly pertinent to the decentralized use of immunoassays by individuals without formal laboratory training. In this situation any one analyte may be determined only occasionally and the most appropriate control methods are those that are used each and every time a test result is produced. Quality controls for some reagents, etc., are already part of some simple to operate pregnancy tests (e.g., Icon [Hybritech] and Unipath [Clearview]), but such measures need to be developed and standardized (Baer and Belsey, 1993).

REFERENCES

Baer DM, Belsey RE. Limitations of quality control in physicians' offices and other decentralized testing situations: the challenge to develop new methods of test validation. Clin Chem 1993;39:9–12.

Bergmeyer HU. Immunoassay standardization. Scand J Clin Investi 1991;51(suppl 205):1–2.

Dudley RA, Edwards P, Ekins R, et al. Guidelines for immunoassay data processing. Clin Chem 1985;31:1264–1271.

Ekins RP. The precision profile: its use in assay design, assessment and quality control. In: Hunter WM, Corrie JET, eds. Immunoassays for Clinical Chemistry. Edinburgh: Churchill Livingstone, 1983;76–105.

Ekins R. Immunoassay standardization. Scand J Lab Investi 1991;51(suppl 205):33–46.

Gosling JP, Middle J, Siekmann L, Read G. Standardization of hapten immunoprocedures: total cortisol. J Clin Invest 1993;53(suppl 216):3–41.

Lensmeyer GL, Wiebe DA, Carlson IH, deVos DJ. Three commercial polyclonal immunoassays for cyclosporine in whole blood compared. 2. Cross-reactivity of the antisera with cyclosporine metabolites. Clin Chem 1990;36:119–123.

Middle J. Report of the UK EQAS for steroid hormones. In: Middle J, ed. Proceedings of the External Quality Assessment Schemes Participants Meeting, 1990. Cardiff: NEQAS for Steroid Hormones, Welsh National School of Medicine 1990;139–155.

Middle J. The state of the art of steroid hormone assays: a UK NEQAS perspective. Communications in Laboratory Medicine, 1992;1:84–113.

Pettersson K, Ding YQ, Huhtaniemi I. An Immunologically anomolous luteinizing hormone variant in a healthy woman. J Clin Endocrinol Metab 1992;74:164–171.

Raggatt PR. Duplicates or singletons?—An analysis of the need for replication in immunoassay and a computer program to calculate the distribution of outlines, error rate and the precision profile from assay duplicates. Ann Clin Biochem 1989;26:26–37.

Raggatt P. Data processing. In: Price CP, Newman DJ, eds. Principles and Practice of Immunoassay. New York: Stockton Press, 1991;190–218.

Rei R, Drake P. The nature of calibrators in immunoassays: are they commutable with test samples? must they be? Scand J Clin Investig 1991;51(suppl 205):47–54.

Rodbard D, Lewald JE. Computer analysis of radioligand assay and radioimmunoassay data. Acta Endocrinol 1970;64:79.

Rodbard D, Munson PJ, DeLean A. Improved curve fitting, parallelism testing, characterisation of sensitivity and specificity, validation and optimisation for radioligand assays. In: Radioimmunoassay and Related Procedures in Medicine. Vienna: Symposium proceedings of the International Atomic Energy Agency, 1977;469–503.

Seth J. Standardization and quality assurance. In: Price CP, Newman DJ, eds. Principles and Practice of Immunoassay. London: Macmillan, 1991;154–189.

Seth J, Ellis AR, Al-Sadie R. The UK EQAS for peptide hormones and related substances: retrospect and prospect. In: Middle J, ed. Proceedings of the External Quality Assessment Schemes Participants Meeting, 1990. Cardiff: NEQAS for Steroid Hormones, Welsh National School of Medicine, 1990;33–40.

Seth J, Ellis AR, Al-Sadie R. Causes of method bias in assays for pituitary gonadotrophins in serum. Communications in Laboratory Medicine 1992;3:25–28.

Seth J, Hanning I. Factors associated with the quality of laboratory performance in the United Kingdom external quality assessment scheme for growth hormone. Clin Chim Acta 1988;174:185–196.

Seth J, Sturgeon CM, Al-Sadie R, Hanning I, Ellis AR. External quality assessment of immunoassays of peptide hormones and tumour markers: principles and practice. Ann Ist Super Sanità 1991;27:443–452.

Stenman U-H, Bidart J-M, Birkin S, Mann K, Nisula B, O'Connor J. Standardization of protein immunoprocedures: chorionic gonadotropin (CG). Scand J Clin Lab Invest 1993;53(suppl 216):42–78.

Sturgeon CM, Seth J, Al-Sadie R. UK EQA for CEA and hCG: aims and achievements. Communications in Laboratory Medicine 1992;1:37–40.

Thienpont L, Siekman L, Lawson A, Colinet E, De Leenheer A. Development, validation and certification by isotope dilution gas chromatography–mass spectrometry of lyophilized human serum reference materials for cortisol (CRM 192 and 193) and progesterone (CRM 347 and 348). Clin Chem 1991;37:540–546.

Thijssen JHH. Immunoassays in endocrinology. Communications in Laboratory Medicine 1992;1:146–151.

Vicari G. External quality assessment programs in Italy. Ann Ist Super Sanità 1991;27:359–363.

Westgard JO, Barry PL, Hunt MR, Goth T. A multi-rule Shewhart chart for quality control in clinical chemistry. Clin Chem 1981;27:493–501.

Whicher JT. Calibration is the key to immunoassay but the ideal calibrator is unattainable. Scand J Clin Invest 1991;51(suppl 205):21–32.

CHAPTER 5

Hypothalamus and Posterior Pituitary

Mary I. Forsling

Vasopressin (VP; also called arginine vasopressin, AVP), the antidiuretic hormone, plays a key role in the maintenance of fluid balance, which depends on appropriate secretion of vasopressin, normal renal responsiveness to the hormone, and on adequate water intake (dependent, in turn on the individual's ability to recognize water deprivation, i.e., thirst). Deficient vasopressin secretion resulting in diabetes insipidus is rare, and inappropriate vasopressin secretion, although also relatively uncommon, is one of the most frequent causes of euvolemic hyponatremia, being seen in 12% to 40% of patients (Anderson, et al., 1985; Gross, et al., 1987).

Prolonged administration of the other neurohypophysial hormone, oxytocin, can also lead to hyponatremia (Fisher, 1985), but this could be due to enhanced sodium excretion (Windle and Forsling, 1991) as well as to water retention. The more established roles of oxytocin are those in lactation and parturition. While there are no defined syndromes associated with overproduction or underproduction of oxytocin, this may be because they have not yet been characterized.

Disturbances of neurohypophysial function are investigated by determinations of plasma and urinary osmolality, in addition to the direct estimation of peripheral hormone concentrations. Measurement of neurophysin, which is secreted in parallel with neurohypophysial hormones, has also been used to monitor posterior pituitary function (Legros, et al., 1975).

NEUROHYPOPHYSIAL HORMONES

Synthesis

Oxytocin and vasopressin are nonapeptides differing only in the amino acid residues in positions 3 and 8 (Fig. 5–1), but these substitutions are sufficient to confer different biologic properties on the molecules. Before release both are stored in the neurohypophysis as insoluble complexes with proteins known as neurophysins, but they

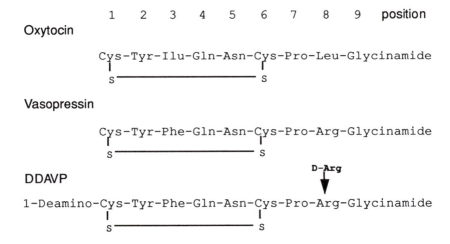

Figure 5–1.   Amino acid sequences of oxytocin, arginine vasopressin, and 1-deamino-(8-D-arginine)-vasopressin (DDAVP).

are synthesized in the magnocellular neurons of the paraventricular and supraoptic nuclei in the form of precursor molecules (mol wt ≈ 20,000). They comprise a signal peptide, a neurophysin (mol wt ≈ 10,000) and the native hormone. The vasopressin precursor, propressorphysin has an additional glycoprotein residue. Once synthesized, the precursor molecules are packaged in neurosecretory granules and transported down the axons to the nerve terminals in the posterior pituitary gland. The active hormone and neurophysin are cleaved from the precursor molecule during transport.

The hormones are released by exocytosis in a process of secretion-stimulus coupling, the action potential for release traveling down the axons of the neurones producing the hormone. The last hormone to be synthesized is the first to be released; hormone not released is stored and may finally be broken down by lysosomal activity. The posterior pituitary contains sufficient vasopressin and oxytocin to last for many days. Vasopressin circulates largely in the unbound form, the volume of distribution being about two thirds of the extracellular space and the half-time of clearance 6 to 8 minutes. The hormones are largely broken down in the kidney and splanchnic region but during pregnancy the placenta produces an enzyme, cysteine aminopeptidase, which cleaves the disulfide bond and successively removes amino acid residues.

Mechanisms of Action

The actions of oxytocin and vasopressin are mediated by membrane bound receptors which have recently been cloned (Kimura, et al., 1992; Morel, et al., 1992). There are two main types of vasopressin receptors: the V1 receptors are found in the blood vessels and produce contraction of the smooth muscle via the phosphatidylinositol system. The V2 receptors, found in the renal collecting ducts and acting via the second messenger cyclic adenosine monophosphate cAMP, produce an increase in the permeability of this region of the tubules thus allowing the reabsorption of water. Oxytocin acts to promote an increase in uterine activity allowing rapid expulsion of its contents, and to promote contraction of the myoepithelial cells promoting milk ejection.

Investigation of the distribution of the various receptor types has been aided by a number of analogs of the neurohypophysial hormones. Many of the analogs have selected potencies; thus 1-deamino-(8-D-arginine)-vasopressin (DDAVP, Desmopressin) (Fig. 5–1) has high antidiuretic activity with little pressor effect (Manning, et al., 1976), whereas N^α-glycyl-glycyl-glycyl-[lys^8]-vasopressin (triglycyl-lysine vasopressin, TGLVP, Glypressin, Terlipressin) exerts its effect largely on blood vessels. Such selective agonists are of obvious therapeutic value as side effects may be reduced. Additionally, both these analogs are much less susceptible to enzymic degradation. Selective V1 and V2 antagonists have been developed as have oxytocin antagonists, the most recent development being nonpeptide antagonists (Saito, et al., 1993).

VASOPRESSIN

Control of Vasopressin Secretion

As might be predicted for a hormone whose main physiologic effect is to promote water retention, the stimuli for the regulation of vasopressin release are associated with altered water content of the extracellular fluid, namely changes in plasma osmolality and volume. Reflecting its vasoconstrictor effects, vasopressin is also released in response to a fall in blood pressure. For descriptive purposes, especially in the context of clinical conditions, factors influencing vasopressin release are classified as osmotic and nonosmotic. The latter are often responsible for inappropriate vasopressin secretion.

Vasopressin release and thirst are controlled by osmoreceptors as originally postulated by Verney (1947), although their exact location has not yet been established, and it is still not clear whether the same set of receptors controls both mechanisms. However, it is generally agreed that the circumventricular organs of the brain play an important role. One possibility is that the magnocellular neurons themselves are sensitive to changes in osmotic pressure and that receptors sensitive to sodium are located in the anteroventral region of the ventricle, providing a permissive input to these neurons.

There is a linear relationship between plasma osmolality and vasopressin (Fig. 5–2), the intercept of a fitted line on the abscissa being termed the osmotic threshold (mmol/kg). It has been shown that both the slope and the intercept of such a line change among normal adults (Thompson and Baylis, 1987), but that there is a high concordance in monozygotic twins (Zerbe, 1985). The osmotic threshold is also in-

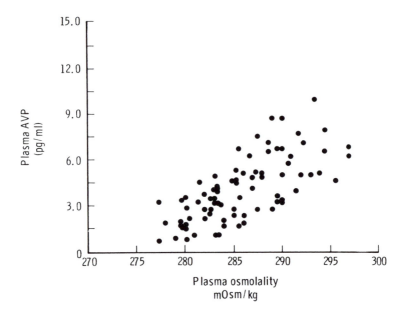

Figure 5–2.   Correlation of plasma vasopressin concentration with plasma osmolality under varying condition of water balance in normal adults. The units for osmolarity cited above (mOsm/kg) are numerically exactly equivalent to the SI units, mmol/kg.

fluenced in women by gonadal steroids, being slightly lower in the midluteal as compared with the midfollicular phase (Baylis, 1985). Aging also influences osmotically controlled vasopressin secretion with an increase in the slope of the osmoregulatory line. While during any short period of the day there is a good correlation between plasma osmolality and plasma vasopressin, this is not true when data are obtained over longer periods (Uhlich, et al., 1975). Plasma vasopressin concentrations, like those of oxytocin, show clear circadian rhythms, being highest during the night and falling during the day. (Montgomery, et al., 1991). This pattern may be disturbed in patients with obstructive sleep apnea (Halpin, et al., 1992) or enuresis (Puri, 1980; Rittig, et al., 1989), but is unaltered by aging.

Of the nonosmotic factors that influence vasopressin release, some, such as blood pressure and plasma volume, reflect total body water. Others are unrelated to fluid balance, vasopressin release being stimulated by changes in blood gas tension, nausea, stress, and pain (Forsling, 1982). The sensitivity of the vasopressin release mechanism is increased by other factors which stimulate vasopressin release, namely a reduction in plasma volume or a decrease in blood pressure. There is in fact a linear increase in plasma vasopressin concentrations with a fall in blood pressure, which appears to contribute to the increased vasopressin concentrations seen during surgery and anesthesia. Relatively large changes in plasma volume are required to influence the concentration of vasopressin, but if an increase in volume is of sufficient magnitude it can overcome a concurrent increase in osmolality (Sagnella, et al., 1987).

Changes of Neurohypophysial Function

Secretion of vasopressin in the newborn is under normal control, although the full renal concentrating capacity is not achieved. During pregnancy there is an increase in plasma volume and a fall in plasma osmolality which should result in very low levels of plasma vasopressin. However, plasma concentrations are maintained, probably through a resetting of the osmoreceptors (Davison, et al., 1984). With aging, there is increased activity of the neurohypophysial system, in contrast with the reduced activity of most other body systems.

TESTS OF VASOPRESSIN FUNCTION

Assays

Sensitive bioassays for vasopressin depending on its antidiuretic action in alcohol-anesthetised, water-loaded rats have been available since around 1960 (Chard and Forsling, 1976; Forsling, 1985), and, combined with an extraction procedure (Forsling, 1974), they can be used to estimate circulating concentrations of vasopressin. A less sensitive pressor assay may be used for the standardization of hormone preparations. Later, sensitive radioimmunoassays (RIAs) were developed (Robertson, et al., 1973; Forsling, 1985), and although some direct assays have been described (Forsling, et al., 1984), an extraction procedure is generally employed.

At normal plasma osmolarity (275 to 295 mmol/kg or mOsm/kg), normal plasma vasopressin lies within the range 0.5 to 1.5 pg/mL (1 to 3 pmol/L), falling to undetectable levels in diabetes insipidus. In the syndrome of inappropriate secretion of vasopressin, concentrations may be elevated, but in the greatest proportion of patients they lie within the normal range, although they are inappropriately high for the concurrent plasma osmolarity (Table 5–1). Relatively few centers offer RIAs for vaso-

Table 5–1 Concentrations of Vasopressin in 100 Patients with Diagnosed Polyuria or Hyponatremia

Number of Patients							
Polyuria (42)					*Hyponatremia (58)*		
Inappropriately low values			Normal values	High values	Low values	Normal values*	High values
Saline infusion test	Water deprivation	Random samples					
5	7	19	7	4	32	20	6

*But inappropriate for concurrent plasma osmolarity.

pressin. Commercially developed kits are available, although some of the tests are not simple to perform. Since the normal circulating concentrations of vasopressin are low and it is often necessary to demonstrate a fall in hormone concentrations or to estimate levels below the normal range, a lower limit of detection of 0.5 pmol/L or better is required; otherwise misclassification errors may occur. A number of in-house assays have lower limits of detection of 0.1 pmol/L, through the use of high affinity antibody, thorough optimization of the assay and exploitation of the extraction step, which effectively increases the concentration of the hormone (Windle and Forsling, 1993).

The low circulating concentrations of the hormone also mean that an extraction procedure is virtually essential. Precipitation methods employing alcohol or acetone are used, but are not entirely satisfactory, nonspecific factors being picked up in both bioassays and immunoassays. Absorption to a solid phase is preferable either with a batchwise technique (Chard, et al, 1970) or Sep Pack columns (La Rochelle, et al, 1980).

Pure preparations of synthetic vasopressin are available, but most kits employ the First International Standard for arginine vasopressin (77/501) as the standard preparation, and it is preferable to express results in terms of such a standard. Although it is possible to raise antibodies against the nonconjugated peptide (Edwards, et al., 1972), most assays employ antibodies raised against vasopressin conjugated to a protein such as thyroglobulin (Forsling, 1985). The labeled preparation employed is ^{125}I-vasopressin with the ^{125}I introduced into the tyrosine in position 2, and this is generally prepared by means of the chloramine T method. However, the lactoperoxidase-catalyzed method (Thorell and Johansson, 1971) may yield label with a lower fraction of damaged molecules. It is relatively easy to separate the small peptide from that bound to antibody by either precipitating the antibody or absorbing the peptide onto charcoal. Most assays have total incubation times of about 48 hours. Urinary assays for the hormone have been described but, with the exception of neonates (Rees, et al., 1983), urinary excretion of vasopressin does not adequately reflect hormone release.

Vasopressin is rapidly destroyed in blood at 37 °C so that samples should be collected on ice and spun at 4 °C. The plasma should be separated and stored in plastic tubes at -20 °C until assay. If for any reason vasopressin is to be determined during pregnancy, enzyme inhibitors should be used (Davison, et al., 1984) since, as already mentioned, the placenta produces an enzyme that cleaves the peptide.

A number of patients with diabetes insipidus treated with Pitressin tannate in oil have developed antibodies to vasopressin (Bisset, et al., 1976) and one should occasionally consider the possibility of interference from antibodies to vasopressin. They may be demonstrated by incubating doubling dilutions of plasma with radioactive label, separating the bound from the free labeled hormone and counting to estimate the fraction bound at each dilution. Comparison with control plasma reveals abnormal levels of specific binding.

Diabetes Insipidus

Diabetes insipidus is just one of the many causes of polyuria, which may be defined as a urine output of greater than 2 L/day, or 30 mL/kg/day. Diabetes insipidus itself may result from failure of vasopressin secretion (central diabetes insipidus) or from renal resistance to the hormone (nephrogenic diabetes insipidus) (Table 5–2). Polyuria may also result from abnormal thirst or persistent water drinking. Other causes are diabetes mellitus, chronic renal failure, metabolic disease such as hypocalcemia or hypokalemia, systemic diseases such as sickle cell anemia, and administration of drugs such as lithium.

An increased urinary volume should first be established, as patients complaining of polyuria may merely be passing urine more frequently. Once polyuria has been confirmed, routine plasma analysis should be performed to exclude conditions such as diabetes mellitus and metabolic abnormalities. Once the common causes of polyuria have been excluded, it is then necessary to distinguish between central and nephrogenic diabetes insipidus and primary polydipsia. Theoretically, combined random measurements of vasopressin and plasma osmolality alone should allow separation of patients with primary polydipsia and diabetes insipidus but, in practice, such measurements are of value in only a limited number of cases (Robertson, 1987), as there is considerable overlap of the reference ranges for the various groups. Values may also be elevated as a result of nonosmotic stimuli. Therefore, as with many of the anterior pituitary hormones, challenge tests are used, namely hypertonic saline infusion or water deprivation.

Table 5–2   Etiology of Diabetes Insipidus

Central diabetes insipidus
    Primary
        Hereditary
        Idiopathic
        DIDMOAD (Wolfram's) syndrome
        Autoimmune
    Secondary
        Trauma
        Tumors
        Diseases, e.g., tuberculosis
        Granulomata
        Vascular, e.g., cerebral aneurysms
        Posthypophysectomy

Nephrogenic diabetes insipidus
    Primary
        Hereditary
        Idiopathic
    Secondary
        Chronic renal disease
        Metabolic disease, e.g., hypokalemia, hypercalcemia
        Drug induced, e.g., lithium
        Loss of concentration gradient on excessive fluid intake (associated with
            psychosis, hypothalamic disease, or drugs)

Hypertonic Saline Infusion

Hypertonic saline infusion was the first test of neurohypophysial function (Carter and Robbins, 1947), a reduced urine flow being noted in healthy individuals but not in those with diabetes insipidus. The preliminary water loading of patients allowed the determination of free water clearance (Moses and Streeten, 1967), which enabled differentiation between primary polydipsia and central diabetes insipidus, but not nephrogenic diabetes insipidus. The natriuresis produced also resulted in further inaccuracies in determining urinary osmolality, which limited the value of the test. However, the development of a sensitive RIA for vasopressin allowed the construction of plots relating plasma vasopressin to plasma osmolality (Fig. 5–3). The relationship is normal in primary polydipsia and nephrogenic diabetes insipidus but not in partial diabetes insipidus, where vasopressin concentrations are below normal for the concurrent plasma osmolality.

The saline infusion test is performed on patients who have been fasted overnight but allowed water to drink. The patient empties the bladder and is weighed. After the patient has rested supine for 30 minutes a basal blood sample is taken via an intravenous cannula for the determination of plasma vasopressin and osmolality. Then hypertonic saline (0.855 mol/L NaCl) is infused for 2 hours at 0.06 mL/kg. Blood pressure is recorded at 15-minute intervals and blood samples taken at 30-minute intervals with a further sample 15 minutes after the end of the infusion. The time of onset of thirst should also be noted. Patients may suck ice during infusion and

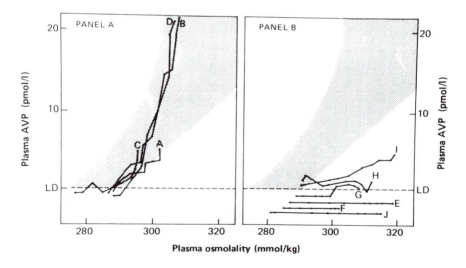

Figure 5–3.   Vasopressin response to hypertonic saline in patients without diabetes insipidus (panel *A*, A–D) and with diabetes insipidus (panel *B*, E–J). (Baylis PH. Posterior pituitary function in health and disease. Clinics in Endocrinology and Metabolism 1983;12:747–770. Reproduced with permission.)

drink after the test, but not large volumes. Measurement of urinary osmolality indicates the renal concentrating ability, thereby distinguishing between primary polydipsia and nephrogenic diabetes insipidus.

The Dehydration Test

The dehydration test was developed to provide an alternative to hypertonic saline infusion (Dashe, et al., 1963). Patients are allowed to ingest nothing for a period of 8 hours during which time they are weighed and urine and plasma osmolality determined regularly. The test must be carried out under careful supervision, and if the patient's body weight falls more than 5% the test is terminated. Under normal conditions the urine osmolality should reach 600 mmol/kg, or more, with a plasma osmolality not exceeding 300 mmol/kg. In diabetes insipidus plasma osmolality is greater than 300 mmol/kg with urinary osmolality remaining below this level. However, patients with primary polydipsia have a loss of interstitial solute in the renal medulla and so will be unable to concentrate the urine maximally. Primary polydipsia may therefore be difficult to distinguish from partial diabetes insipidus. Diagnosis may also be complicated by the fact that patients with partial diabetes insipidus may be relatively sensitive to vasopressin (Robertson, 1987) and that renal resistance to vasopressin is not complete. Plasma vasopressin determinations are again of value. At the end of the water deprivation test DDAVP may be given intravenously in a dose of 2 μg intravenously, or intranasally in a dose of 20 mg, and further urine samples analyzed to reveal the renal responsiveness (Baylis, 1981). Fluid intake should be restricted to twice the volume of urine passed during fluid restriction to avoid the development of hyponatremia.

The possibility of using nonosmotic stimuli of vasopressin release such as hypovolemia or hypotension (Robertson, et al., 1976) or hypoglycemia (Baylis, et al., 1981) has been investigated. However, patients with diabetes insipidus can secrete vasopressin in response to such stimuli. Therefore, although these stimuli cannot be used for the differential diagnosis of polyuria they may be used to identify osmoreceptor dysfunction.

The Syndrome of Inappropriate Vasopressin Secretion

The characteristic features of the syndrome of inappropriate antidiuresis (SIAD) or inappropriate vasopressin secretion were set down by Bartter and Schwartz in 1967 (Table 5–3). In addition, certain other tests may be performed to confirm the diagnosis. Water loading has been used when investigating moderate hyponatremia and is of value in confirming absence of continued inappropriate antidiuresis following treatment of an underlying causative disorder. A water load of 5 mL/kg is administered and normally more than 90% of the load is excreted in 4 hours with the urine osmolality being reduced to less than 100 mmol/kg. The etiology of inappropriate vasopressin is described in Table 5–4.

Table 5–3   Criteria for the Diagnosis of Inappropriate Vasopressin Secretion

- Decreased effective plasma osmolality (pOsm <275 mmol/kg or corrected plasma Na$^+$<135 mmol/L)
- Urine Na$^+$concentration inappropriately high for concurrent plasma osmolality
- Elevated urine Na$^+$with normal salt and water intake
- Absence of edema
- Normal thyroid, adrenal, and renal function (including recent diuretic therapy)
- Confirmation supplied by:
  Plasma vasopressin inappropriately high for concurrent plasma osmolality
  Improvement following fluid restriction

Plasma vasopressin may also be determined and a concentration which is inappropriately elevated relative to plasma osmolarity supports a diagnosis of SIAD. However, vasopressin determination does not always provide conclusive evidence, as its concentration remains within the normal range (see Table 5–1) or may even, depending on the assay employed, be below the level of detection. Final confirmation of the diagnosis may be provided by an elevation of plasma osmolality on fluid restriction, although a similar response may be seen in proximal types of dilutional disorders.

Table 5–4   Etiology of Inappropriate Vasopressin Secretion

Tumors
  Pulmonary or mediastinal
  Nonchest

Central nervous system disorders
  Mass lesions
  Infectious/inflammatory
  Degenerative
  Other, e.g., subarachnoid hemorrhage and trauma

Respiratory disorders*
  Infections
  Mechanical/ventilatory

Other diseases
  Hypothyroidism, acute intermittent porphyria, cirrhosis, others

Drugs
  Chlorpropamide, vinblastine, others

Surgery
  Administration of high doses of vasopressin or its analogs

*Possibly as a result of the accompanying hypoxia and hypercapnia. (Rees L, et al. Causes of hyponatremia in the first week of life in preterm infants. I. Arginine vasopressin secretion. Arch Dis Child 1984;59:423–429.)

OXYTOCIN

Oxytocin has two main systemic effects, acting to stimulate uterine contractions and milk ejection. It may not be important in the initiation of parturition, but its increase at the time of delivery (Chard, 1985) suggests a specific function at this time, namely, retraction of the uterus thus providing natural hemostasis. It also plays a significant role in lactation and has been shown in some species to have a number of other actions, for example, influencing maternal behavior and sodium excretion. It is used in the induction of labor, but if prolonged infusions are given they may result in hyponatremia. Since oxytocin is synthesized in the same hypothalamic nuclei as vasopressin, it has been suggested that there may be deficient oxytocin production in central diabetes insipidus. However, plasma oxytocin concentrations are within the physiologic range in pregnant women, even when there is total vasopressin deficiency (Shangold, et al., 1983), and normal labor and milk ejection have been reported (Chau, et al., 1969).

Biologically active oxytocin has been determined using the milk ejection reflex in the lactating rat (Chard and Forsling, 1976). A less sensitive assay, which may be used in the standardization of preparations, is the rat uterus assay. RIAs for oxytocin are available in a small number of laboratories and there are a few kits on the market. However, such assays have no routine clinical applications and are for research purposes only.

REFERENCES

Anderson RJ, Chung H-M, Klage R, Schrier RW. Hyponatraemia: prospective analysis of its epidemiology and the pathogenic role of vasopressin. Ann Intern Med 1985; 102:164–168.

Bartter FC, Schwartz WB. The syndrome of inappropriate secretion of antidiuretic hormone. Am J Med 1967;42:790–806.

Baylis PH. Disorders of antidiuretic hormone secretion. Med Int 1981;1:249–252.

Baylis PH. Posterior pituitary function in health and disease. Clin Endocrinol Metab 1983;12:747–770.

Baylis PH. Vasopressin secretion during the menstrual cycle. In: Cowley AW, Liard J-F, Ausiello DA eds, Vasopressin: Cellular and integrative Functions. New York: Raven Press 1985:273–280.

Baylis PH, Zerbe RL, Robertson GL. Arginine vasopressin response to insulin-induced hypoglycaemia in man. J Clin Endocrinol Metab 1981;53:935–940.

Bisset GW, Black A, Hilton RJ, Jones NF, Montgomery M. Polyuria associated with an antibody to vasopressin. Clin Sci Mol Med 1976;50:277–283.

Carter AC, Robbins J. The use of hypertonic saline infusions in the differential diagnosis of diabetes insipidus and psychogenic polydipsia. J Clin Endocrinol 1947;7:753–766.

Chard T. Oxytocin, physiology and pathophysiology. In: Baylis PH, Padfield PL, eds. Posterior Pituitary. New York: Marcel Dekker, 1985:361–390.

Chard T, Boyd NRH, Forsling ML, McNeilly AS, Landon J. The development of a radioimmunoassay for oxytocin: the extraction of oxytocin from plasma and its measurement during parturition in the human and goat. J Endocrinol 1970;48:223–243.

Chard T, Forsling ML. Bioassay and radioimmunoassay of oxytocin and vasopressin. In: Antoniades HN, ed. Hormones in Human Blood. New York: Academic Press, 1976; 486–516.

Chau SS, Fitzpatrick RJ, Jamieson B. Diabetes insipidus and parturition. Br J Obstet Gynaecol 1969;76:444.

Dashe AM, Cramm RE, Crist CA, Habener JF, Solomon DH. A water deprivation test for the differential diagnosis of polyuria. JAMA 1963;185:699–703.

Davison JM, Gilmore EA, Durr J, Robertson GL, Lindheimer MD. Altered osmotic threshold for vasopressin secretion and thirst in human pregnancy Am J Physiol 1984; 246:F105–F109.

Dunn H, Brennan TJ, Nelson AE, Robertson GL. The role of blood osmolality in regulating vasopressin secretion in the rat. J Clin Invest 1973;52:3212–3219.

Edwards CRW, Chard T, Kitau MJ, Forsling, ML, Landon J. The development of a radioimmunoassay for vasopressin: production of antisera and labelled hormone; separation techniques; specificity and sensitivity of the assay in aqueous solution. J Endocrinol 1972;52:279–288.

Fisher BM. Water intoxication and oxytocin. Br Med J 1985;290:637.

Forsling ML. Extraction of neurohypophysial hormones for bioassay. J Physiol 1974;241:35P–36P.

Forsling ML. Antiduiretic Hormone, vol 5. Montreal:Eden Press, 1982.

Forsling ML. Measurement of vasopressin in body fluids. In: Baylis PH, Padfield PL, eds. Posterior Pituitary. New York: Marcel Dekker, 1985;161–192.

Forsling ML, Henneberry H, Slater JDH. A solid phase radioimmunoassay for vasopressin. J Physiol 1984;349:2P.

Gross PA, Pehrisch H, Rascher W, Schomig H, Hackenthal E, Riz EL. Pathogenesis of clinical hyponatraemia observations of vasopressin fluid intake in 100 hyponatraemic medical patients. Eur J Clin Invest 1987;17:123–129.

Halpin DMG, Kemp D, Treacher DF, Forsling ML, Cameron I. The effects of acute and chronic hypoxia on the secretion of vasopressin, renin and aldosterone. Thorax 1992;47:846.

Kimura T, Tanizawa D, Mori K, Brownstein MJ, Okayama H. Structure and expression of a human oxytocin receptor. Nature 1992;356:526–529.

La Rochelle FT, North WG, Stern P. A new extraction of AVP from blood; the use of octadecasilyl-silica. Pflugers Arch 1980;387:79–81.

Legros JJ, Franchimont P, Burger H. Variations of neurohypophysial function in normally cycling women. J Clin Endocrinol Metab 1975;41:54–59.

Manning M, Balaspiri L, Moehring J, Haldar J, Sawyer WH. Synthesis and some pharmacological properties of deamino [4-threonine, 8-D-arginine] vasopressin and deamino [8-D arginine] vasopresin and deamino arginine vasopressin. J Med Chem 1976; 19:842–845.

Montgomery H, Windle RJ, Treacher DF, Forsling ML. Daily rhythms of plasma neurohypophysial hormone concentration in man. J Physiol 1991;438:252P.

Morel A, O'Carroll A-M, Brownstein MJ, Lolait SJ. Molecular cloning and expression of a rat V1a arginine vasopressin receptor. Nature 1992;346:523–526.

Moses AM, Streeten DHP. Differentiation of polyuric states by measurement of responses to changes in plasma osmolalities induced by hypertonic saline infusions. Am J Med 1967;42:368–377.

Puri VN. Urinary levels of antidiuretic hormone in nocturnal eneuresis. Indian Pediatr 1980;17:675–676.

Rees L, Brook CGD, Forsling ML. Continuous urine collection in the study of vasopressin in the new born. Hormone Res 1983;28:134–140.

Rees L, Brook CGD, Shaw JCL, Forsling ML. Causes of hyponatremia in the first week of life in preterm infants. I. Arginine vasopressin secretion. Arch Dis Child 1984;59:423–429.

Rittig S, Knudsen B, Nøgaard JP, Pedersen E.B, Djurhus JC. Abnormal patterns of plasma vasopressin and urine output in patients with enuresis. Am J Physiol 1989; 256:F664–F671.

Robertson GL. Physiology of ADH secretion. Kidney Int 1987;32(suppl 21):520–526.

Robertson GL, Athar S. The interaction of blood osmolality and blood volume in relating plasma vasopressin in man. J Clim Endocrinol Metab 1976;42:613–620.

Robertson GL, Mahr EA, Athar S. Development and clinical application of a new method for the radioimmunoassay of arginine vasopressin in human plasma. J Clin Invest 1973;52:2340–2352.

Robertson GL, Shelton RI, Athar S. The osmoregulation of vasopressin. Kidney Int 1976;10:25–37.

Sagnella GA, Markandu NA, Shore AC, Forsling ML, MacGregor GA. Plasma atrial natriuretic peptide: its relationship to changes in sodium intake, plasma renin activity and aldosterone in man. Clin Sci 1987;72:25–30.

Saito T, Fujisawa G, Tsuboik F, Okada K, Ishikawa S–e. Nonapeptide vasopressin antagonist and its application to the correction of experimental hyponatraemia. Regul Pept 1993; 45: 295–298.

Shangold MM, Freeman R, Kumaresan P. Plasma oxytocin concentrations in a pregnant woman with total vasopressin deficiency. Obstet Gynecol 1983;61:662–667.

Thompson CJ, Baylis PH. Reproducibility of osmotically stimulated thirst and vasopressin release. J Endocrinol 1987;112(suppl): Abstract 69.

Thorell JI, Johansson BG. Enzymic oxidation of polypeptide with ^{125}I to high specific activity. Biochim Biophys Acta 1971;251:363–369.

Uhlich E, Weber P, Groschel-Stewart U, Ruschlau T. Radioimmunoassay of arginine vasopressin in human plasma. Horm Metab Res 1975;7:503–507.

Verney EB. The antidiuretic hormone and the factors which determine its release. Proc R Soc Lond [Biol] 1947;135:25–106.

Windle RJ, Forsling ML. The renal actions of oxytocin in the conscious rat. J Physiol Pharmacol 1991;42:417–425.

Windle RJ, Forsling ML. Variations of oxytocin secretion over the 4-day oestrus cycle of the rat. J Endocrinol 1993;136:305–311.

Zerbe RL. Genetic factors in normal and abnormal regulation of vasopressin secretion. In: Schrier RW, ed. Vasopressin. New York: Raven Press, 1985;213–220.

CHAPTER 6

The Somatotropic Axis

Bruno Barenton and
Wieland Kiess

Growth hormone (GH, somatotropin) and a family of peptide hormones referred to as insulin-like growth factors (IGFs, somatomedins) are the most important stimulants of skeletal and somatic growth.

GH is secreted by somatotroph cells which are mainly located in the lateral parts of the anterior pituitary gland (Fig. 6–1). Two hypothalamic peptides regulate the synthesis and secretion of GH. Growth hormone releasing hormone (GHRH) stimulates while somatostatin (somatotropin release inhibiting factor, SRIF) inhibits GH synthesis and secretion. In the circulation, GH is complexed to a binding protein corresponding to the extramembranous portion of the cellular GH receptor. The GH receptor is a monomeric transmembranous protein that lacks tyrosine kinase activity.

The IGF family consists of two related peptides, IGF-I (somatomedin-C) and IGF-II, of similar chemical structure which exhibit growth promoting actions and complement the metabolic effects of insulin. IGF-I is GH dependent and mediates most of the biologic effects of this hormone. IGF-II is much less GH dependent and is thought to play an important role during embryonic and fetal development.

The IGFs bind to specific binding proteins (IGFBPs) which are present in blood, in extracellular fluids, in intracellular membrane vesicles, and are also associated with the cellular matrix. At least six classes of IGFBPs have already been purified and cloned and it is not certain that all of the existing IGFBPs have been discovered yet. Although the role of each of the IGFBPs is not understood, there is evidence showing that they may modulate IGF action.

IGFs are involved in most of the cellular aspects of growth, development, and aging. They are present in many tissues early in embryogenesis. They promote the clonal expansion of stem cell populations and subsequent tissue formation. They participate with other growth factors with respect to the determination and differentiation of numerous fetal tissues and organs, whatever their embryonic origin. In postnatal life, IGFs are still highly concentrated in tissues, such as epiphyseal growth-plate cartilage and the gonads, which continue to undergo rapid growth and

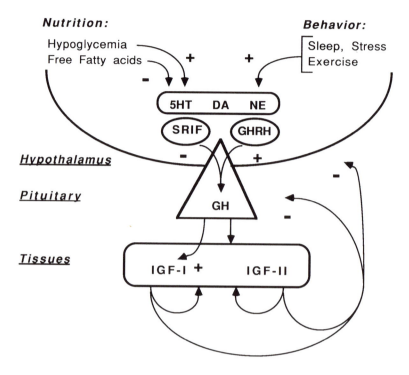

Figure 6–1. The somatotropic axis. Abbreviations: 5HT, 5-hydroxytryptophan; DA, dopamine; NE, norepinephrine;SRIF, somatotropin (growth hormone), release inhibiting factor; GHRH, growth hormone releasing hormone; GH, growth hormone; IGF-I and IGF-II, insulin-like growth factor-I and -II.

differentiation. IGFs also play an important role in tissue wound healing and nerve regeneration.

Since IGFs circulate in the blood, they may act upon distal target organs in an endocrine fashion. There is strong evidence indicating that IGFs are paracrine factors regulating growth and development of neighboring cell types. It has also been demonstrated in many cell lines that the IGFs act through an autocrine mode of action which involves several intracrine interactions and regulatory processes.

The biologic actions of the IGFs are mediated through two types of cellular receptors. The IGF-I receptor, a complex of proteins with $\alpha_2\beta_2$ quaternary structure, is similar to the insulin receptor and bears tyrosine kinase activity. It is thought to mediate most of the biologic effects of both IGF-I and IGF-II. The IGF-II/mannose-6-phosphate receptor is a monomer which has a small cytoplasmic domain lacking tyrosine kinase activity, similar to other cycling receptors. In addition to IGF-II, it binds lysosomal enzymes bearing mannose-6-phosphate residues. This receptor targets lysosomal enzymes to lysosomes. Its role in mediating IGF-II action on cellular growth and differentiation is highly controversial.

All these features of IGF biology have been extensively reviewed (Humbel, 1990; Rechler and Nissley, 1990; Shimasaki and Ling, 1991). A basic understanding of IGF biology is important to appreciate the relevance of IGF levels in regard to pathophysiology.

CHEMICAL AND BIOLOGIC PROPERTIES

Hypothalamic Factors

The hypothalamic factors GHRH and SRIF are secreted into the portal vessels linking the hypothalamus and the pituitary gland. Their synthesis and release are controlled by various neurotransmitters including norepinephrine (NE), dopamine (DA), and serotonin (5-HT) (Fig. 6–1). Human GHRH is a peptide of 40 or 44 amino acids (mol wt 4545 or 5040, respectively) which exerts a tonic stimulatory effect on GH secretion. Recombinant GHRH is available for diagnostic and treatment purposes. SRIF is secreted as a monomer of 14 amino acids (SRIF-14, mol wt 1638) or as a dimer (SRIF-28). SRIF inhibits both basal and GHRH-induced GH secretion, and increases the episodic time interval between GH peaks. In addition to its role in the central nervous system, SRIF also has extensive inhibitory hormonal properties in the gut (see Chap. 11).

Growth Hormone

In the human, two GH genes have been identified on chromosome 17. The *GH-N* gene encodes for pituitary GH while the *GH-V* gene is predominantly expressed in placental tissues. Both genes encode for prohormones. Secreted GH consists of heterogeneous molecular species. The predominant form is a single-chain polypeptide of 191 amino acids (mol wt 21,500) with two disulfide bridges. The most important variant has 176 residues (mol wt 20,000). It is generally found at very low concentration but it may prevail in rare cases of growth failure. Other structural variants such as big-GH corresponding to a GH dimer and the GH-binding protein complex, and abnormal less-active forms of GH may be found in the blood. GHRH injections and other provocative tests do not change the ratios of the molecular forms of GH.

GH is an anabolic hormone which has intermediary metabolic effects on fat tissue and skeletal muscle, regulating protein synthesis, fat mobilization, and carbohydrate metabolism. GH promotes longitudinal bone growth directly by stimulating the differentiation of precursor cells from the epiphyseal growth plate and, indirectly, by controlling local IGF-I production.

Insulin-Like Growth Factors

Protein and Gene Structure

The structures and amino acid sequences of the IGFs are highly homologous to those of proinsulin. The IGF polypeptide chain has five distinct domains and contains three intramolecular disulfide bonds. The human IGF polypeptides are resistant to acid pH and are not glycosylated.

IGF-I has 70 amino acids (Table 6–1) and its gene, located on chromosome 12, consists of a number of introns and five exons that encode large precursor proteins. Different IGF-I mRNA transcripts are generated by alternative splicing, for example, IGF-IA and an IGF-IB mRNA. Interestingly, GH seems to exert selective regulatory effects on the different IGF-I mRNA transcripts in different tissues. In addition to GH, other hormones such as estrogens, prolactin, and various growth factors have been described as regulating IGF-I mRNA levels. Nonhormonal factors modulating IGF-I gene expression include all of the following: fasting, streptozocin induction of diabetes, ischemic injury of skeletal muscle, and renal hypertrophy following diabetes induction or unilateral nephrectomy.

Truncated IGF-1 lacking the first three residues of the B domain (des(1-3)IGF-I) has been isolated from fetal brain extracts. Des(1-3)IGF-I variant has greatly reduced affinity for the IGF binding proteins and is much more potent in stimulating some IGF-induced biologic functions than is normal IGF-I.

IGF-II has 67 amino acids (Table 6–1) and its gene is located on chromosome 11. Eight exons are responsible for the transcription of a large precursor protein. Through the use of alternative promoters different mRNA transcripts are generated. IGF-II gene expression has been shown to undergo very little variation through the influence of GH or during fasting and is very high during fetal life. Recently, it has been shown that targeted disrupture of the IGF-II gene in transgenic mice leads to the

Table 6–1   Properties of Insulin-Like Growth Factor-I and -II

	IGF-I	*IGF-II*
Gene localization	Chromosome 12	Chromosome 11
Molecular weight	7649 dalton	7471 dalton
Source	Hepatic, renal, connective tissues	Hepatic, embryonal tissue, plexus chorioideus, tumors
Regulation	GH, nutritional factors, insulin	Fetal growth factor
Serum concentration	170–350 ng/ml (age dependent)	570–650 ng/ml
Receptor	IGF-I receptor heterotetramer	IGF-II/M6P receptor, $\alpha_2\beta_2$ heterotetrameric receptors
Second messenger	Tyrosine phosphorylation	G-proteins (?)
Biologic action	Anabolic, insulin-like, mediator of GH action	Fetal growth, development of the central nervous system, insulin-like
Pathophysiology	High levels in acromegaly; low levels in GH deficiency, liver disease, and malnutrition	High levels in some tumors, hypoglycemia syndromes; low levels in liver disease

generation of dwarf animals at birth (DeChiara, et al., 1990), indicating that IGF-II plays a major role in fetal growth and development.

Biologic Properties

Both IGFs are potent growth factors and important regulators of metabolic home-ostasis (Table 6–2). In vitro, IGFs are potent mitogens for cells in culture. Frequently, they act in concert with other growth factors such as platelet-derived growth factor (PDGF), epidermal growth factor (EGF), fibroblast growth factor (FGF), and trans-forming growth factor-α (TGF-α) and -β (TGF-β). The IGFs stimulate [^{35}S]sulfate uptake into chondrocytes and [^{3}H]thymidine incorporation into DNA of most cells. They also exert strong stimulatory effects upon glucose uptake, amino acid uptake, and ion fluxes in many cells. Both IGFs also suppress GH secretion, and insulin and C peptide secretion.

In vivo, IGF-I acts as the mediator of GH action (Table 6–2) and directly pro-motes longitudinal bone growth. Extraosseous effects of IGF-I include the enhance-ment of renal function (filtration rate, plasma flow, and creatinine clearance) and of vascular tone; the stimulation of erythropoiesis and an increase of thymus size and thymus cell content. IGF-I also decreases glucose plasma levels and increases lipid mobilization. The in vivo action of IGF-II is less well defined, although it seems to be clear that it exerts similar effects to IGF-I, although at much higher concentrations.

Insulin-Like Growth Factor Binding Proteins

According to recent recommendations, the six IGFBPs which have been presently characterized should be numbered and designated as IGFBP-1, IGFBP-2, etc. (Table 6–3). Comparisons of the sequence homologies between the six IGFBPs have shown that all contain highly conserved, cysteine-rich regions. IGFBP-1 and IGFBP-2 also contain Arg-Gly-Asp (RGD) sequence, which renders them capable of attaching to

Table 6–2 Biologic effects of the Insulin-Like Growth Factors

In Vivo	*In Vitro*
Promotion of longitudinal bone growth	Stimulation of glucose uptake
Antilipolytic effect	Stimulation of protein synthesis
Suppression of GH secretion	Stimulation of DNA synthesis
Suppression of insulin and C-peptide secretion	Stimulation of RNA synthesis
	Stimulation of mitogenesis in cell culture
Stimulation of creatinine clearance	Stimulation of cellular differentiation
Stimulation of renal plasma flow	Stimulation of ion fluxes
Stimulation of glomerular filtration rate	Stimulation of extracellular matrix synthesis
Stimulation of erythropoiesis	
Stimulation of glucose disposal	
Effect on thymus architecture and thymus size and cell content	

Table 6–3   Classification and Characterization of Human IGF Binding Proteins

	Mol Wt (kDa)*	AA†	Glyco‡	RGD§	Ka^II(nM^{-1})		Source	Regulation	Physiology	Pathology	RIA
					IGF-I	IGF-II					
IGFBP-1	28–31	234	O-gly	Yes	5	10	Amnion, placenta, fetal tissue	Insulin	Modulation of IGF action	Diabetes, fetal growth retardation?	Yes
IGFBP-2	32	289	No	Yes	1	20	CNS, serum	GH-insulin, IGF, glucose fasting	Blunts IGF action, morphogenesis	Diabetes, malnutrition	Yes
IGFBP-3#	47–53	264	N-gly	No	10	10	Serum, liver, various tissues	GH, IGFs, nutrition, corticoids	IGF-reservoir enhances and blunts IGF action	GH deficient, liver disease, short stature	Yes
IGFBP-4	24–25	237	N-gly	No	20	20	Osteosarcoma, carcinoma, serum, atretic graafian follicle	PTH, cAMP	Inhibitor of IGF action	Cancer	No
IGFBP-5	29	252	No	No	30	30	CSF, serum, osteosarcoma, various tissues	IGF-I	?	?	No
IGFBP-6	34	216	O-gly	No	0.8	100	CSF, serum, various tissues	?	?	?	Yes

*Apparent molecular weight on electrophoresis.
†AA, Number of amino acids.
‡Glyco, Potential N-linked or O-linked glycosylation sites.
§RGD, Arg-Gly-Asp sequence.
^{II}Ka, Apparent affinity constant.
#IGFBP-3 is associated with an 80-Kd acid-labile subunit (ALS) to form a 150-Kd complex in the serum.
Data as reviewed by Shimasaki and Ling (1991), Blum (1992), and Kiefer, et al. (1992).

cellular membranes. Thus, IGFBPs are excellent candidates as local regulators of IGF action.

Otherwise the IGFBPs are a rather heterogeneous group, some of which are highly glycosylated (IGFBP-3), and some of which lack carbohydrate additions (IGFBP-2, IGFBP-5). IGFBP-3 has a rather complex structure being made up of an acid-labile subunit (ALS) and the GH-dependent IGF binding subunit. After binding of IGF-I or IGF-II, these two IGFBP-3 subunits form a large molecular weight complex (mol wt 150,000) which can be recovered after chromatography of plasma under neutral conditions. IGFBP-1 levels are very high in amniotic fluid and in placental tissues. Nutritional factors, insulin, and corticoids are known regulators of IGFBP-1 expression. IGFBP-2 is the predominant IGFBP species in the cerebrospinal fluid and in the central nervous system. IGFBP-2 expression is also modulated by glucose and/or insulin.

Only small amounts of IGF might be present in free form and the IGFBPs prolong the biologic half-lives of the IGFs. On the other hand, IGFBPs delay and blunt the biologic effects of the IGFs by slowly releasing small amounts of free IGFs which are capable of binding to IGF receptors. Both inhibitory and stimulatory effects of the IGFBPs on IGF-induced biologic functions have been described. The relative ratios between the IGFs and the different IGFBPs might discriminate among the respective actions of IGF-I and IGF-II, and thus determine their bioactivity in a given tissue.

LABORATORY MEASUREMENTS

Growth Hormone Releasing Hormone and Somatotropin Release Inhibiting Factor

Recombinant peptides and specific antibodies are available to set up radioimmunoassays for both GHRH and SRIF. In particular, there are several commercial kits to measure SRIF after plasma extraction with a sensitivity of 5 to 25 pg/mL. Except in the case of pancreatic tumors, there is no clinical interest in assaying these peptides because the diagnosis of growth disorders that involve alteration of GHRH or SRIF secretion is better achieved with GH provocative tests.

Growth Hormone

Two bioassays, based on GH effects on either body weight gain or on the widening of the cartilage growth plate of the tibia of hypophysectomized rats, have been used to standardize purified and recombinant GH preparations (Bangham, 1986). These bioassays are not suitable for clinical measurement of GH in the serum because they have low sensitivity and are time-consuming.

Immunoassays for GH (radioimmunoassay [RIA], immunoradiometric assay [IRMA], immunoenzymatic assay, and immunofluorometric assay) allow the measurement of circulating levels of the hormone in large numbers of samples. A multicenter study of several commercial kits revealed that a part of the variability in GH assays was due to technical human factors. Differences between kits also exist in regard to the estimation of large molecular weight forms of GH (Chatelain, et al., 1990). There is a need to define the assay criteria for the estimation of free, bound, or total GH, GH dimers, GH variants, and GH related hormones.

Receptor assays for GH are useful tools in evaluating the bioactivity of plasma immunoreactive GH, as well as in the estimation of the GH related hormone, placental lactogen. Membrane preparations from tissues such as rabbit liver (Tsuhima and Friesen, 1973) or viable cells such as IM9 lymphoblasts (Rosenfeld and Hintz, 1980) can serve as sources of GH receptors.

Insulin-Like Growth Factors

Bioassays

The biologic activities of the IGFs depend on their relative concentrations but also on the presence of IGFBPs. The estimation of IGF bioactivity is very relevant because it provides information as to the equilibrium between IGFs and their IGFBPs, and integrates the activity of other components, such as insulin or IGF inhibitors (Phillips and Unterman, 1984), which may also interfere with the IGF system. The standard method to estimate IGF bioactivity is to measure [^{35}S]sulfate incorporation into pieces of cartilage in response to dilutions of a pool of plasma containing known concentrations of standard IGF and unknown plasma samples. A less laborious method has been developed using pelvic cartilage rudiments from 12-day old chick embryos (Hall, 1972). In this assay, IGF-I and IGF-II are equipotent in stimulating [^{35}S]sulfate incorporation (Froesch, et al., 1976). The measurement of [^{3}H]thymidine incorporation into DNA may complement the analysis of [^{35}S]sulfate incorporation in cartilage. [^{3}H]Thymidine has also been used to assay IGF mitogenic activity in several other tissue systems such as embryo fibroblasts (Morell and Froesch, 1973).

Assays

Separation Procedures.   In order to avoid pitfalls generated by the presence of IGFBPs in biologic fluids and tissues, several removal procedures have been proposed.

The standard method is acid-ethanol extraction (Daughaday, et al., 1980). Some of the residual IGFBPs can be removed by recentrifugation of the precipitate that forms after a few hours at $-20\,^{\circ}$C (Breier, et al., 1991). While it does not remove all of the IGFBPs, this method is not time-consuming and is suitable for routine assays of biologic fluids rich in proteins, such as serum. In contrast, it cannot be used for the analysis of IGF in cell culture–conditioned media and other body fluids such as milk.

Several alternative methods are used such as formic acid-acetone extraction, which may be convenient for measuring IGFs in tissue extracts (Lee, et al., 1991), or solid phase extraction (Silbergeld, et al., 1986) using C18 Sep Pak minicolumn (Waters, Millipore Division, Milford, MA), which are supplied with some commercial IGF-I kits. Gel chromatography under acidic conditions using Bio-Gel P60 (Daughaday, et al., 1987) or high performance liquid chromatography (HPLC) with a gel permeation column (Protein-Pak 125 [Waters]) (Scott, et al., 1985) is considered the most effective way to remove the IGFBPs. However, this technique is time-consuming for clinical purposes and the recovery of IGFs may vary. To our knowledge, ultrafiltration of acidified samples (Canalis, et al., 1991) with a 20,000 mol wt cutoff filtration device (UFP 1 LGC, Millipore, Bedford, MA) is a good method. It may also be used for the assay of free IGFs in unacidified samples.

Saturation of IGFBPs with the *other* IGF is an alternative to IGF/IGFBP separation (Mohan, et al., 1990). Samples (50 μL) are preincubated for 30 minutes before the assay with 50 μL of either IGF-I (400 ng/mL) for the IGF-II assay, or IGF-II (100 ng/mL) for the IGF-I assay. The technique requires very specific assays (with no cross-reactivity between IGF-I and IGF-II) and must be validated according to the kind of sample and the concentration of IGFBPs. Indeed, samples containing high concentrations of IGFBPs and exhibiting very high affinity for IGF-II would be unlikely to become saturated by IGF-I. No specific [^{125}I]IGF binding activity should remain detectable in the sample after saturation.

Immunoassays and Other Binding Assays. Immunoassay kits (RIA, IRMA) for IGF-I are widely available commercially. The least detectable quantity of IGF-I is generally around 0.2 ng/mL. The use of des(1-3)IGF-I as radioligand, which binds poorly to the IGFBPs, has been reported to resolve the interference of residual IGFBPs in the IGF-I RIA (Bang, et al., 1991).

To date the best antibody against IGF-II commercially available is a monoclonal antibody for rat IGF-II (Sera-lab, Crawley Down, Sussex, UK). It allows the setting up of a reliable RIA (Asakawa, et al., 1990), but its price may be prohibitive for clinical purposes and routine measurements. Therefore, measuring IGF-II by a sensitive radioreceptor assay is still a good alternative to RIA. This technique requires plasma instead of serum samples. Radioreceptor assays with human placental membranes, in which the IGF-I receptor is present, should be avoided. Using rat liver membranes as matrix, we developed an assay which allows the measurement of 0.5 ng/mL of IGF-II (Barenton, et al., 1987). Alternatively, binding protein assays with IGFBPs harvested from biologic fluids exhibiting preferential affinity for IGF-II, as in cerebrospinal fluid (CSF) (Binoux, et al., 1986), may be more sensitive but they are also less specific, and CSF is difficult to collect and, therefore, not easily available for routine clinical measurements.

Insulin-Like Growth Factor Binding Protein Analyses

There is increasing interest in measuring IGFBPs for clinical purposes. Both qualitative and quantitative aspects of IGFBPs should be considered, as both the nature and the concentration of IGFBP species can be determined. The identification of all IGFBP species is achieved by ligand blotting and immunoblotting (Hossenlopp, et al., 1986). Binding assays and RIA have been developed for quantitative IGFBP measurements (Table 6–3).

PHYSIOLOGIC LEVELS AND PROVOCATIVE TESTS

Growth Hormone, Insulin-Like Growth Factor, and Insulin-Like Growth Factor Binding Protein Levels

The secretion of GH is episodic in nature. Therefore, a randomly taken blood sample often estimates the baseline GH level (about 1 ng/mL) but does not reflect the actual pattern of secretion. In children, GH is normally secreted in 6 to 9 pulses over 24 hours with an increasing peak amplitude (from 5 to 20 ng/mL) during the sleep period. Thus, the evaluation of spontaneous GH secretion requires a 24-hour profile of blood samples taken at short intervals.

In the human, IGF-I plasma concentrations are age dependent. Until 6 years of age, IGF-I plasma levels are low, usually less than 50 ng/mL. With advancing puberty IGF-I increases and remains relatively constant throughout adulthood. There is a good correlation between plasma IGF-I level and bone maturation (bone age). In old age there is a small but clear decrease in IGF-I plasma concentration. The normal IGF-I plasma concentrations throughout adult life are 170 to 350 ng/mL (Kiess, et al., 1993) or 110 to 320 ng/mL (Blum, 1992), as determined by classic RIA. These values vary somewhat with the method used to separate the IGFs from IGFBPs and also depend on the antibody used in the RIA.

IGF-II plasma levels are relatively constant in the human. In the newborn, the IGF-II level is about 200 to 250 ng/mL and in adults is around 570 to 650 ng/mL (Kiess, et al., 1993) or 400 to 570 ng/mL (Blum, 1992).

Human blood contains rather large amounts of IGFBP-3. Although IGFBP-3 levels also vary from less than 1 mg/mL at birth to around 2.5 to 3.5 mg/L throughout childhood, IGFBP-3 plasma concentrations are less age dependent than are IGF-I levels. Blum (1992) has published centile tables of reference plasma concentrations for IGF-I, IGF-II and IGFBP-3, which may prove very useful for physicians.

Reference values for IGFBP-1 and IGFBP-2 plasma concentrations have been less well defined owing to the scarcity of appropriate antisera and the small number of laboratories that have been able to establish potent and reliable RIAs. Usually, plasma levels for IGFBP-1 vary around 20 to 400 ng/mL in the newborn and decline with age reaching levels of 10 to 90 ng/mL in the adult (Hall, et al., 1988). IGFBP-2 plasma concentrations in the adult are in the range of 90 to 210 ng/mL, but are fourfold higher in cord blood (Clemmons, et al., 1991).

Concentrations of the IGFs and their binding proteins have also been measured in milk, urine, seminal plasma, and follicular fluid. Until now the clinical relevance of such measurements has not been proved. However, in view of the autocrine-paracrine mechanisms of IGF action it may well be of greater importance and biologic relevance to know the local levels of IGFs and IGFBPs than their plasma concentrations.

Growth Hormone Testing

Growth Hormone Provocative Tests

The integrity of normal GH secretion rates can be evaluated by measuring GH output during a predetermined period of time where GH plasma levels are assessed every 20 or 30 minutes from 12 (overnight) to 24 hours. The results can then be analyzed using deconvolution analysis (Toutain, et al., 1988) or an appropriate olgorithm for the characterization of hormone pulses such as in the PULSAR program (Merriam and Wachter, 1982).

Physical exercise has been shown to stimulate GH release. Thus, a defined exercise test such as working a cycle ergometer at 2 W/kg body weight for 10 minutes and sampling blood for GH determination at 0 and 15 minutes after beginning the exercise can be performed to estimate physiologic GH release. Pharmacologic tests are being used extensively to determine the capacity of the pituitary to synthesize and release GH. Table 6–4 summarizes the most widely used pharmacologic GH stimulation tests. It is generally agreed that at least two of these tests should be carried out before a diagnosis of GH deficiency is made. In all provocative tests an increase of GH plasma levels above 10 ng/mL is considered sufficient to exclude the diagnosis of GH deficiency. The clinical importance of GHRH in testing the pituitary reserve of GH is doubtful. However, the accuracy, sensitivity, and specificity of the other GH

Table 6–4 Pharmacologic Growth Hormone Provocative Tests

Pharmacologic agent	Dosage and Application	Blood Sampling (min)	Possible Side Effects
Glucose	1.75 g/kg, PO, in water	−30, 0, 30, 60, 90, 120, 180	—
Arginine HCl	0.5 g/kg (max. 30 g), IV, 10% arginine HCl in 0.9% NaCl over 30 min	−30, 0, 15, 30, 45, 60, 90, 120	Shock
Insulin	0.05–0.1 IU/kg, IV, only after blood glucose determination	−30, 0, 15, 30, 45, 60, 90, 120	Hypoglycemia, shock
Clonidine	0.15 mg/m², PO	−30, 0, 30, 60, 90, 120, 150	Hypotension, weakness
L-Dopa	PO: 125 mg (to 15 kg) 250 mg (15–35 kg) 500 mg (>35 kg)	−30, 0, 30, 60, 90, 120	—
GHRH	1 µ/kg, IV	−30, 0, 15, 30, 45, 60, 90, 120	—

Data as reviewed by Ranke MB, Haber P. GH stimulation tests. In: Ranke MB, ed. Functional Endocrinologic Diagnostics in Children and Adolescents. Mannheim: J&J Verlag, 1992;61–75. *PO*, per os (orally); *IV*, Intra Venous.

provocative tests are considered to range between 80% and 100%. In any case of GH deficiency neuroradiologic investigations are required.

Growth Hormone Suppression Tests

The most valuable test in the diagnosis of GH hypersecretion (such as in acromegaly) is the glucose tolerance test (Table 6–4). The patient should be fasting and resting for at least 12 hours. High GH levels which do not decrease below 2 ng/mL within 60 to 120 minutes of an appropriate glucose load are diagnostic for acromegaly (Frisch and Waldhauser, 1992). Provocative tests of GH secretion can add to the diagnosis. Neuroradiologic investigations are of the utmost importance.

Insulin-Like Growth Factor Provocative Tests

The somatomedin-generation test has been designed to assess the ability of an individual to respond biochemically to the administration of exogenous GH when plasma IGF-1 and IGFBP-3 levels are already known to be much lower than normal. GH is given at a dose of one IU/m^2 subcutaneously every night for 7 days. IGF-I and IGFBP-3 plasma concentrations are measured before the administration of GH (baseline) and 12 to 24 hours after the last GH injection. The difference in IGF-I levels before and after treatment should exceed 50 ng/mL, and that in IGFBP-3 levels should reach normal plasma levels (1 to 3.5 mg/L). This test has been especially useful in the evaluation of children with suspected Laron type dwarfism or GH insensitivity syndrome and the syndrome of bioinactive GH.

PATHOLOGIC CHANGES AND CLINICAL APPLICATIONS

Growth Hormone Deficiency and Acromegaly

GH deficiency is characterized by low plasma levels of GH, IGF-I, IGF-II and IGFBP-3 (Table 6–5). However, low IGF-I and IGFBP-3 levels can by no means be

Table 6–5   IGF-I, IGF-II, and IGFBP-3 Plasma Concentrations in Human Disease

	IGF-I	*IGF-II*	*IGFBP-3*
GH deficiency	Low	Low	Low
Acromegaly	High	Normal	High
Hypothyroidism	Low	Normal	Low
Liver disease	Low	Low	Low
Chronic renal failure	(Low)	(High)	High
IDDM*	Low	Normal	High
Chronic malnutrition	Low	Normal	Low
Fasting	Low	Normal	(Normal)

* Insulin- dependent diabetes mellitus

considered to be specific for GH deficiency because they are already low in infants and young children, and low concentrations also occur in several other growth disorders (Fig. 6–2). Since IGFBP-3 levels are less age dependent than are IGF-I levels, IGFBP-3 concentrations can serve as an additional diagnostic parameter in the initial characterization of GH-deficient children. The measurement of IGF-II in short chil-

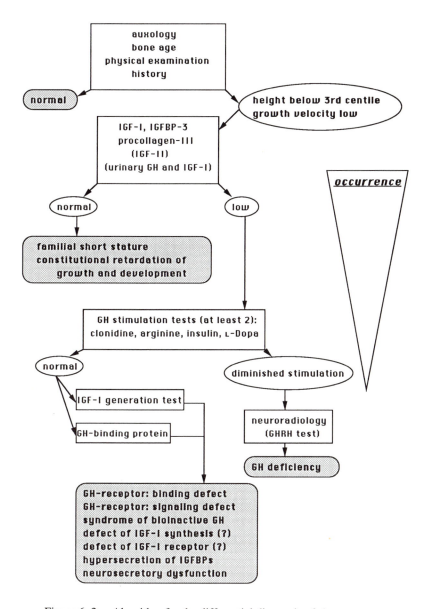

Figure 6–2. Algorithm for the differential diagnosis of short stature.

dren may be helpful, because IGF-II plasma levels are low in GH deficiency but tend to be normal in other growth deficiency states. Long-term treatment with recombinant GH is generally used to restore normal growth, but treatment with GHRH is of increasing interest (Thorner, et al., 1990).

In acromegaly, a disease which is characterized by elevated GH secretion, IGF-I and IGFBP-3 levels very accurately reflect the activity of disease (Table 6–5). Both IGF-I and IGFBP-3 are excellent tools to supervise treatment protocols in acromegalic patients. IGF-II levels have been reported to be normal in acromegaly.

Laron Type Dwarfism

Children with Laron type dwarfism are usually characterized by severe growth failure, abnormal features, microphallus, high pitched voice, and the occurrence of hypoglycemia early in life. It is caused by deletions or mutations within the GH receptor gene or its signaling cascade. Therefore despite high concentrations of GH, the levels of IGF-I and IGFBP-3 are extremely low. Application of exogenous GH does not lead to an elevation of the low IGF-I and IGFBP-3 plasma concentrations. Only recently treatment has become feasible for affected individuals, as the administration of recombinant IGF-I is thought to correct both the growth failure and metabolic derangements in such patients (Walker, et al., 1991).

Bioinactive Growth Hormone

Very rarely patients have been described who do not grow despite normal levels of radioimmunologically detectable GH and normal GH receptor status (Fig. 6–2). Such patients also have low IGF-I, IGF-II, and IGFBP-3 levels. It is thought that such patients synthesize GH molecules that are biologically inactive. Treatment consists of the administration of GH.

Precocious and Delayed Puberty

Unlike IGF-II levels, both IGF-I and IGFBP-3 levels are closely linked with bone age and thus reflect sexual maturation. In precocious puberty, both IGF-I and IGFBP-3 levels are elevated for chronologic age but are normal when assessed for bone age, which is accelerated. In delayed puberty, IGF-I and IGFBP-3 are low for chronologic age but again appropriate for bone age, which is retarded.

Hypothyroidism

Hypothyroidism usually leads to decreased IGF-I and IGFBP-3 plasma levels (Table 6–5). This might add to, or actually cause, the severe growth retardation that is commonly seen in children with hypothyroidism. For patients with suspected combined endocrine deficiencies it is important to bear in mind that in hypothyroid patients low IGF-I and IGFBP-3 levels do not necessarily reflect GH deficiency (Blum, 1992).

Hyperprolactinemia

High levels of prolactin (PRL) seem to be capable of stimulating IGF-I and IGFBP-3 synthesis even when there is GH deficiency. This is thought to reflect the weak somatotropic effect of PRL and a weak cross-reactivity to the hormone with the GH receptor. It is possible that in some children with craniopharyngioma who grow despite a severe GH deficiency at a normal rate, PRL acts as the somatotropic hormone in lieu of GH. Usually in hyperprolactinemic patients normal or slightly elevated IGF-I and IGFBP-3 levels prevail.

Insulin-Dependent Diabetes Mellitus

Insulin-dependent diabetes mellitus (IDDM) induces a defect in IGF-I synthesis in peripheral tissues. Thus IGF-I levels are usually depressed, but GH secretion is enhanced and IGF-II levels are normal (Table 6–5). In addition, the IGF-I response to exogenous GH administration is blunted. During the onset of diabetes high serum and tissue concentrations of IGFBP-I and IGFBP-2 have been found both in humans and rats (Batch, et al., 1991; Flyvbjerg, et al., 1992).

Liver and Kidney Disease

Since liver tissue is the major source for circulating IGF-I, IGF-II and IGFBP-3, it is not surprising that low serum concentrations of these proteins are found in hepatic disease (Blum, 1992; Jaeggi-Groisman, et al., 1992). In addition, very often patients with liver disease are in a catabolic state which adds to their impaired synthesis of IGFs and IGFBP-3 (Table 6–5). Conventional parameters of liver function such as blood coagulation tests and cholinesterase activity are significantly correlated with IGF-I, IGF-II, and IGFBP-3 levels.

In chronic renal failure, disorders of growth are very common. Usually, in kidney failure IGF-II plasma concentrations are normal or even elevated and IGF-I levels are normal to low. In contrast, low molecular weight forms of IGFBP-3 and possibly of other IGFBPs are very high. This may reflect a decrease in renal clearance of such proteins or may be a consequence of the development of the metabolic derangement which occurs in renal failure.

Malnutrition and Malabsorption

IGF-I levels but not IGF-II levels decline rapidly during fasting (Table 6–5). IGF-I concentrations tend to stay low in caloric and protein malnutrition and in malabsorption states. Children with celiac disease may have blunted GH response to provocative tests or GH levels may be normal with low IGF-I levels. In patients with nutritional deficiency based on GH resistance, IGF-I rises on a gluten-free diet but not after GH injection. Since IGFBP-3 is less sensitive to fasting and catabolic states than is IGF-I, the measurement of IGFBP-3 may aid in the diagnostic differentiation between GH deficiency and growth failure due to undernutrition and malabsorption disorders.

Cancer

High plasma levels of IGF-II have been found in patients with endothelial cancers, which causes the development of hypoglycemia. In addition, IGF-II is thought to play a major role in the development and growth of some childhood tumors such as Wilms' tumor, rhabdomyosarcoma, and also in hepatoblastoma. It has been clearly established that the cancer tissues actually express large copy numbers of the IGF-II gene and occasionally also synthesize large amounts of IGF-II at the local level. IGF-I levels have been shown to be higher in women with mammary carcinomas. However, this may simply reflect the fact that such women very often tend to be obese. Thus, somewhat elevated IGF-I levels may be a consequence of their nutritional status rather than a correlate of their cancer growth.

Wound Healing and Nerve Regeneration

In patients suffering from major burns or polytrauma, low-serum IGF-I levels have been measured. Both multiple organ failure involving the liver and catabolism and malnutrition may add to the rapid decline of IGF-I in these patients. It has been suggested that GH and/or IGF-I may be helpful adjuncts in the treatment of major wounds or nerve lesions. Such treatment modalities would be administered both systemically and locally.

REFERENCES

Asakawa K, Hizuka N, Takano K, Fukuda I, Sukegawa H, Shimuze K. Radioimmunoassay for insulin-like growth factor II (IGF-II). Endocrinol Jpn 1990;37:607–614.

Bang P, Eriksson U, Sara V, Wivall I-L, Hall K. Comparison of acid ethanol extraction and acid gel filtration prior to IGF-I anf IGF-II radioimmunoassays: improvement of determinations in acid ethanol extracts by the use of truncated IGF-I as radioligand. Acta Endocrinol 1991;124:620–629.

Bangham DR. Standards for growth hormone. In: Raiti S, Tolman RA, eds. Human Growth Hormone. New York: Plenum Medical, 1986;229–240.

Barenton B, Guyda HJ, Goodyer CG, Polychronakos C, Posner BI. Specificity of insulin-like growth factor binding to type II IGF receptors in rabbit mammary gland and hypophysectomized rat liver. Biochem Biophys Res Commun 1987;149:555–561.

Batch JA, Baxter RC, Werther G. Abnormal regulation of IGFBPs in adolescents with insulin-dependent diabetes. J Clin Endocrinol Metab 1991;73:964–968.

Binoux M., Lassarre, C, Gourmelen MJ. Specific assay for insulinlike growth factor (IGF) II using the IGF binding proteins extracted from human cerebrospinal fluid. Clin Endocrinol Metab 1986;63:1151–1155.

Blum WF. Insulin like growth factors and their binding proteins. In: Ranke MB, ed. Functional Endocrinologic Diagnostics in Children and Adolescents. Mannheim: J & J Verlag, 1992;102–117.

Breier BH, Gallaher BW, Gluckman PD. Radioimmunoassay for insulinlike growth factor-I: solutions to some potential problems and pitfalls. J Endocrinol 1991;128:347–357.

Canalis E, Centrella M, McCarthy TL. Regulation of insulin-like growth factor-II production in bone cultures. Endocrinology 1991;129:2457–2462.

Chatelain P, Bouillat B, Cohen R, et al. Assay of growth hormone levels in human plasma using commercial kits: analysis of some factors influencing the results. Acta Paediatr Scand 1990;(suppl)370:56–61.

Clemmons DR, Snyder DK, Busby WH. Variables controlling the secretion of IGFBP-2 in normal human subjects. J Clin Endocrinol Metab 1991;73:727–733.

Daughaday WH, Mariz IK, Blethen SL. Inhibition of access bound somatomedin to membrane receptor and immunobinding sites: a comparison of RRA and RIA of somatomedin in native and acid ethanol-extracted serum. J Clin Endocrinol Metab 1980;51:781–788.

Daughaday WH, Starkey RH, Saltman S, Gavin JR III, Mills-Dunlap B, Heath-Monnig E. Characterization of serum growth hormone (GH) and insulin-like growth factor in active acromegaly with minimal elevation of GH. J Clin Endocrinol Metab 1987;65:617–623.

DeChiara TM, Efstratiadis A, Robertson EJ. A growth-deficiency phenotype mice carrying an insulin-like growth factor II gene disrupted by targeting. Nature 1990;345:78–80.

Flyvbjerg A, Kessler U, Dorka B, Funk B, Orskov H, Kiess W. Transient increase in renal IGF binding proteins during initial kidney hypertrophy in experimental diabetes in rats. Diabetologia 1992;35:589–693.

Frisch H., Waldhauser F. GH suppression: diagnosis of GH excess. In: Ranke MB, ed. Functional Endocrinologic Diagnostics in Children and Adolescents. Mannheim: J & J Verlag, 1992;119–127.

Froesch ER, Zapf J, Audhya TK, Ben-Porath E, Segen BJ, Gibson KD. Nonsuppressible insulin-like activity and thyroid hormones: major pituitary-dependent sulfation factors for chick embryo cartilage. Proc Natl Acad Sci USA 1976;73:2904–2908.

Hall K. Human somatomedin. Acta Endocrinol 1972;70(suppl 163):1–45.

Hall K, Lundin G, Povoa G. Serum levels of the low molecular weight form of IGFBP in healthy subjects and patients with GH deficiency, acromegaly and anorexia nervosa. Acta Endocrinol (Copenh) 1988;118:321–326.

Hossenlopp P, Seurin D, Segovia-Quinson B, Hardouin S, Binoux M. Analysis of serum insulin-like growth factor binding protein (BPs) using Western blotting: use of the method for titration of the binding proteins and competitive binding studies. Anal Biochem 1986;154:138–143.

Humbel RE. Insulin-like growth factors I and II. Eur J Biochem 1990;190:445–462.

Jaeggi-Groisman S, Kiess W, Kessler U, Christomanou H, Froesch ER. IGFs in lysosomal storage disease. Eur J Pediatr 1992;151:29–31.

Kiefer MC, Schmid C, Waldvogel M, et al. Characterization of recombinant insulin-like growth factor binding protein 4, 5, and 6 produced in yeast. J Biol Chem 1992; 267: 12692–12699.

Kiess W, Kessler U, Schmitt S, Funk B. GH and IGF-I: basic aspects. In: Flyvbjerg A, Orskov H, Alberti K, eds. GH and IGF-I in diabetic complications. Chichester, England: John Wiley Publishers, 1993:1–21.

Lee W-H, Bowsher RR, Apathy JM, Smith MC, Henry DP. Measurement of insulin-like growth factor-II in physiological fluids and tissues. II. Extraction and quantification in rat tissues. Endocrinology 1991;128:815–822.

Merriam GR, Wachter KW. Algorithms for the study of episodic hormone secretion. Am J Physiol 1982;243:E310–E318.

Mohan S, Bautista CM, Herring SJ, Linkhart TA, Baylink DJ. Development of valid methods to measure insulin-like growth factor-I and -II in bone cell-conditioned medium. Endocrinology 1990;126:2534–2542.

Morell B, Froesch ER. Fibroblasts as an experimental tool in metabolic and hormone studies. II. Effects of insulin and nonsuppressible insulin-like activity (NSILAs) on fibroblasts in culture. Eur J Clin Invest 1973;3:119–123.

Phillips LS, Unterman TG. Somatomedin activity in disorders of nutrition and metabolism. Clin Endocrinol Metab 1984;13:145–189.

Ranke MB, Haber P. GH stimulation tests. In: Ranke MB, ed. Functional Endocrinologic Diagnostics in Children and Adolescents. Mannheim: J & J Verlag, 1992;61–75.

Rechler MM, Nissley SP. Insulin like growth factors. In: Sporn MB, Roberts AB, eds. Handbook of Experimental Pharmacology, vol 95/I. Peptide Growth Factors and Their Receptors. Heidelberg: Springer-Verlag, 1990;263–367.

Rosenfeld RG, Hintz RL. Modulation of homologous receptor concentrations: sensitive radioassay for human growth hormone in acromegalic, newborn and stimulated plasma. J Clin Endocrinol Metab 1980;50:62–69.

Scott CD, Martin JL, Baxter RC. Production of insulin-like growth factor I and its binding protein by adult rat hepatocytes in primary culture. Endocrinology 1985;116:1094–1101.

Shimasaki S, Ling N. Identification and molecular characterization of insulin-like growth factor binding proteins (IGFBP-1,-2,-3,-4,-5,-6). Prog Growth Factor Res 1991;3:243–266.

Silbergeld A, Litwin A, Bruchis S, Varsano I, Laron Z. Insulin-like growth factor-I, -IGF-I) in healthy children, adolescents and adults as determined by a radioimmunoassay specific for the 53-70 peptide region. Clin Endocrinol 1986;25:67–74.

Thorner MO, Vance ML, Rogol AD, et al. Growth hormone releasing hormone and growth hormone-releasing peptide as potential therapeutic modalities. Acta Paediatr Scand 1990;(suppl)367:29–32.

Toutain PL, Laurentie M, Autefage A, Alvinerie M. Hydrocortisone secretion: production rate and pulse characterization by numerical deconvolution. Am J Physiol 1988;255:E688–E695.

Tsuhima T, Friesen HG. Radioreceptor assay for growth hormone. J Clin Endocrinol Metab 1973;37:334–337.

Walker JL, Ginalska-Malinowska M, Romer TE, Pucilowska JB, Underwood LE. Effects of the infusion of IGF-I in a child with GH insensitivity syndrome (Laron dwarfism). New Engl J Med 1991;324:1483–1488.

CHAPTER 7

Pituitary-Adrenal Function

Lawrence V. Basso and
James P. Gosling

The adrenal gland is virtually four endocrine glands in one—three associated with the cortex and the fourth with the medulla. Correspondingly, the cortex is in three layers: the outer glomerulosa secretes aldosterone while the fasciculata is the source of cortisol (hydrocortisone, Kendall's "compound F," Reichstein's "substance M"). Both the fasciculata and the inner reticularis secrete androgens and estrogens.

The endocrine medulla, located as its name implies at the interior of the gland, is an essential part of the sympathochromaffin system. Because the present methods (fluorimetric, radioenzymatic, high performance liquid chromatography [HPLC]) for determination of epinephrine, norepinephrine and their metabolites, are not immunoassays, it is not appropriate to discuss the endocrinology of the adrenal medulla here. However, the best methods in use involve extensive sample pretreatment (Rosano, et al., 1991) and simpler immunoassay methods have been described that offer promise for the future (Linuma, et al., 1986; Oishi, et al., 1988). This development has been hindered by difficulties in raising antibodies with adequate specificity and affinity. In addition, immunoassay of chromogranin A may help in the diagnosis of pheochromocytoma (O'Connor, et al., 1984). Stein and Black (1990) described a simplified approach to the diagnosis of pheochromocytoma.

HYPOTHALAMIC-PITUITARY-ADRENAL SYSTEM

The secretion of adrenocorticotropic hormone (ACTH) is under two main controls. Corticotropin-releasing hormone (CRH), a 41-amino-acid peptide, is the primary stimulator of ACTH release but vasopressin and catecholamines act synergistically with it (Watabe, et al., 1988; Tomori, et al., 1989). Second, cortisol inhibits ACTH release, by acting directly on both the pituitary and the hypothalamus.

The hypothalamic-pituitary-adrenal (HPA) system is easily suppressed by exogenous glucocorticoids. When treatment (e.g., 30 mg/day prednisone for 2 years) is stopped, ACTH levels begin to rise after 3 to 6 months; subsequently adrenal atrophy

115

slowly reverses and cortisol returns to normal with suppression of ACTH to normal levels (an additional 3 to 5 months).

Circadian Rhythm

CRH is secreted by the hypothalamus with diurnal variation. The consequent diurnal ACTH and cortisol concentrations show maximal levels in early morning with declining levels through the day leading to minimal secretory activity in the evening, and reattainment of maximal levels during late sleep. Circadian rhythms of the other adrenocortical steroids are not as marked. Changes in plasma cortisol are dependent on selective amplitude control of secretory bursts of ACTH occurring at regular 40-minute intervals (Veldhuis, et al., 1990). Diurnal HPA activity is not affected by short-term changes in sleeping-waking pattern or on feeding times.

Most Cushing's syndrome patients exhibit altered cortisol circadian variation, sometimes with the pulsatility (which may be decreased or increased) occurring above a higher basal level. Pulsatile release is dampened in cases of adrenal adenoma. Normal variations of ACTH and cortisol are sensitive to changes in sleep pattern and age (Sherman, et al., 1985).

The Effects of Stress

When significant stress is experienced, other control mechanisms are overridden, diurnal variation is disrupted, ACTH immediately increases and peaks within minutes, and cortisol peaks shortly after. A wide variety of nonspecific stresses have profound effects, many of which are mediated by ACTH and cortisol. These include surgical stress, trauma, exercise, (Luger, et al., 1987), hypoglycemia, and depression (Rubin, 1991).

Adrenocorticotropic Hormone

Proopiomelanocortin (POMC) is a polypeptide synthesized in the anterior lobe of the pituitary and at other sites (Fig. 7–1). It contains the sequences of ACTH and other biologically active peptides.

In the anterior pituitary POMC is degraded by specific peptidases to give ACTH, N-terminal glycopeptide, and β-lipotropin, the biologic functions of which are unknown; however, these can be further degraded to yield γ-melanocyte-stimulating hormone (γ-MSH) and β-endorphin. ACTH has 39 amino acid residues (mol wt 4500), but full biologic activity is associated with the 24 residues near the N-terminal, and even the first 10 exhibit some activity. Forty percent of ACTH is post-translationally modified by the addition of a phosphate moiety. Circulating ACTH has a half-life of 10 to 15 minutes.

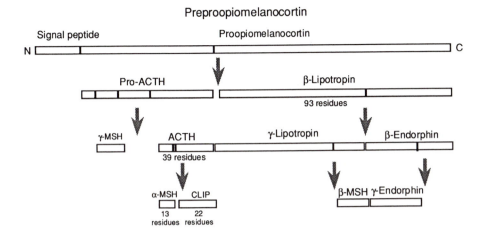

Figure 7–1. Proopiomelanocortin (POMC) is a 265 amino acid polypeptide synthesized in the anterior lobe and the intermediate lobe cells of the pituitary, in the arcuate nucleus of the hypothalamus, in the gonads, and in the gastrointestinal tract; where the peptides derived from POMC may have neurotransmitter and paracrine functions. It contains the sequences of ACTH and at least six other active peptides. POMC is the predominant adrenocortictropin related peptide in cerebrospinal fluid (Tsigos et al., 1993).

The cleavage sites (I) are Arg-Lys, Lys-Arg, or Lys-Lys and additional specificity of cleavage is conferred by neighboring amino acid residues. The further cleavage of ACTH and β-lipotropin occurs mainly in the pars intermedia. Other abbreviations used are MSH, melanocyte stimulating hormone; and CLIP, cortioctropin-like intermediary peptide.

Blood for ACTH assay should always be collected in plastic or siliconized glass tubes with heparin, as it is inactivated by untreated glass. Since, even at −20°C, plasma slowly loses ACTH activity, it should be separated by cold centrifugation and the assay carried out as soon as possible. Radioimmunoassay (RIA) and, increasingly, two-site immunometric assays with a combination of antibodies specific to different parts of the molecule, are normally used to determine ACTH. Longer established RIA have a sensitivity of 10 to 20 ng/L, while immunometric assays have detection limits less than 10 ng/L (Raff and Findling, 1989; Gibson, et al., 1989). Immunometric assays employ solid phase antibody against the carboxyl terminal region (e.g., residues 34 to 39) and labeled antibody against the amino terminal (e.g., residues 1 to 17), or vice versa (sp-Ab–ACTH–Ab-^{125}I). Therefore, only entire ACTH molecules (residues 1 to 39) are detected. An immunoradiometric assay (IRMA) has been found to be more effective than an RIA in detecting ACTH suppression after dexamethasone administration (Sharp, et al., 1992).

However, in actively secreting tumors (either pituitary or ectopic) etiologic for Cushing's syndrome, many biologically active ACTH fragments as well as parts of the POMC molecule that would not be detected by a two-site assay such as IRMA, may be secreted (Raff and Findling, 1989). Therefore, an immunometric assay for

ACTH may report a level much lower than the effective biologic activity. Lower specificity, competitive immunoassays with polyclonal antibodies may give results more representative of ACTH activity but the actual levels estimated may be highly method- or antibody-dependent.

In the early morning ACTH levels are 11 to 18 nmol/L (50 to 80 pg/mL) and in the late afternoon, at the nadir of secretion, they drop to a 4.5 nmol/L (20 pg/mL). While β-endorphin and/or β-lipotrophin, which are secreted with ACTH (Veldhuis, et al., 1990), have greater stability and a longer half-life in blood than ACTH (Kuhn, et al., 1989), the measurement of these peptides has never gained wide acceptance.

ACTH stimulates and maintains the adrenal cortex, but excess ACTH secretion causes hyperplasia of the entire cortex, as in Cushing's disease. It stimulates the synthesis of cortisol but has much less effect on androgen and aldosterone production. Hyperpigmentation found in disorders of excess ACTH maybe due to ACTH itself or to the γ-MSH also released from POMC.

Cortisol and Related Steroids

Figure 7–2 outlines the synthesis of the adrenal steroids. About 20 to 25 mg of cortisol (10 to 12 mg/m^2) are released daily. The peak plasma cortisol in the morning varies between 190 and 500 nmol/L (7 and 18 μg/dL) with an average of 275 to 330 nmol/L (10 to 12 μg/dL), while the nadir in the late afternoon is 55 to 250 nmol/L (2 to 9 μg/dL). Normal concentrations at 10 PM are generally less than 110 nmol/L (< 4μg/dL).

Immunoassays with nonisotopic labels such as enzymes (Tunn, et al., 1990) are becoming more popular and tritiated cortisol is now rarely used as label in RIAs. Polyclonal antibodies are presently used in most commercial assays. Most commercial immunoassays for cortisol employ a label which is "site" and "bridge" homologous with the immunogen used to raise the antibody, and both label and immunogen are usually linked via the 3-position. The Batch No 1150 antibody (Scottish Antibody Production Unit, Carluke, Scotland), which was raised in sheep against cortisol-3-carboxymethyloxime-bovine serum albumin, was cited as a highly specific antibody (Moore, at al., 1985). It had cross-reactions of 0.6%, 0.2%, and 22% with 11-deoxycortisol, corticosterone and prednisolone, respectively, but this level of potential interference from prednisolone is still excessive. Although antibodies raised against immunogens linked to cortisol via other sites are usually resistant to prednisolone, they often bind strongly to cortisol metabolites.

Hashimoto, et al. (1989) highlighted the possibilities of misinterpretation of results from cortisol procedures with different types of antibodies. For one patient, later diagnosed as having 17 α-hydroxylase deficiency, a kit with antibody against cortisol-21-hemisuccinate-bovine serum albumin gave high readings while another kit with antibody against immunogen with a 3-link indicated (correctly) low levels of cortisol. However, for an unconscious patient not known to be on prednisolone treatment because no medical history was available, the former kit gave a correct result and the latter indicated elevated concentrations of cortisol.

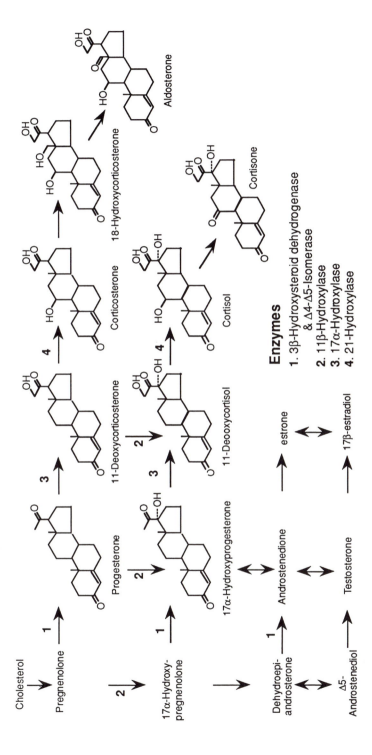

Figure 7–2.   The synthesis of cortisol and related hormones. This diagram overlaps with that of Figure 9.1, which employs the same numbering system for the enzymes.

Plasma cortisol assays now rarely have an initial extraction step and are carried out with the "direct" addition of sample to the assay mixture. Direct assays are more prone to interference, but extraction assays are sometimes imprecise. Automated, liquid chromatographic methods for cortisol determination are also available (Turnell, et al., 1988).

Newer immunoassays for cortisol and other steroids will increasingly be validated against reference methods such as isotope-dilution gas chromatography mass spectrometry (ID-GCMS) (Tunn, et al., 1990). Human serum reference materials for cortisol, certified by means of ID-GCMS, are available for use by assay developers and individual users (Thienpoint, et al., 1991). Gosling, et al. (1993) reviewed cortisol immunoassays at length and made comprehensive recommendations for improving their standardization (see also Chap. 4).

Cortisol in the circulation is about 90% bound by corticosteroid-binding globulin (CBG) and about 7% by albumin, leaving 3 to 5% free. Immunoassays for CBG are available and normal levels are 39.9 to 45 mg/L (Pugeat, et al., 1989). Conditions that alter the concentrations of binding proteins can indirectly alter total hormone levels. CBG may be elevated congenitally, in hyperthyroidism, depression, starvation, anorexia nervosa, hepatitis, or pregnancy, and after estrogen administration (Orbach and Schussler, 1989). It may be depressed congenitally, in some cases of obesity, in hypothyroidism, nephrotic syndrome, or multiple myeloma.

Although not widely utilized, it is possible to measure plasma free cortisol by an equilibrium dialysis technique in patients with CBG abnormalities. Normal plasma free cortisol blood levels are 33 to 39 nmol/L (1.2 to 1.4 µg/dL) (Robin, et al., 1978). Salivary cortisol determinations (normal morning level is 11 nmol/L, 0.4 µdL) are considered to be a good measure of the plasma free cortisol (Laudat, et al., 1988).

Despite the associated inconvenience, the determination of unconjugated (free) cortisol in 24-hour urine samples is considered a good screening test for the evaluation of adrenal hyperfunction (Burch, 1982). The normal range is not altered by obesity and a normal value is less than 276 nmol/day (100 µq/day). Immunoassays for urinary cortisol have almost completely replaced colorimetric methods for the determination of 17-hydroxycorticosteroids (Porter-Silber chromogens). The immunoassays are sometimes carried out without an extraction step, but routine extraction is necessary (Huang and Zweig, 1989).

Immunoassays for other glucocorticoids are commercially available, including corticosterone, 11-deoxycortisol and 11-deoxycorticosterone (Wheeler, 1993).

Sex Steroids

Table 7–1 show the percent adrenal contribution to the production rates for the most important sex steroids. The relative importance of the adrenal gland as a source of sex steroids is particularly evident with respect to the production of all androgens and even of progesterone during the follicular phase in the female, and some andro-

Table 7–1 Total Production Rates and Adrenal Contributions to the Major Circulating Steroids

Steroid	Mean Blood Production Rate (mg/24h)		Adrenal Contribution (%)	
	Male	*Female*	*Male*	*Female*
Cortisol	20	16	100	100
11-Deoxycortisol	0.4	0.4	100	100
Aldosterone	0.1	0.1	100	100
Corticosterone	4	4	100	100
Progesterone	0.3	0.5	—	60
17α-Hydroxyprogesterone	1.6	1	10	10
DHEA	16	16	>90	>90
DHEA sulfate	10	8	>90	>90
Δ^5-Androstenediol	1.4	1	50	80
Δ^4-Androstenedione	2	3.4	70	50
Testosterone	7	0.2	1.5	50
Estrone	0.1	0.1	40	40
Estradiol-17β	0.03	0.1	10	4

Data from Pescovitz OH, et al. Synthesis and secretion of corticosteroids. In: Becker KL, ed. Principles and Practice of Endocrinology and Metabolism. Philadelphia: JB Lippincott, 1990;579–591.

gens (e.g., dehydroepiandrosterone [DHEA] and DHEA sulfate) and estrogens in the male. In the postmenopausal, agonadal woman the principle source of estrogens is via aromatization of adrenal testosterone and androstenedione to estradiol and estrone, respectively. Commercial immunoassay kits are available for the determination of androstenediol glucuronide, androstenedione, DHEA, DHEA sulfate, estrone, 17α-hydroxypregnenolone, and 17α-hydroxyprogesterone (Wheeler, 1991) (see also Chap. 9).

RENIN-ANGIOTENSIN-ALDOSTERONE AXIS

The main control of the adrenocortical glomerulosa, where aldosterone is synthesized, is through the renin-angiotensin-aldosterone (RAA) axis. This cascade control system, which consists of the active components renin, angiotensin II (A-II, an octapeptide) and aldosterone, regulates blood pressure homeostasis, blood volume, and sodium-potassium balance.

Renin and prorenin are both released from the kidney by a drop in volume perfusion and by a decrease in sodium concentration perfusion. Prorenin is also secreted by extrarenal tissues (e.g., the ovaries) and some tumors, and extrarenal prorenin can contribute to high levels of total plasma renin in women with hyperstimulated ovaries or during pregnancy. Renin is secreted fully activated but prorenin accounts for more than 90% of the total plasma renin.

Renin (mol wt 40,000) secreted by the juxtaglomerular apparatus of the kidney, is an aspartyl protease that specifically cleaves angiotensin I (A-I, a decapeptide) from angiotensinogen, an α_2-globulin (mol wt 65,000), which is synthesized in the liver. A-I is converted to A-II, chiefly in the lung, by a ubiquitous, angiotensin-converting enzyme (ACE) (mol wt 200,000). ACE is increased in some forms of granulomatous lung disease such as sarcoidosis and can be blocked by captopril-type drugs. While A-I is relatively inactive, A-II is a potent vasoconstrictor, stimulates aldosterone release, and also exerts feedback inhibition of renin release from the kidney. By a loss of a further residue from the amino terminus, A-II can be converted to angiotensin III (A-III). The physiologic function of A-III is not fully defined, but it is capable of stimulating aldosterone secretion. RIAs for the measurement of A-I and A-II are commercially available.

Plasma Renin Activity

Renin has a half-life of 15 minutes and plasma renin activity (PRA) is expressed as ng A-I generated per L of plasma per second (ng/L/second) or, alternatively, as ng/mL/hour. The assay of PRA was described in detail by Sealey (1991).

PRA determination by enzyme kinetic assay is sensitive and reflects the capacity of plasma to generate A-I. Because ACE activity in plasma is not limiting, PRA is equivalent to the capacity to generate A-II. Inaccurate results may be obtained if the patient was taking an ACE-inhibiting drug, cryoactivation of prorenin occurs during handling and storage, if A-I is degraded or converted to A-II, or if there is inadequate control of the pH during A-I generation (renin is unstable at pH < 8.0 at 37°C). Because the endogenous angiotensinogen becomes used up by higher renin activities, incubation times should be adjusted with 18 hours for activities less than 1 µg/L/hours, 15 minutes for activities greater than 70 µg/L/hours and 3 hours for intermediate activities (Sealey, 1991).

Before sampling for PRA determination, the patient should be on moderate sodium intake, have given the previous day, a 24-hour urine sample for sodium determination, and have been ambulatory for 30 minutes. Plasma should be prepared with EDTA at room temperature and, if longer term storage is necessary, quickly frozen and thawed. Blood or plasma should never be stored on ice or in a refrigerator, conditions which cause activation of prorenin. Incubation at 37 °C to allow A-I formation is carried out in the presence of neomycin to inhibit bacterial growth, phenylmethyl sulfonyl fluoride (PMSF) to inhibit converting enzyme, and maleic acid to reduce pH to 5.7. A pH of 5.7 is favorable for renin formation, stabilizes renin when it is formed, and facilitates inhibition of converting enzyme (Sealey, 1991). However, some commercial kits recommend a pH of 6.0 and blood collection into precooled tubes.

The RIA for A-I of Sealey (1991) is carried out in liquid phase and makes use of polyethylene glycol as a separation agent. In principle other labeling substances than ^{125}I, or labeled antibody, could be used. The samples from the first incubation may be stored frozen before analysis. A range of commercial A-I RIA kits, configured for PRA measurement are available.

After an overnight rest the supine PRA is about 0.1 to 0.4 ng/mL/second (0.5 to 1.6 ng/mL/hour) if the patient had been on a 120 mEq salt diet. After an upright period of 4 hours there is a normal two- to fivefold increase in PRA which parallels a simultaneous increase in plasma aldosterone. Both PRA and aldosterone levels should always be interpreted relative to the salt intake of the patient as established by a 24-hour urine sodium determination after, if possible, some days on a stable salt intake.

Prorenin has been reported to increase in patients with diabetes mellitus who are prone to develop nephropathy (Wilson and Leutscher 1990) and may be determined by measuring active renin, and then total renin, after converting prorenin to renin by limited proteolysis with trypsin (Sealey, 1991).

In addition, immunometric assays have been developed for the direct measurement of renin (Sanofi Diagnostic Pasteur, France), prorenin (Schumacher, et al., 1992) and total renin (e.g., Matinlauri, et al., 1994). The concentrations of total renin and renin are highly correlated and the direct determination of one or the other may replace completely the measurement of PRA.

Aldosterone and Related Steroids

Although aldosterone is the major mineralocorticoid, cortisol and most of the major corticosteroids possess mineralocorticoid activity which can become evident under conditions of excess secretion. The normal level of aldosterone is very dependent on posture and sodium chloride status. With patients on an ad libitum salt diet (usually >120 mEq/day) after an overnight recumbency, plasma aldosterone levels are 55 to 330 pmol/L (2 to 12 ng/dL). After 4 hours upright the concentration increases to at least 2 to 5 times the recumbent value (Malchoff, et al., 1989). On a low sodium diet (20 to 40 mEq NaCl per day) the plasma aldosterone is 2 to 5 times that for medium or high salt intake. Aging does not decrease the plasma aldosterone level but the response to posture and a low sodium diet is blunted (Hegstadt, et al., 1983). Aldosterone is very dependent on total body potassium and hypokalemia can drastically reduce aldosterone output even in patients with aldosterone producing tumors. The other important mineralocorticoid predominantly secreted by the glomerulosa is 18-hydroxycorticosterone (Gomez-Sanchez, et al., 1987). It responds to posture, low sodium diet, and ACTH much like aldosterone.

While there are wide fluctuations in the amount, about 30% of aldosterone is free, with CBG, red blood cells, and albumin binding most of the remainder. In some respects all the aldosterone can be considered to be "free" since it dissociates easily and rapidly from its binding proteins.

Before determination the steroid is generally extracted from plasma. As with other steroids, aldosterone is determined by competitive immunoassay, with nonisotopic labels (e.g., Stabler and Siegel, 1991) slowly supplanting radioiodinated labels.

DISORDERS OF ADRENOCORTICAL FUNCTION

Adrenocortical Hyperfunction

Hypercortisolism is manifested clinically as Cushing's syndrome which is either ACTH dependent (75% of cases) or ACTH independent (25% of cases). Excess ACTH secretion may be due to a pituitary basophilic adenoma (Cushing's disease, or pituitary Cushing's syndrome) or ectopic ACTH or (CRH) secretion by a nonpituitary tumor. Etiologic disorders of the adrenal gland that are ACTH independent include adrenal carcinoma (60%) and adenoma (40%). Figure 7–3 presents a scheme for the diagnosis of patients with suspected Cushing's syndrome. Adrenal function studies can only be reliably carried out in the presence of normal thyroid function (Kamilaris, et al., 1987).

The dexamethasone suppression test, a test of the feedback control of the HPA system, depends on the administration of the potent cortisol agonist, dexamethasone, to repress ACTH release and, hence, cortisol secretion. The amount of dexamethasone given, and the timing and number of administrations, vary greatly. In recent years shorter tests for use in an outpatient setting have been designed and are now very widely used. Usually such tests (e.g., Kaye and Crapo, 1990) involve a blood sample for the determination of cortisol by immunoassay drawn at 8 AM, a dose of 1 to 2 mg or (8 mg for a high dose test) of dexamethasone given at 11 PM, with a second blood sample drawn at 8 AM the following morning. Resistance to suppression is indicated by plasma cortisol greater than 138 nmol/L ($>$ 5 μg/dL). Orth (1991) claimed that for confirmation of hypercortisolism a 2-day test, with multiple dosing of dexamethasone and measurement of urinary unconjugated (free) cortisol and plasma cortisol, is more reliable.

A high dose dexamethasone (8 mg) suppression test partially suppresses ACTH secretion and thus cortisol production in most patients with Cushing's disease, but has no effect in most patients with ectopic ACTH syndrome, (oat cell cancer, carcinoid, thymoma, islet cell tumor), in which ACTH secretion is usually autonomous), or adrenal Cushing's syndrome (adrenal adenomas, carcinomas), in which ACTH secretion is already suppressed (Leinung, et al., 1990; Orth, 1991).

A modified suppression test with intravenous administration of dexamethasone has recently been evaluated and reported as clearly distinguishing Cushing's disease from other forms of Cushing's syndrome (Biemond, et. al., 1990; Miller and Crapo, 1994).

The ACTH blood level, which is usually normal or borderline high in Cushing's disease, is elevated in the ectopic ACTH syndrome and low in patients with adrenal adenomas or functioning carcinomas (Kaye and Crapo, 1990; Orth, 1991). Occasionally patients with ectopic ACTH secretion have normal ACTH levels and can show suppression at a high dose of dexamethasone (thereby resembling Cushing's disease) (Findling, 1990).

To distinguish patients with Cushing's disease from those with ectopic ACTH secretion (who may display similar symptoms), the effect of CRH administration on ACTH may be investigated. However, to clearly identify the origin of the measured

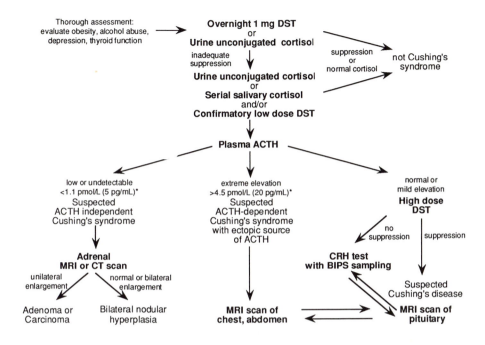

Figure 7–3.   The differential diagnosis of Cushing's syndrome commences with a confirmation of cortisol hypersecretion by:(1) showing resistance to inhibition of adrenal cortisol secretion by low doses of dexamethasone (dexamethasone suppression test, DST); (2) increased daily urinary secretion of cortisol, or (3) lack of a normal nocturnal nadir in plasma cortisol concentration. There is much variation from clinic to clinic in how this is done.

With the advent of improved immunoassays for ACTH most cases of hypercortisolism can now be classified as ACTH dependent or ACTH independent on the basis of plasma ACTH concentration but, because of the pulsatile nature of ACTH release and the biologic potency of ACTH fragments, ACTH determinations may have to be repeated.

Although the result of a high dose DST alone may be sufficient to indicate Cushing's disease, additional confirmatory information may be obtained from CRH testing with bilateral inferior petrosal sinus (BIPS) sampling and/or MR scanning of the adrenals, chest, abdomen, or pituitary.

ACTH, ACTH monitoring during bilateral, inferior petrosal sinus (BIPS) samplings with CRH stimulation is advised (Findling, et al., 1991; Oldfield, et al., 1991; Tabarin, et al., 1991). Although requiring a skilled team to place the catheters correctly and process and label several sets of duplicate blood samples, etc., IPSS is advocated as a routine procedure for appropriate patients in some centers (Oldfield, et al., 1991). Imaging techniques (magnetic resonance and computed tomography) are also important in exact diagnosis.

Although not used routinely, RIA for CRH can be used to demonstrate elevated CRH in patients with CRH-secreting tumors (Rückert, et al., 1990).

Adrenocortical Hypofunction

Figure 7–4 summarizes an approach to the diagnosis of suspected adrenocortical hypofunction. There are two general classes of adrenal insufficiency, primary (Addison's disease), caused by damage to the adrenal gland itself, and secondary, associated with abnormal hypothalamic-pituitary function leading to deficient or absent ACTH secretion. Primary adrenal failure is due to autoimmune destruction (70%), tuberculosis (up to 20%), or one of a variety of other causes including fungal infections, adrenal hemorrhage, and acquired immune deficiency syndrome (AIDS). The most common causes of secondary disease are adrenal suppression by exogenous

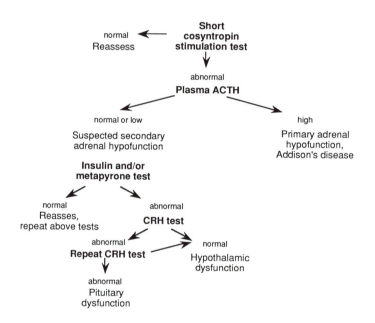

Figure 7–4.   The diagnosis of adrenocortical hypofunction. If a patient arrives with a probable diagnosis of acute adrenal insufficiency, a blood sample for later cortisol determination may be taken but treatment must be started at once and the performance of further tests can await stabilization of the acute condition. In other cases the initial diagnosis may be based on a low level of cortisol determined in a timed plasma sample.

However, the investigation proper begins with a short cosyntropin stimulation test and an abnormal response indicates adrenal insufficiency. Localization of the defect may be conveniently performed by estimating the plasma ACTH with a modern immunometric assay, a high level indicating Addison's disease. The finding of a low or normal ACTH concentration may be followed by testing the entire hypothalamic-pituitary-adrenal axis with a metapyrone or insulin test. MR or CT scanning of the pituitary and hypothalamus to examine for space-occupying lesions of these organs should be undertaken in patients who prove to have secondary adrenal failure.

glucocorticoids used in the treatment of inflammatory disorders, and complications occurring after treatment of Cushing's syndrome.

Serum cortisol levels in the healthy basal state, as well as normal 24-hour urinary unconjugated cortisol excretion, overlap with those in adrenal insufficiency, and therefore the short ACTH stimulation test is widely used as the primary test for hypofunction. In this, a plasma sample for basal cortisol determination is taken, then injection, intravenous or intramuscular, of 250 μg cosyntropin (synthetic β1-24 ACTH, Synacthen, Cortrosyn), and further samples for cortisol measurement are taken after 30 and 60 minutes. A normal pattern of concentrations is a basal cortisol concentration equal to or greater than 140 nmol/L (5 μg/dL); a maximum concentration greater than 490 nmol/L (18 μg/dL); and an incremental change of greater than 190 nmol/L (7 μg/dL) (May and Carey, 1985). The test may be performed at any time of the day and during any day of the menstrual cycle (Azziz et al., 1990). A negative response indicates primary adrenocortical insufficiency, but the response can be normal in patients with secondary insufficiency (Cunningham et al., 1983).

Plasma ACTH level, determined by means of a reliable assay, can be used to locate the level of the defect. Standard RIAs for ACTH have proved inadequate for this application, but modern two-site immunometric assays appear to be suitable (Gibson, et al., 1989).

The metapyrone test can be used to assess the adequacy of the entire hypothalamic-pituitary-adrenal axis (Streeten, et al., 1984), but is now less often used. Metapyrone, an inhibitor of 11β-steroid hydroxylase, causes reduced blood cortisol levels and consequently reduced feedback inhibition of the pituitary, normally leading to increased ACTH secretion and elevated 11-deoxycortisol levels.

The insulin test is another test of the entire hypothalamic-pituitary-adrenal axis, but one which is potentially dangerous. It must be performed under close medical supervision, with glucose and cortisone available for immediate infusion if necessary (Moore, et al., 1985), and is now very rarely used in children in the United Kingdom after two recent deaths. At about 9 AM a baseline sample is taken, the fasting patient is injected with insulin, and serum samples are taken at 30, 60, 90 and 120 minutes for glucose, cortisol, and usually growth hormone measurements. Interpretation of the results is complex and involves a consideration of a range of clinical symptoms as well as cortisol concentrations, which peak to greater than 550 nmol/L at 60 to 90 minutes in healthy persons.

Congenital Enzymatic Defects

The most common defect of adrenal steroid biosynthesis is deficiency of 21-hydroxylase (White, et al., 1987) (see Fig. 7–2). In the classic form virilization is apparent in newborn girls and in boys during childhood. With the late-onset form hirsutism develops in early adulthood. A cryptic form with mild 21-hydroxylase deficiency also exists in which there are no symptoms of the disease.

In affected babies basal serum 17-hydroxyprogesterone is high (60 to 300 nmol/L; 2000 to 10,000 ng/dL) and is used as the basis for perinatal screening, whereas in late-onset and cryptic forms it is normal or slightly high (3 to 6 nmol/L; 100 to 200 ng/dL) (preferably measured in the follicular phase of the menstrual cycle). However, 1 hour after 2 μg of cosyntropin is administered there is a three- to sixfold stimulation of 17-hydroxyprogesterone, as compared with a twofold increase in normal subjects. New and Speiser (1986) summarized these data in a nomogram. Fetal diagnosis of 21-hydroxylase deficiency is by determination of 17-hydroxyprogesterone in midgestational, amniotic fluid.

Other congenital enzymatic defects are all rare. Both 17-hydroxylase and 11-hydroxylase deficiency are associated with hypertension because their immediate precursors affected are potent mineralocorticoids. Another unusual defect is 3β-hydroxysteroid dehydrogenase deficiency which sometimes presents as hirsutism in adults. Diagnosis is by measurement of specific steroids distal to the enzymatic block, sometimes combined with a cosyntropin stimulation test.

Hyperaldosteronism and Hypoaldosteronism

Detailed consideration of the diagnosis of the many disorders resulting in hyperaldosteronism (often with associated hypokalemia and hypertension) or hypoaldosteronism (with associated hyperkalemia, etc.) is beyond the scope of this chapter. Less than 2% of all hypertensives have autonomous overproduction of aldosterone.

Hypertension resulting from a definable pathogenesis is rare and screening by aldosterone and/or PRA determinations is not justified, unless indicated by hypokalemia or hyperkalemia and a detailed physical assessment of the patient. Primary aldosteronism is typified by hypokalemia, alkalosis, hypertension, low or suppressed PRA, and high plasma aldosterone, and results mainly from one of three disorders: aldosterone producing adenoma (APA), idiopathic hyperaldosteronism, or glucocorticoid suppressible hyperaldosteronism. Secondary aldosteronism is also associated with hypokalemia, alkalosis, and raised PRA and aldosterone, but there may or may not be associated hypertension. Either may be found in chronic renal disease and other chronic conditions, but if hypertension is present the cause may be a renin secreting tumor. Correspondingly, aldosterone deficiency may also be primary, caused by adrenocortical dysfunction, or secondary, when the cause is related to inadequate stimulation of adrenal aldosterone secretion (i.e., inadequate renin secretion which may occur in long-standing diabetes mellitus).

In all of the above conditions an initial diagnosis is aided by measurements of plasma aldosterone and PRA. Recently it has been claimed that all disorders of the renin-angiotensin-aldosterone axis can be diagnosed by measuring aldosterone (pmol/L) and PRA (ng/mL/hour) in random plasma samples (McKenna, et al., 1991). An elevated or normal aldosterone level with a raised aldosterone/PRA ratio (>920) was found to be diagnostic of primary aldosteronism and an elevated aldosterone level (>2000 pmol/L) with a normal ratio indicated secondary aldosteronism. Primary and secondary deficiencies are associated with low aldosterone levels and low or normal aldosterone/PRA ratios, respectively.

For the differential diagnosis of primary aldosteronism, an appropriate test is saline loading (Aretega, et al., 1985), by which 1 to 2 L of saline is infused over 1 to 4 hours with plasma aldosterone, 18-hydroxydeoxycorticosterone, and cortisol measured before and during infusion (Biglieri, 1991). Patients with an aldosterone producing adenoma have aldosterone levels which are not suppressed to less than 280 pmol/L (10 ng/dL), while patients with idiopathic hyperaldosteronism have suppressed levels of 140 to 280 pmol/L (5 to 10 ng/dL) as opposed to normal subjects (< pmol/L). If the ratios of aldosterone to cortisol and 18-hydroxydeoxycorticosterone to cortisol are both greater than 3 this indicates an aldosterone producing adenoma with a high degree of certainty (Biglieri, 1991). If after saline loading, excessive aldosterone secretion is demonstrated, then the next step is to differentiate an aldosterone producing adenoma (effectively treatable by adrenalectomy) from idiopathic hyperaldosteronism (treated medically) (Young, et al., 1990). Bilateral sampling of the adrenal venous outflow before and after ACTH administration with corticosteroid determination is claimed to be a definitive diagnostic procedure. In an aldosterone producing adenoma the aldosterone/cortical serum ratio is elevated on the side containing the adrenal tumor, while it is markedly suppressed on the contralateral side (Noth, et al., 1985). However, bilateral adrenal nodular hyperplasia can resemble an aldosterone producing adenoma because one of the adrenal glands can be producing most of the aldosterone.

REFERENCES

Aretega E, Klein R, Biglieri E. Use of the saline infusion test to diagnose the cause of primary aldosteronism. Am J Med 1985;79:721–727.

Azziz R, Bradley E, Huth J. Acute adrenocorticotropin (1-24-ACTH) adrenal stimulation in eumenorrheic women: reproducibility and effect of ACTH dose, subject weight, and sampling time. J Clin Endocrinol Metab 1990;70:1273–1279.

Biemond P, de Jong FH, Lomberts SW. Continuous dexamethasone infusion for seven hours in patients with Cushing's syndrome. Ann Int Med 1990;112:738–742.

Biglieri E. Spectrum of mineralocorticoid hypertension. Hypertension 1991;17:251–261.

Burch W. Urinary free cortisol determination. JAMA 1982;247:2002–2004.

Cunningham S, Moore A, McKenna J. Normal cortisol response to corticotropin in patients with secondary adrenal failure. Arch Intern Med 1983;143:2276–2279.

Findling J. Eutopic or ectopic adrenocorticotrophic hormone-dependent Cushing's syndrome, a diagnostic dilemma (editorial). Mayo Clin Proc 1990;65:1377–1380.

Findling JW, Kehoe ME, Shaker JL, Raff H. Routine inferior petrosal sinus sampling in the differential diagnosis of adrenocorticotropin (ACTH)-dependent Cushing's syndrome: early recognition of the occult ectopic ACTH syndrome. J Clin Endocrinol Metab 1991;73:408–413.

Gibson S, Pollock A, Littley M, Shalet S, White A. Advantages of IRMA over RIA in the measurement of ACTH. Ann Clin Biochem 1989;26:500–507.

Gomez-Sanchez C, Upcavage R, Zager P. Urinary 18-hydroxycortisol and its relationship to the excretion of other adrenal steroids. J Clin Endocrinol Metab 1987;65:310–314.

Gosling JP, Middle J. Siekmann L, Read G. Standardization of immunoprocedures: total cortisol. Scand J Clin Invest 1993;53(suppl 216):3–41.

Hashimoto T, Matsubara F, Takeda R. Reservations regarding assessment of data obtained with commercially available cortisol radioimmunoassay kits. Clin Chem 1989;35: 2153–2154.

Hegstadt R, Brown R, Jiang N. Aging and Aldosterone. Am J Med 1983;74:442–448.

Huang CM, Zweig M. Evaluation of a radioimmunoassay for urinary cortisol without extraction. Clin Chem 1989;35:125–126.

Kamilaris T, DeBold C, Pavlou S. Effect of altered thyroid hormone levels on hypothalamic pituitary adrenal function. J Clin Endocrinol Metab 1987;65:994–999.

Kaye T, Crapo L. The Cushing syndrome: an update on diagnostic tests. Ann Intern Med 1990;112:434–444.

Kuhn J, Proeschel M, Seurin D. Comparative assessment of ACTH and lipotropin plasma levels in the diagnosis and follow-up of patients with Cushing's syndrome: a study of 210 cases. Am J Med 1989;86:678–684.

Laudat M, Cerdas S, Fournier C. Salivary cortisol measurement: a practical approach to assess pituitary adrenal function. J Clin Endocrinol Metab 1988;66:343–348.

Leinung M, Young W, Whitaker M. Diagnosis of corticotropin-producing bronchial carcinoid tumors causing Cushing's syndrome. Mayo Clin Proc 1990;65:1314–1321.

Linuma K, Ikeda I, Ogihara T, Hashizume K, Kurata K, Kumahara Y. Radioimmunoassay of metanephrine and normetanephrine for the diagnosis of pheochromocytoma. Clin Chem 1986;32:1879–1883.

Luger A, Deuster P, Kyle S. Acute hypothalamic pituitary adrenal responses to the stress of treadmill exercise. New Eng J Med 1987;316:1309–1320.

Malchoff C, Rosa J. DeBold C. Adrenocorticotropin-independent bilateral macronodular adrenal hyperplasia. J Clin Endocrinol Metab 1989;68:855–860.

Matinlauri I, Eskola JU, Aalto M, Koskinen P, Irjala K. Time-resolved immunofluorometric assay of total renin in human plasma and follicular fluid. Clin Chem 1994;40:74–79.

May M, Carey R. Rapid adrenocorticotropic hormone test in practice. Am J Med 1985;79:679–684.

McKenna TJ, Sequeira SJ, Heffernan A, Chambers J, Cunningham S. Diagnosis under random conditions of all disorders of the renin-angiotensin-aldosterone axis, including primary hyperaldosteronism. J Clin Endocrinol Metab 1991;73:952–957.

Miller J, Crapo L. The biochemical diagnosis of hypercortisolism. The Endocrinologist 1994;4:7–15.

Moore A, Aitken R, Burke C, Gaskell S, Groom G, Holder G, Selby C, Wood P. Cortisol assays: guidelines for the provision of a clinical biochemistry service. Ann Clin Biochem 1985;22:435–454.

New M, Speiser P. Genetics of adrenal steroid 21-hydroxylase deficiency. Endocr Rev 1986;7:331–349.

Noth R, Glaser S, Palmaz J. Cosyntropin stimulation in adrenal vein testing for aldosteronoma. West J Med 1985;142:92–95.

O'Connor D, Bernstein K. Radioimmunoassay of chromogranin A in plasma as a measure of exocytotic sympathoadrenal activity in normal subjects and patients with pheochromocytoma. New Eng J Med 1984;311:764–770.

Oishi S, Sasaki M, Ohno M, Sata T. Urinary normetanephrine and metanephrine measures by radioimmunoassay for the diagnosis of pheochromocytoma: utility of 24-hour and random 1-hour determinations. J Clin Endocrinol Metab 1988;67:614–618.

Oldfield EH, Doppman JL, Nieman LK, et al. Petrosal sinus sampling with and without corticotropin-releasing hormone for the differential diagnosis of Cushing's syndrome. N Engl J Med 1991;325:897–905.

Orbach O, Schussler G. Increased serum cortisol binding in chronic active hepatitis. Am J Med 1989;86:39–42.

Orth DN. Differential diagnosis of Cushing's syndrome (editorial). New Engl J Med 1991;325:957–959.

Pescovitz OH, Cutler GB Jr, Loriaux DL. Synthesis and secretion of corticosteroids. In: Becker KL, ed. Principles and Practice of Endocrinology and Metabolism. Philadelphia, JB Lippincott, 1990;579–591.

Pugeat M, Bonneton A, Perrot D. Decreased immunoreactivity and binding activity of corticosteroid-binding globulin in serum in septic shock. Clin Chem 1989;35:1675–1679.

Raff H, Findling J. A new immunoradiometric assay for corticotrophin evaluated in normal subjects and patients with Cushing's syndrome. Clin Chem 1989;35:956–960.

Robin P, Predine J. Milgrom E. Assay of unbound cortisol in plasma. J Clin Endocrinol Metab 1978;46:277–283.

Rosano TG, Swift TA, Hayes LW. Advances in catecholamine and metabolite measurements for the diagnosis of pheochromocytoma. Clin Chem 1991;37:1854–1867.

Rubin RT. The hypothalamic-pituitary-adrenal-cortical axis in mental disorders. J Clin Endocrinol Metab 1991;72:253–259.

Rückert Y, Rohode W, Furkert J. Radioimmunoassay of corticotropin-releasing hormone. Exp Clin Endocrinol 1990;96:129–137.

Schumacher M, Nanninga A, Delfs T, Mukhopadhyay AK, Leidenberger FA. A direct immunoradiometric assay for human plasma prorenin: concentrations in cycling women and in women taking oral contraceptives. J Clin Endocrinol Metab 1992;75:617–623.

Sealey JE. Plasma renin activity and plasma prorenin assays. Clin Chem 1991;37:1811–1819.

Sharp AM, Walters CA, Wong SD, Caterson ID. IRMA and RIA compared for assessing dexamethasone suppression of corticotropin in plasma (Technical brief). Clin Chem 1992;38:149.

Sherman B, Wysham C, Pfohl B. Age related changes in the circadian rhythm of plasma cortisol. J Clin Endocrinol Metab 1985;61:439–442.

Stabler TV, Siegel AL. Chemiluminescence immunoassay of aldosterone in serum. Clin Chem 1991;37:1987–1989.

Stein PP, Black HR. A simplified diagnostic approach to pheochromocytoma. Medicine 1990;70:46–66.

Streeten D, Anderson G, Dalakos TG. Normal and abnormal function of the hypothalamic-pituitary-adrenocortical system in man. Endocr Rev 1984;5:371–394.

Tabarin A, Greselle JF, San-Galli F, et al. Usefulness of the corticotropin-releasing hormone test during the bilateral inferior petrosal sinus sampling for the diagnosis of Cushing's disease. J Clin Endocrinal Metab 1991;73:53–59.

Thienpont L. Siekman L, Lawson A, Colinet E, De Leenheer A. Development, validation and certification by isotope dilution gas chromatography-mass spectrometry of lyophilized human serum reference materials for cortisol (CRM 192 and 193) and progesterone (CRM 347 and 348). Clin Chem 1991;37:540–546.

Tomori N, Suda T, Nakagami Y. Adrenergic modulation of ACTH responses to insulin induced hypoglycemia and corticotropin releasing hormone. J Clin Endocrinol Metab 1989;68:87–92.

Tsigos C, Crosby SR, Gibson S, Young RJ, White A. Proopiomelanocortin is the predominant adrenocorticotropin-related peptide in human cerobrospinal fluid. J Clin Endocrinol Metab 1993;76:620–624.

Tunn S, Pappert G, Willnow P, Kreig M. Multicentre evaluation of an enzyme-immunoassay for cortisol determination. J Clin Chem Clin Biochem 1990; 28:929–935.

Turnell DC, Cooper JDH, Green B, Hughes G, Wright DJ. Totally automated liquid-chromatographic assay for cortisol and associated glucocorticoids in serum, with use of ASTED ™ sample preparation. Clin Chem 1988;34:1816–1820.

Veldhuis JD, Iranmanesh A, Johnson ML, Lizarralde G. Amplitude, but not frequency, modulation of adrenocorticotropin secretory bursts give rise to the nyctohemeral rhythm of the corticotropic axis in man. J Clin Endocrinol Metab 1990;71:452–463.

Watabe T, Tanaka K, Kumagae M. Role of endogenous arginine vasopressin in potentiating corticotropin releasing hormone stimulated corticotropin secretion in man. J Clin Endocrinol Metab 1988;66:1132–1137.

Wheeler MJ, ed. Steroid and Thyroid Hormones, vol 2, part 2. In: Seth J, ed. The Immunoassay Kit Directory, Series A: Clinical Chemistry. Norwell MA: Kluwer Academic Publishers, 1993.

White P, New M, Dupont B. Congenital adrenal hyperplasia. New Engl J Med 1987;316:1519–1586.

Wilson DM, Leutscher JA. Plasma prorenin activity and complications in children with insulin-dependent diabetes mellitus. N Engl J Med 1990;323:1101–1106.

Young W, Hogan M, Klee G. Primary aldosteronism. Mayo Clin Proc 1990;65:96–110.

CHAPTER 8

Pituitary-Thyroid Function

Lawrence V. Basso and
James P. Gosling

Thyroid secretions are vital to growth and development in children and in the adult and have major effects on virtually every organ system. After diabetes mellitus, abnormalities of thyroid function constitute the most common disorders seen by endocrinologists. The prevalence of hypothyroidism is high, especially in women. Below 60 years of age it is close to 1% of the total adult female population but later it can be 6% or greater (Spaulding, 1987). One study found elevated levels of thyroid-stimulating hormone (TSH, thyrotropin) (indicating primary hypothyroidism) in 13.2% of an otherwise healthy elderly population (Rosenthal, et al., 1987). The prevalence of hyperthyroidism is about 0.3% to 3% of the population (Robuschi, et al., 1987). The symptoms and signs of thyroid disease are frequently subtle or misleading, which makes the competent use of thyroid function tests exceedingly important.

BIOCHEMISTRY OF THYROID RELATED HORMONES

The synthesis of the thyroid hormones triiodothyronine (T_3) and thyroxine (T_4) is unusual. Under the influence of a peroxidase, iodine, actively concentrated in the thyroid gland, inserts into tyrosine residues of immature thyroglobulin, a 660,000 mol wt glycoprotein with 110 tyrosines. Mono- and diiodotyrosines become coupled by a peroxidase-dependent reaction leaving dehydroalanines at the donor residues. This gives 4 to 8 T_4 or T_3 per mature thyroglobulin, which is packaged in vesicles and extruded into the colloid space of the thyroid follicle. After reuptake, thyroglobulin is digested by proteases and peptidases giving many mono- and diiodinated tyrosines, which are recovered and the iodine recycled, and T_4 and T_3, which are secreted by means of phagocyte-assisted reverse endocytosis into capillaries at the base of the thyroid cell. Some thyroglobulin is also secreted.

Figure 8–1 indicates how T_4 is converted to T_3 and to physiologically inactive reverse T_3 (rT_3), both of which occur in virtually all peripheral tissues, and Table 8–1

133

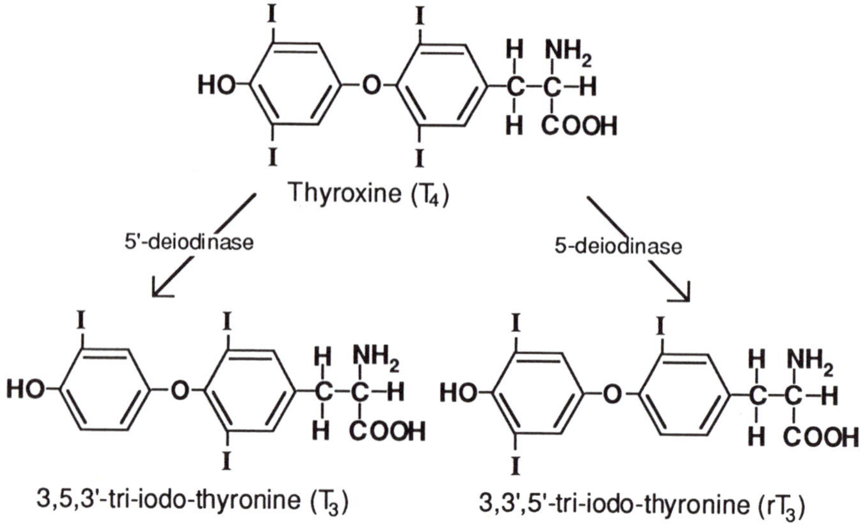

Figure 8–1.   The conversion in peripheral tissues of T_4 to physiologically active T_3 and inactive rT_3.

gives their normal concentrations, etc. The relatively high serum concentration of T_4 is mainly because T_3 has a much shorter half-life, and the greater distribution of T_3 is due to the much higher concentration of its free form in serum (0.3% versus 0.03% for T_4). The thyroid secretes about 5 µg of T_3 per day and the additional 30 µg comes from peripheral T_4 conversion.

T$_4$ binds to several proteins in the blood (Bartalena, 1990) and the free form (0.03%) is traditionally held to be the physiologically important form of the hormone, with the binding proteins serving three functions: (1) maintenance of a large pool with a constant free hormone concentration, (2) ensuring an even distribution of hormone among peripheral cells, and (3) minimizing hormone loss by renal filtration. However, the "free hormone hypotheses," as it is called, is now being questioned (Ekins, 1992), but its practical relevance with respect to T_4 is still strongly supported (Midgely, 1993).

Table 8–1   Serum Concentrations, Half-Lives, Production, and Clearance Rates for Thyroid Hormones in the Normal 70-kg Adult

Hormone	Serum Concentration nmol/L (ng/dL)	Serum Free Concentration pmol/L (ng/dL)	Half-life in Blood (days)	Production Rate (µg/day)	Metabolic Clearance Rate (L/day)
T$_4$	58–161 (4500–12,500)	10.3–29.7 (0.8–2.3)	7–10	90–100	1.18
T$_3$	1.23–3.39 (80–220)	2.00–8.47 (0.13–0.55)	1–1.5	30–35	23.6
rT$_3$	0.123–0.539 (8–35)	All free	0.25	25–35	110

Thyroxine is bound by thyroxine-binding globulin (TBG) (75%), thyroid binding prealbumin (TBPA, 15%), and albumin (10%). Any change in TBG concentration leads to an altered total T_4 concentration. For instance, if TBG is low, total T_4 is low but the concentration of free T_4 (FT_4) may be normal. A much greater percentage of T_3 is free because the affinity of both TBG and TBPA is much less than for T_4.

Mechanisms of Action of Thyroid Hormones and TSH

T_4 has low activity and is effectively a prohormone with selective deiodination giving rise to inactive rT_3 or highly active T_3, the genomic effects of which are mediated by a 55,000 mol wt nuclear receptor. T_3 enters the nucleus directly and binds to the receptor which in turn binds to specific DNA sequences, termed thyroid responsive elements. These are located beside a range of thyroid responsive genes and modulate DNA-dependent RNA synthesis. These genes code for the synthesis of a diverse set of proteins including enzymes necessary for metabolism of protein, fat and carbohydrate, β-adrenergic receptors and insulin-like growth factor-I (IGF-1). In this way T_3 can induce specific effects and increased general metabolism and growth.

TSH is a 28,000 mol wt glycoprotein composed of two subunits (α and β). The α-subunit is the same in LH, FSH, and MCG, while the β-subunit is specific for TSH. TSH acts by binding to specific receptors on the surface of thyroid cells and stimulates cAMP synthesis, which activates protein kinases which, in turn, promotes maintenance of the thyroid gland and stimulates the synthesis and release of thyroid hormones.

Hypothalamic-Pituitary-Thyroid Axis

A large number of controlling factors are known to participate in the regulation of thyroid hormone secretion (Fig. 8–2), with feedback inhibition of TSH release by circulating T_4 and T_3 concentrations being one of the most important. This inhibition is exponential so that when the FT_4 concentration falls by half, the TSH concentration increases about 100-fold and, conversely, if free T_4 doubles, TSH concentration falls dramatically. However, such control responses occur with rapid and slow phases and, in a normal patient on a suppressive dose of L-thyroxine, it takes about 4 to 8 weeks before the hypothalamic-pituitary axis is normalized after this is stopped.

THYROID FUNCTION TESTS

Tests Involving Iodothyronines

Total T_3, rT_3 and T_4

The standard method for quantifying total levels of the thyroid hormones is radioimmunoassay (RIA). RIA is especially appropriate for these analytes because radiolabeling is simply a matter of substituting with [125]I. However, other competitive

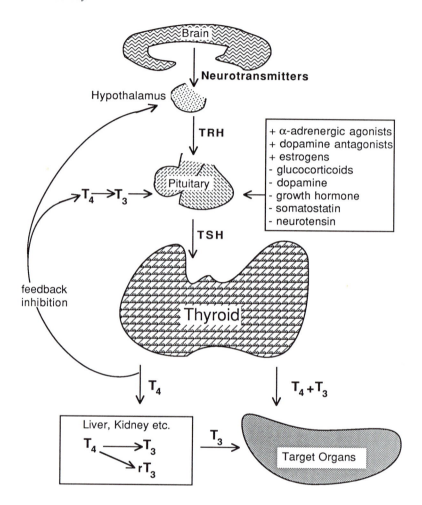

Figure 8–2.   The brain-hypothalamic-pituitary-thyroid axis. Thyrotropin releasing hormone ([TRH], tripeptide pyroglutamyl-histidyl-prolinamide) is synthesized in the paraventricular nucleus of the hypothalamus, travels down nerve endings to the median eminence and reaches the thyrothropes of the anterior pituitary by means of the portal capillary plexus. On binding to specific cell-surface receptors, TRH stimulates tonically the thyrotrophs to synthesize and secrete TSH by means of a Ca^{2+} dependent process. In addition, TRH increases glycosylation of TSH molecules rendering them more biologically active (Magner, 1990).

Many factors modulate TSH release (see box) and, even if not all are physiologically important, their effects can be highly significant if pharmacological amounts are administered.

immunoassays with enzyme, luminescent, and fluorescent labels are commercially available.

Total T_4 in newborn children can be up to 190 nmol/L (15 μg/dL); from 3 months to 13 years it is about 130 nmol/L (10 μg/dL), with a range of 90 to 180 nmol/L (7 to 14 μg/dL); and from 25 to 90 years it is about 96 nmol/L (7.5 μg/dL), with a range of 58 to 161 nmol/L (Table 8–1). This is in contrast to the total T_3 blood level which decreases with advancing age so that while for a 20-year-old person 3.2 nmol/L (210 ng/dL) is normal, this level may also be found in an 80-year-old person with hyperthyroidism. In 95% of cases of hyperthyroidism both the T_4 and T_3 are elevated. However, in early hyperthyroidism (especially Graves' disease), or patients with autonomous nodules or iodine deficiency (Laurberg, 1984), T_3 alone may be elevated (T_3 toxicosis). Measurement of rT_3 seems to have no practical value in the evaluation of thyroid disease.

T_3 Uptake Test and Free Thyroid Index

The resin T_3 uptake (T_3U) test does not measure T_3 and, although by convention T_3 is the tracer, it is the binding of T_4 that is of interest. In effect a tracer amount of ^{125}I-T_3 is used to measure the relative distribution of the T_3 tracer between binding proteins in the patient's serum and a nonspecific resin. Increasing numbers of unoccupied binding sites in the sample give decreasing resin uptake and vice versa. It is generally reported as a percent (normal range 22% to 34%) but some laboratories report it as a ratio such as patient T_3U:control T_3U. T_3U is inversely proportional to TBG concentration (normal adult range is 12 to 30 mg/L).

However, the T_3U should never be used as the sole measure of thyroid function and must be combined with a total T_4 measurement to give the FT_4 index ($FT_4I=$ total $T_4 \times \%T_3U$). The normal FT_4I range is 1.0 to 4.3 units and this is an indirect estimate of FT_4 levels.

Free Thyroxine

Free thyroxine (FT_4) has a normal range in blood of 10 to 30 pmol/L (0.8 to 2.3 ng/dL), and it is measured by a range of methods (Ekins, 1990).

1. *Equilibrium dialysis RIA* (Nelson and Tomel, 1988). Generally, sample is diluted and mixed with a small amount of ^{125}I-T_4 in a dialysis cell. The protein bound T_4 (T_4 and ^{125}I-T_4) remains in the original compartment whereas the FT_4 diffuses across a semipermeable membrane. At equilibrium (generally 24 hours) a sample of the solution containing FT_4 is taken for analysis and the ^{125}I count allows calculation of the fraction of T_4 which was free to cross the membrane. The total T_4 is determined separately by RIA, and the FT_4 calculated. Equilibrium dialysis methods, though considered to be reliable, are expensive and are primarily used for research and method validation.
2. *Two-step, free-hormone immunoassays.* A very small amount of anti-T_4 antibody is immobilized on the well of a test tube. Patient serum is added and allowed to interact for a short period of time (30 minutes) and then removed (first step) and the test tube is washed before addition of radiolabeled tracer (^{125}I-T_4) and the test continued as for a competitive immunoassay (second step). Therefore, the serum is left in contact with the immobilized antibody to allow a portion of the FT_4 to bind but not so long that the equilibrium is shifted, releasing

further T_4 from the TBG, etc. In general, two-step FT_4 immunoassays agree well with equilibrium dialysis (Nuutila, et al., 1990).

3. *One-step free-hormone immunoassays.* These assays utilize a labeled analog of T_4, which, together with anti-T_4 antibody is added to the patient's serum as in a single-step, competitive immunoassay. Their ability to measure FT_4 and not total T_4 is based on the assumption that the T_4 analog tracers used bind only to the anti-T_4 antibody reagent and not to serum T_4 binding proteins. However, most analog tracers used have been demonstrated to show some binding to other serum proteins such as albumin and there have been many reports of anomalous results in severe nonthyroidal illness when albumin is very low, in analbuminemia, and when autoantibodies against T_4 are present (Ekins, 1990). For example, in patients with nonthyroidal systemic illness and in pregnant women, free T_4 levels determined by analog methods are significantly low as compared with two-step methods and equilibrium dialysis (Csako, et al., 1990). This controversy has led to increased emphasis being placed on thorough assay validation, and newer non-isotopic one-step procedures, some with labeled antibody, appear to be more resistant to anomalous conditions.

In a practical sense, two-step assays are better for hospitalized patients, but a good analog FT_4 assay or an FT_4I should be adequate for nonpregnant, ambulatory attendees of outpatient clinics.

Table 8–2 summarizes the levels of thyroid hormones found in three congenital states with increased blood thyroid binding proteins. Note that these patients are euthyroid and FT_4 is normal despite anomalous total T_4, T_3 and even FT_4I. Therefore, these conditions are not detected if FT_4 is used as the sole determinant of thyroid function. In contrast, patients with abnormally low TBG, while also euthyroid, exhibit hypothyroxinemia.

Thyroid-Stimulating Hormone

TSH measurement has become the most important of the thyroid function tests (Klee and Hay, 1987). RIAs for thyroid-stimulating hormone have detection limits of about

Table 8–2   Thyroid Hormone Levels in Some Congenital Conditions with Increased Blood Binding Proteins

Congenital Condition	Mode of Inheritance	T_4	T_3	T_3U	FT_4I	FT_4
Increased TBG	X-linked	High	High	Low	Normal/high	Normal
Increased albumin	Autosomal dominant	High	Normal	Normal	Normal/high	Normal
Increased TBPA	Not known	Normal	Normal	Normal	Normal/high	Normal

0.4 mIU/L and previously TSH levels were used only in the evaluation of hypothyroidism. Currently, TSH immunoradiometric assays (IRMAs) routinely have detection limits of at least 0.1 mIU/L and so-called third-generation immunometric assays, many with nonisotopic labels, can detect 0.005 to 0.01 mIU/L (McConway, et al., 1989; Spencer, et al., 1990), enabling their use to diagnose hyperthyroidism as well as hypothyroidism. The newer assays are faster and can be run in as little as 2 hours, in contrast to conventional RIA (48 hours). No laboratories participating in the United Kingdom external quality assessment scheme for TSH now use RIA.

Interference by sample constituents in immunoassays has always existed but recently it has become more widely recognized and understood. With respect to TSH immunoassays, heterophilic antibodies in general and (human) antimouse antibodies (HAMA), induced, for example, after immunoscintigraphy with mouse monoclonal antibodies, are of greatest relevance. In some immunometric assays for TSH both (monoclonal) antibodies are derived from mice, and therefore HAMA in a sample can link labeled and immobilized antibodies and result in a false TSH determination that is abnormally high. Theoretically this can be offset by adding mouse IgG to the assay to saturate any HAMA present but, to be effective, this IgG may have to come from the same strain of mice which produced the reagent antibodies, and it may not be feasible to add sufficient mouse IgG to be always effective (Kricka, et al. 1990). This phenomenon and the necessity to guard against it, will become much more important with the increasing use of diagnostic or therapeutic products that include mouse, as opposed to human or humanized antibodies.

The normal TSH range is 0.25 to 6.70 mIU/L and Figure 8–3 shows data obtained by means of two newer TSH assays and samples from euthyroid, hypothyroid, and hyperthyroid patients as well as patients with the sick euthyroid syndrome (Parnham and Tarbit, 1987). All hyperthyroid patients and some sick euthyroid patients had levels of TSH below 0.1 mIU/L, and all hypothyroid patients had levels of TSH above 6 mIU/L. Therefore, the new TSH assays allow reliable diagnosis of thyroid status with a single test in most clinical circumstances. There is little question that TSH concentration is the most sensitive indicator of thyroid hypofunction, and TSH analysis of dried blood spots taken from newborn infants is used to screen routinely for neonatal hypothyroidism.

For the thyrotropin releasing hormone (TRH) stimulation test a bolus intravenous administration of about 200 μg of TRH is preceded and followed by blood sampling for TSH assay. One sample at +20 or 30 minutes or a series of samples at 30-60-minute intervals for 2 to 3 hours may be taken. In euthyroid subjects the maximal increase in TSH is 2 to 35 mIU/L. This test is used in the functional evaluation of the hypothalamic-pituitary-thyroid axis and, occasionally, in the assessment of mild hyperthyroidism.

The new TSH assays also enable the evaluation of L-thyroxine replacement therapy in hypothyroid patients. For the treatment of primary hypothyroidism, a correct replacement dose results in TSH in the normal range (0.25 to 6.7 mIU/L) (Ross, 1988). However, in patients with thyroid cancer it may be important to give doses of L-thyroxine that severely suppress TSH (< 0.1 mIU/L).

A further range of pathological conditions are characterized by inappropriate TSH secretion (Table 8–3).

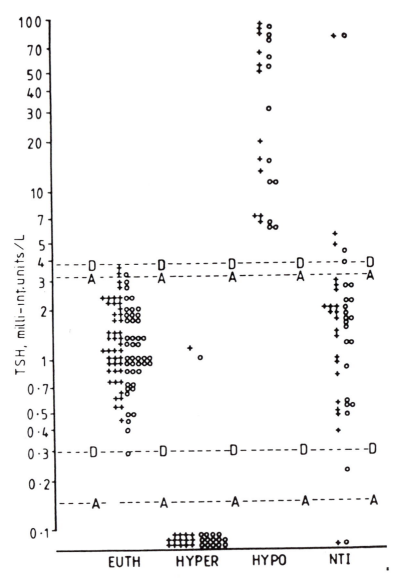

Figure 8–3.   Two modern nonisotopic immunometric assays were used to determine TSH levels in serum samples from persons defined clinically as euthyroid, hyperthyroid, hypothyroid, or with nonthyroidal illness by the Delfia (O) (LKB Wallac, Turku, Finland, detection limit 0.02 mIU/L) and Amerlite (+) (Amersham International, Amersham, Bucks, England, detection limit 0.04 mIU/L) methods. Delfia supplier quoted reference interval, D—D; Amerlite supplier quoted reference interval A—A. (Parnham AJ, Tarbit IF. 'Delfia' and 'Amerlite': Two sensitive nonisotopic immunoassay systems for assay of thyrotropin compared. Clin Chem 1987;33:1421–1424. Reproduced with permission.)

Table 8–3   Some Pathologic Conditions Characterized by Inappropriate
TSH Levels

	Pathologic condition		
Symptom	*Generalized Thyroid Hormone Resistance[†]*	*Partial Thyroid Hormone Resistance**	*Pituitary TSH-Secreting Tumor[‡]*
Metabolic status	Euthyroid	Hyperthyroid	Hyperthyroid
Goiter	Present	Present	Present
T_4 and FT_4 level	Increased	Increased	Increased
TSH level	Normal/increased	Increased	Increased/normal
TSH response to TRH	Increase[§]	Increase	Minimal increase
α Subunit:TSH ratio	<1	<1	>1
TSH suppression by T_3	Yes	Yes	Minimal suppression

[†]In generalized thyroid hormone resistance the exact defect is unknown but there appears to be diminished binding of T_3 to a mutant thyroid receptor (Menezes-Ferreira MM, et al. J Clin Endocrinol Metab 1984;59:1081–1087).

*Partial thyroid hormone resistance is limited to the pituitary gland and is caused by defective T_4 to T_3 conversion or by a mutant receptor limited to the pituitary thyrotrophs.

[‡]Tumors of the pituitary thyrotrophs may hypersecrete TSH with associated clinical hyperthyroidism (Gesundheit N, et al. Ann Intern Med;1987;111:827–835). α Subunit is often hypersecreted and there is usually no response to TRH.

[§]Sarne D, et al. J Clin Endocrinol Metab 1990;70:1305–1310.

Thyroglobulin

Thyroglobulin has become an important tumor marker for papillary-follicular thyroid cancer but, since it can be suppressed by exogenous thyroid hormone, it is accurately measured in patients with diagnosed or suspected thyroid cancer only when all exogenous thyroid suppressive therapy is stopped and the serum TSH level has returned to greater than 0.25 mIU/L. This is conveniently done just prior to a ^{131}I total body scan when the patient has been off suppressive treatment for 5 to 6 weeks. A wide range of RIA and two-site immunometric assays for thyroglobulin measurement are commercially available. Normally thyroglobulin should be less than 60 µg/L and in athyroidal patients it should be less than 2 µg/L. Another common problem is the simultaneous presence of anti-thyroglobulin autoantibodies and samples should be screened for these.

Autoantibodies

Autoimmune thyroid diseases represent a very wide spectrum of abnormalities from Graves' thyrotoxicosis to the impaired thyroid function of Hashimoto's thyroiditis. However, low level titers of autoantibodies against a wide range of proteins are found in many healthy people and these increase with age with respect to both incidence and level.

Antibodies directed against thyroid cellular elements including microsomal proteins (anti-M) (mainly thyroid peroxidase [TPO]) and thyroglobulin (anti-Tg) are characteristic of Hashimoto's thyroiditis. These patients may be euthyroid, hypothyroid (reduced T_4, T_3, and elevated TSH) or, more rarely, thyrotoxic (elevated T_4, T_3, and suppressed TSH). Measurement of anti-M antibodies is the more sensitive test for Hashimoto's thyroiditis and approximately 90% of patients have positive titers that are quite high, often exceeding 1:2000, whereas only about 50% of affected patients have positive titers of anti-Tg.

The most common method for determining these autoantibodies is hemagglutination with sensitized erythrocytes coated with thyroid microsomal membranes or thyroglobulin. The result is reported as a titer of the highest dilution of a patient's serum that causes agglutination. A very high titer (for example 1:10,000) is diagnostic of Hashimoto's thyroiditis.

Newer immunoassays with labeled antigen or labeled antibody are also available. In the labeled antigen assays, either purified thyroglobulin or microsomal membrane fractions labeled with ^{125}I (or an enzyme) are incubated with the patient's serum and, after incubation, the labeled antigen-antibody complexes are precipitated with a second antibody ($[^{125}I\text{-Ag}-\textbf{Ab}-\text{Ab}]_n$). In the labeled antibody procedure, antigen is immobilized on test tubes and incubated with the patient's serum in the initial step (sp-Ag-**Ab**). After a washing, a labeled antibody is added that is directed against immunoglobulins (sp-Ag-**Ab**-Ab-enz). The specificity of the test may be improved by using a labeled antibody specific for a certain class or subclass of immunoglobulin (e.g., anti-human IgG or IgM). In the future, all assays for anti-M antibodies may employ TPO as antigen, to make them more specific (Kaufman, et al., 1990). These autoantibodies are also found in most hyperthyroid patients with an autoimmune etiology, and the presence of anti-M antibody is helpful in diagnosing Graves' disease.

Measurement of the autoantibodies with TSH "activity" that are etiologic factors in Graves' disease (Grubeck-Loebenstein, et al., 1988) is not widespread. A radioreceptor assay can determine the inhibition of ^{125}I-TSH interaction with the receptor (human or porcine thyroid membranes) produced by the antibody present in the patient's serum thyroid receptor antibody (TRAb), where TRAb is expressed as percent inhibition (Davies, et al., 1983; McNamara, et al., 1993). Greater than 10% to 20% inhibition is considered positive. Alternatively, microbioassay for thyroid stimulating immunoglobulin (TSI) can be used to quantify the ability of patient serum to increase the amount of cAMP released by cells of a rat thyroid cell line (FRTL-5) (Morris, et al., 1988). Most laboratories would expect the TSI to be at least 130% above the control in order to be positive.

The practical diagnostic and prognostic value of determining TRAb and TSI has been questioned (Davies, 1988). However, if the patient with Graves' disease is pregnant her antibodies, after crossing the placenta, may cause neonatal hyperthyroidism. A high titer in the third trimester can indicate the possibility of hyperthyroism in the newborn at birth.

Autoantibodies against T_4 and T_3 are found chiefly in patients with autoimmune thyroid disease (Rhys, et al., 1990). Their main relevance is that they can interfere in assays for T_4 or T_3 but, if present, a tube containing no added antibody but only tracer and patient serum should show marked binding of tracer. A recent report described the finding in a patient of endogenous antibodies that bound fluorescein-T_4 conjugate. They resulted in apparently undetectable levels of T_4 when it was measured by an immunoassay with this conjugate (Ritter, et al., 1993).

Radionuclide Studies

The radioiodine uptake (RAI uptake) test is still useful in diagnosing different types of hyperthyroidism, rare organification defects, and iodine deficiency hypothyroidism. Five μCi of ^{131}I or 20 μCi of ^{123}I is given orally and the percent incorporated in the neck determined after 24 hours. Normal RAI uptake is 8% to 30% with the upper limit of 30% not being exceeded in 24 hours. However, the upper limit is geographically dependent, as it depends on dietary iodine, with lower RAI uptake associated with higher intakes of iodine.

High RAI uptake is associated with hyperthyroidism, for example, Graves' disease, toxic nodular goiter, rare TSH-secreting pituitary tumor, and some cases of autoimmune thyroiditis. Normal or low RAI uptake is associated with hyperthyroidism. Examples include subacute thyroiditis (very low when active), silent thyroiditis (very low when active), iodide induced hyperthyroidism (Jod-Basedow effect), Graves' disease with iodide excess, factitious hyperthyroidism, and rare, functioning thyroid cancers.

Inherited disorders of thyroid hormone metabolism have been thoroughly reviewed by Lever, et al. (1983). Deficiency of thyroid peroxidase, which oxidizes iodide and enables its incorporation into thyroglobulin, is characterized by a positive perchlorate discharge test. After loading the thyroid with [131]I (or ^{123}I), perchlorate (which inhibits the inorganic iodine trapping mechanism and releases free iodine) is given and the thyroid gland monitored for 2 hours. A 5% or greater (often 10% to 50%) fall in thyroid ^{123}I content suggests a defect in iodine organification.

THYROID FUNCTION IN HEALTH AND DISEASE

Pregnancy and the Fetus

TBG rises in the first trimester with resultant rises in total T_4 and T_3 (Price, et al., 1989), and albumin tends to fall during pregnancy. Therefore FT_4 and free T_3 (FT_3) are higher than normal as determined by equilibrium dialysis techniques, and FT_4 should be determined by two-step methods until simpler methods are accepted as valid. Human chorionic gonadotropin (hCG) may contribute to this relative hyperthyroid state and one study equated 27,000 to 128,000 IU of hCG to 1 mIU of TSH (Yoshikawa, et al., 1989). During pregnancy TSH levels drop from 1.48 to 0.8 mIU/L.

Every pregnant woman with a history of thyroid disease should have her serum FT_4 and basal TSH levels measured. If she is receiving therapy this should be adjusted to keep FT_4 and TSH within normal limits for pregnancy.

Fetal thyroid status can be monitored by the new technique of cordocentesis (ultrasound-guided blood sampling from the umbilical cord) (Utiger, 1991). T_4, TSH, and TRH appear in the fetus about 10 weeks of gestation and thereafter total T_4 increases gradually. Low T_4 levels produce a substantial, though limited, rise in TSH (Thorpe-Beeston, et al., 1991). T_4 to T_3 conversion is limited but there is a 10-fold increase in the T_3:T_4 ratio from 30 weeks of gestation to 1 month after birth.

Thyroid Function During Nonthyroidal Systemic Illness

Up to 50% of intensive care patients and many patients with systemic illness exhibit abnormalities of thyroid function without having thyroid disease. This is part of a vast readjustment of the entire neuroendocrine system in which blood levels of sex steroids, LH, FSH, and IGF-1 are all diminished, while cortisol, prolactin, and renin are increased. Such thyroid abnormalities make the diagnosis of thyroidal disease very difficult (Chopra, et al., 1983) and are often referred to as the sick euthyroid syndrome. Examples of thyroid hormone levels in these patients include

1. *High total T_4.* This has been described in acute systemic and psychiatric illness (Kleinhaus, et al., 1988). Generally the elevated total, and often free T_4, is transient and the diagnosis of hyperthyroidism should be pursued only if persistent. The elevated T_4 in these circumstances appears to be due to decreased metabolic clearance and/or decreased peripheral conversion of T_4 to T_3.
2. *Normal T_4, low T_3.* With systemic illness peripheral iodothyronine metabolism is altered giving increased rT_3, which may be useful because it leads to partial hypometabolism at times of great stress. Accordingly, in the patient with true hyperthyroidism and serious systemic illness, T_4 may be elevated but with normal or even low T_3. Other causes of the low T_3, high rT_3 combination include pregnancy, starvation (Burger, et al., 1987), chronic liver disease, antithyroid drugs, steroids, β blockers, and contrast agents. Thyroid hormone levels in acquired immune deficiency syndrome (AIDS) are unique with a progressive decline in rT_3, an elevation of TBG, but normal T_3, which may be the cause of the frequently observed weight loss (Lopresti, 1989).
3. *Low T_4 and low T_3.* With increasing severity of illness, especially in intensive care patients, T_4 falls and there is an inverse relationship between the severity of illness and T_4 concentration. The FT_4I is also low, but FT_4 is high when determined with equilibrium dialysis (Csako, et al., 1990), and therefore should be determined only with reliable methods (Midgley, 1990). The reason for the low T_4 is unknown but tumor necrosis factor may be implicated (Mooradian, et al., 1990).
4. *Abnormal TSH levels.* About 3% of hospitalized patients have TSH values less than 0.1 mIU/L (Wehmann, et al., 1985) and nearly 4% have values greater than 7 mIU/L; examples of TSH levels less than 0.01 mIU/L and greater than 20 mIU/L have been found. A high TSH is usually observed in the recovery phase

of systemic illness. Nonetheless, a TSH level greater than 20 mIU/L is almost certainly due to hypothyroidism. In addition, TSH in most sick euthyroid patients is greater than 0.005 mIU/L, whereas in almost all truly hyperthyroid patients it is less than 0.005 mIU/L. Furthermore, in the sick euthyroid syndrome TRH administration stimulates TSH 7 to 10 times (e.g., from 0.01 to 0.1 mU/mL), while in true hyperthyroidism the increase is much smaller or absent.

Strategies in the Evaluation of Thyroid Function

The analysis of thyroid function tests must take into account several factors for a proper interpretation. They include age and nutritional status; drugs the patient may

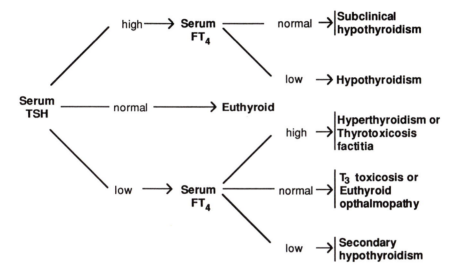

Figure 8–4.   Diagnostic scheme for patients exhibiting no obvious systemic illness and who may be described as ambulatory. Here the single best screening test is a TSH blood sample obtained with a modern assay (Surks, et al., 1990). If the TSH is normal, then the patient is euthyroid and no further testing is necessary. If the TSH is high (>7 mU/mL), then primary hypothyroidism is verified. A FT_4 test (either by a one- to two-step method) or a FT_4I may then be performed. If the FT_4 is low (<10 pmol/L, 0.8 ng/dL), overt primary hypothyroidism is diagnosed. If normal, subclinical hypothyroidism (Cooper, 1987) is suspected and although such patients may be asymptomatic, they need to be followed closely for the development of overt disease.

If TSH is low (<0.2 mIU/L), this is consistent with either hyperthyroidism or, more rarely, secondary hypothyroidism due to either hypothalamic or pituitary disease (Ross, et al., 1988,1989). An elevated FT_4 or T_3 verifies the diagnosis of hyperthyroidism. Occasionally TSH may be suppressed by an elevated T_3 alone. These patients are hyperthyroid but are secreting mainly T_3 from the thyroid (T_3 toxicosis). If the FT_4 is low, this raises the possibility of secondary hypothyroidism.

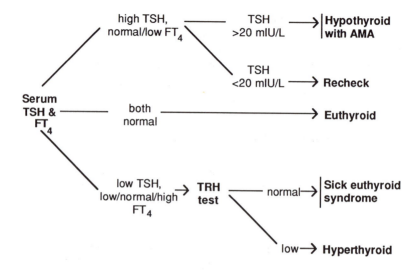

Figure 8–5.   Diagnostic scheme for patients with general systemic illness who are seen in intensive care wards, or in inpatient clinics. If concentrations of both TSH and FT$_4$ are normal, the patient can be considered to be normal and euthyroid. If the TSH is greater than 20 mIU/mL and the FT$_4$ is less than or equal to normal, this is certainly consistent with primary hypothyroidism. If the TSH is suppressed, the FT$_4$ is high and a TRH test assay shows no stimulation, hyperthyroidism is diagnosed. If the TSH is suppressed with a normal or slightly low FT$_4$ and a TRH test shows stimulation of TSH, this is consistent with the sick euthyroid syndrome or with hypothalamic disease. In other such patients who are recovering from systemic illness, TSH may be greater than 10 mIU/L and these patients need to be checked later when recovered from the primary illness. Antimicrosomal antibodies (anti–M antibodies, AMA) should be tested for.

be using; prior studies involving radiographic contrast agents; and the coexistence of systemic nonthyroidal illness.

The Ambulatory Outpatient.   Here the single best screening test for thyroid function is the determination of TSH concentration in serum or plasma, further classification of any abnormalities present is facilitated by a later determination of FT$_4$ (Fig. 8–4).

The Hospitalized Patient.   For the sick patient both TSH and FT$_4$ (by a two-step method) should be measured (Szabolcs, 1990) (Fig. 8–5). If possible do not check thyroid function in patients on drugs such as corticosteroids and dopamine, which are known to suppress TSH release (see also Table 8–4).

Hypothyroid Patient.   The most common cause of primary hypothyroidism is autoimmune thyroiditis associated with anti-M antibodies. If a normal or suppressed TSH level is associated with a low FT$_4$ or FT$_4$I, secondary hypothyroidism must be suspected. A suppressed response in a TRH test would point to a possible pituitary lesion, and a positive response in a hypothyroid patient to hypothalamic disease, so

Table 8–4   Some Drugs That Influence Thyroid Hormone and TSH Levels

Mechanism	Drugs	T_4	FT_4	T_3	TSH
Decreased TBG	Androgens, danazol, L-asparaginase	Low	Low/ normal	Low/ normal	Normal
Decreased TBG plus decreased T_4 to T_3 conversion	Glucocorticoids	Low	Low	Low	Low
Increased TBG	Estrogens, methadone, heroin, clofibrate, perphezine, 5-fluorouracil	High	Normal	High/ normal	Normal
Inhibited TGB binding	Salicylate	Normal	High	Normal	
	Furosemide	Normal	Normal	Normal	
Decreased TSH	Dopamine	Low	Low	Low	Low
Increased TSH (transient)	Metoclopramide	Normal	Normal	Normal	High
Decreased T_4 to T_3 conversion	Propanalol	High/ normal	High/ normal	Low	Normal
	Cholecystographic contrast dyes	High/ normal	High/ normal	Normal	
Decreased T_4 synthesis and T_4 to T_3 conversion	Propylthiouracil (acute)	Low	Low	Low	
Decreased thyroid hormone synthesis	Sulfonamide, 6-MP, phenylbutazone, aminoglutethimide	Low	Low	Low/ normal	High
Decreased thyroglobulin synthesis and breakdown	Excess iodide	Low	Low	Low/ normal	Normal
Decreased T_4 and T_3 release	Lithium carbonate	Low	Low	Low/ normal	High
Decreased T_4 catabolism and conversion to T_3	Amiodarone	High	High	Normal/ low	
	Phenytoin	Low	Low	Normal	Normal
Decreased iodide uptake	Nitroprusside	Low	Low	Low/ normal	High
Increased hepatic binding	Phenobarbital	Normal	Normal	Normal	Normal
Bind T_4 and T_3 in GI tract	Cholestyramine, cholestipol	Low	Low	Low	Low

that a TRH test should always be followed by magnetic resonance imaging of the hypothalamic area and by further testing of anterior pituitary function.

Hyperthyroid Patient.   If hyperthyroidism is strongly suspected, T_3 should be measured. A combination of high FT_4 and T_3 virtually diagnoses hyperthyroidism (Fig.

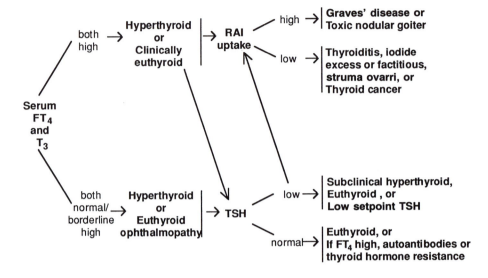

Figure 8–6.   The measurement of total T_3 is necessary for the exact diagnosis of patients with suspected hyperthyroidism and a combination of high FT_4 and T_3 is consistent with hyperthyroidism, with an RAI uptake test being necessary for the identification of less common causes.

In low setpoint TSH syndrome, TSH levels may be suppressed at lower blood levels of FT_4. This may occur in Graves' disease with clinical euthyroidism, euthyroid ophthalmopathy, or following radioiodine treatment of Graves' disease (Browlie, 1990). If FT_4 and/or T_3 are markedly elevated with a normal or increased TSH, then autoantibodies to T_4 and/ T_3, the thyroid resistance syndrome, as well as a TSH-secreting pituitary tumor must be considered.

8–6), with an RAI uptake test being necessary for the identification of less common causes. If FT_4 and T_3 are normal or borderline high in the face of clinical hyperthyroidism, a TRH administration test is often useful.

REFERENCES

Bartalena L. Recent achievements in studies on thyroid hormone binding proteins. Endocr Rev 1990;11:47–65.

Browlie BEW. Frequency and significance of suppressed sensitive TSH levels in euthyroid patients with a history of hyperthyroidism. Acta Endocrinol 1990;122:623–627.

Burger AG, O'Connell M, Scheidegger K, Woo R, Danforth E. Mono-iododination of tri-iodothyronine during low and high calorie diets. J Clin Endocrin Metab 1987; 65:829–834.

Chopra I, Hershman J, Pardridge W. Thyroid function in non-thyroidal illness Ann Intern Med 1983;98:945–957.

Cooper DS. Subclinical hypothyroidism. JAMA 1987;258:246–247.

Csako G, Zweig M, Ruddel M, Glickman J, Kestner J. Direct and indirect techniques for free thyroxine compared in patients with non-thyroidal illness. Clin Chem 1990;36:645–650.

Davies TF. Thyroid stimulating hormone receptor antibodies. [editorial] Mayo Clinic Proc 1988:736–739.

Davies TF, Platzer M, Schwartz A, Freidman E. Functionality of thyroid stimulating antibodies assessed by cryopreserved human thyroid cell bioassay. J Clin Endocrinol Metab 1983;57:1021–1027.

Ekins RP. Measurement of free hormones in blood. Endocr Rev. 1990;11:5–46.

Ekins RP. The free hormone hypothesis and measurement of free hormones. Clin Chem 1992;38:1289–1293.

Gesundheit N, Petrick PA, Nissim M. Thyrotropin-secreting pituitary adenomas: clinical and biochemical heterogeneity. Annals Intern Med 1987;111:827–835.

Grubeck-Loebenstein B, Londei M, Greenall C, et al. Pathogenetic relevance of HLA class II antigens expressing thyroid follicular cells in nontoxic goiter and in Graves' disease. J Clin Invest 1988;81:1608–1614.

Kaufman KD, Filetti S, Seto P, Rapaport B. Recombinant human thyroid peroxidase generated in eukaryotic cell: a source of specific antigen for the immunological assay of antimicrosomal antibodies in the sera of patients with autoimmune thyroid disease. J Clin Endocrinol Metab 1990;70:724–728.

Klee GG, Hay ID. Assessment of sensitive TSH assays for an expanded role in thyroid function testing: proposed criteria for analytic performance and clinical utility. J Clin Endocrinol Metab 1987;64:461–471.

Kleinhaus N, Faber J, Kahana L, Schneer J, Scheifeld M. Euthyroid hyperthyroxemia due to a generalized 5'-deiodinase defect. J Clin Endocrinol Metab 1988;66:634–688.

Kricka L, Schmerfeld-Pruss D, Senior M, Goodman B, Kaladas P. Interference by human antimouse antibody in two-site immunoassays. Clin Chem 1990;36:892–894.

Laurberg P. Mechanism governing the relative proportions of thyroxine and 3,5,3'-triiodothyronine in thyroid secretion. Metabolism 1984;33:379–389.

Lever EG, Medeiros-Neto GA, DeGroot LJ. Inherited disorders of thyroid metabolism. Endocr Rev 1983;4:213–235.

Lopresti J, Fried J, Spencer C, Nicoloff J. Unique alteration of thyroid hormone indices in the acquired immunodeficiency syndrome (AIDS). Ann Intern Med 1989;110:970–975.

Magner JA. Thyroid-stimulating hormone: biosynthesis, cell biology, and bioactivity. Endocr Rev 1990;11:354–385.

McConway MG, Chapman RS, Beastall GH, et al. How sensitive are the immunometric assays for thyrotrophin? Clin Chem 1989;35:289–291.

McNamara EM, Perillieux I, Billing JK, et al. Radioreceptor assay (RRA) for TSH receptor autoantibodies (TRAbs). [abstract] Clin Chem 1993;39:1271.

Menezes-Ferreira MM, Eil C, Wortsman J, Weintraub BD. Decreased nuclear uptake of 125-iodine tri-iodothyronine in fibroblasts from patients with peripheral thyroid hormone resistance. J Clin Endocrinol Metab 1984;59:1081–1087.

Midgley JEM. The free hormone hypothesis and measurement of free hormones. Clin Chem 1993;39:1342.

Midgley J, Sheehan C, Christofides N, Fry J, Browing D, Mardell R. Concentrations of free thyroxin and albumin in serum in severe nonthyroidal illness: assay artefacts and physiological influences. Clin Chem 1990;36:765–771.

Mooradian AD, Reed RL, Osterweil D, Schiffman R, Scuderi P. Decreased serum triiodothyronine is associated with increased concentrations of tumor necrosis factor. J Clin Endocrinol Metab 1990;71:1239–1242.

Morris J, Hay I, Nelson R, Jiang N. Clinical utility of thyrotropin receptor antibody assays: comparison of radioreceptor and bioassay methods. Mayo Clin Proc 1988;63:707–717.

Nelson J, Tomel R. Direct determination of free thyroxin in undiluted serum by equilibrium dialysis radioimmunoassay. Clin Chem 1988;34:1737–1744.

Nuutila P, Koshinen P, Irkala K, et al. Two new two-step immunoassays for free thyroxine evaluated: solid phase radioimmunoassay and time-resolved fluoroimmunoassay. Clin Chem 1990;36:1355–1360.

Parnham AJ, Tarbit IF. 'Delfia' and 'Amerlite': Two sensitive nonisotopic immunoassay systems for assay of thyrotropin compared. Clin Chem 1987;33:1421–1424.

Price A, Griffiths H, Morris BW. A longitudinal study of thyroid function in pregnancy. Clin Chem 1989;35:275–278.

Rhys J, Henley R, Shankland D. Concentrations of free thyroxin and free triiodothyronine in serum of patients with thyroxin and triiodothyronine-binding autoantibodies. Clin Chem 1990;36:470–473.

Ritter D, Stott R, Grant N, Nahm MH. Endogenous antibodies that interfere with fluorescence polarization assay but not with radioimmunoassay or EMIT™. Clin Chem 1993; 39:508–511.

Robuschi G, Safran M, Braverman LE, Gnudi A, Roti E. Hyperthyroidism in the elderly. Endocr Rev 1987;8:142–153.

Rosenthal M, Hunt W, Garry P, Goodwin J. Thyroid failure in the elderly: microsomal antibodies as discriminant for therapy. JAMA 1987;258:209–214.

Ross D. Subclinical hypothyroidism: possible danger of overzealous thyroxine replacement therapy. Mayo Clin Proc 1988;63:1233–1299.

Ross DS, Ardisson LJ, Meskell MJ. Measurement of thyrotropin in clinical and subclinical hyperthyroidism using a new chemiluminescent. J Clin Endocrinol Metab 1989; 69:686–688.

Sarne D, Sobieszczyk S, Ain K, Refetoff S. Serum thyrotropin and prolactin in the syndrone of generalized resistance to thyroid hormone: response to thyrotropin-releasing hormone stimulation and short term tri-iodothyronine suppression. J Clin Endocrinol Metab 1990;70:1305–1310.

Spaulding SW. Age and the thyroid. Endocrinol Metabolic Clin of North America 1987;16:1013–1016.

Spencer CA, Lopresti JS, Patel A, et al. Applications of a new chemiluminometric thyrotropin assay to subnormal measurement. J Clin Endocrinol Metab 1990;70:453–460.

Surks M, Chopra I, Mariash C, Nicoloff J, Solomon D. American Thyroid Association guidelines for use of laboratory tests in thyroid disorders. JAMA 1990;263:1529–1532.

Szabolcs I. Value of screening for thyroid dysfunction in hospitalized elderly patients. Horm Metabo Res 1990;22:298–302.

Thorpe-Beeston J, Nicolaides KH, Felton CV, Butler J, McGregor AM. Maturation of the secretion of thyroid hormone and thyroid stimulating hormone in the fetus. New Engl J Med 1991;324:532–536.

Utiger RD. Recognition of thyroid disease in the fetus (editorial). New Engl J Med 1991;324:559–562.

Wehmann RE, Gregerman MD, Burns WH, Sarel R, Santos GW. Suppression of thyrotrophin in the low thyroxine state of severe non-thyroidal illness. New Engl J Med 1985;312:546–552.

Yoshikawa N, Nishikawa M, Horimoto M, et al. Thyroid stimulating activity in sera of normal pregnant women. J Clin Endocrinol Metab 1989;69:891–895.

CHAPTER 9

Reproduction

Randolph Linde and
James P. Gosling

Endocrine regulation of reproduction involves the hypothalamus, the pituitary, the gonads, and a wide range of target tissues. While male reproductive function is relatively stable, in females it is cyclic and profoundly different during pregnancy. In addition, reproductive endocrine function changes greatly with development, growth, maturation, and aging. Inevitably, each of these stages and states has associated abnormalities.

HORMONES OF REPRODUCTION AND THEIR ASSAYS

Steroid Hormones and Related Analytes

The steroid hormones secreted by the gonads, and by the placenta during pregnancy, determine and regulate reproductive function. They determine function by modulating a wide range of genes in primary and secondary sexual tissues and in general somatic tissues, thereby deciding sexual capacity and characteristics. They regulate function as important feedback inhibitors of hypothalamic and pituitary reproductive activities. The synthesis of the principal sex steroids is shown in Figure 9–1.

The routine determination of reproductive steroids is by means of reagent-limited immunoassays, which generally use labeled hapten. Most often labels are made from a derivative of the steroid such as progesterone-11α-hemisuccinate conjugated to a labeling molecule such as [^{125}I]iodohistamine or horseradish peroxidase. ^{125}I is still the most popular labeling substance, but enzymes, europium ion-chelates, and luminescent compounds are also used in labels. The antibodies employed are mostly polyclonal and are usually raised against an immunogen that is bridge and site homologous with the label. The antibody is often passively adsorbed to tubes or microtiter wells or covalently coupled to microbeads, which may be magnetizable (sp-Ab). Adsorption to solid phase may be indirect, as via a second antibody such as

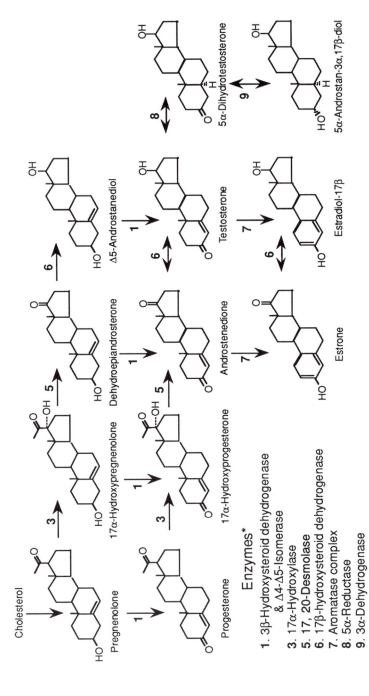

Figure 9–1.   The synthesis of the gonadal hormones and related steroids. This diagram overlaps with that of Figure 7–2, which employs the same numbering system for the enzymes.

sheep anti-rabbit IgG if the antisteroid antibody was raised in rabbit (sp-SAb-RAb) (see also Chaps. 2 and 7).

Most commercial steroid assays involve no preliminary extraction or purification of the serum or other sample, although such convenience may be at the price of susceptibility to general or metabolite interference.

Immunoassays for steroidal contraceptive agents such as ethinyl estradiol and norethindrone have been developed and are used in pharmacodynamic studies, etc. (e.g., Zacur, et al., 1991).

Progesterone

Progesterone levels are most often measured in investigations of ovarian function in order to gauge the adequacy of luteinization and to confirm that ovulation has taken place. Progesterone is generally determined once or twice in serum samples taken during the luteal phase, as estimated from the date of the last menstruation. Alternatively, progesterone may be determined in saliva samples taken by the patient herself so that daily variations may be determined and short, as well as deficient, luteal phases may be confidently recognized (Tallon, et al., 1984; Finn, et al., 1988; Finn, et al., 1990). Determination of progesterone levels on every third day permits diagnosis of fine defects of luteal function from the analysis of as few as four saliva samples per cycle (Finn, et al., 1992). However, commercial immunoassays for progesterone and other steroids are rarely validated for the analysis of saliva samples.

Estradiol-17β

Estradiol-17β is the principal estrogen in humans and its peripheral concentration is a useful indicator of follicular development. Clinically, it is determined to aid diagnosis of female infertility and the menopause, and to monitor superovulation treatments for assisted conception procedures. Analytically, it is one of the most demanding hormones (Hershlag, et al., 1992) because a highly sensitive assay with a range of 50 to 2000 pmol/L (14 to 545 ng/L) is needed for infertility investigations, but for in vitro fertilization (IVF) monitoring the range is 0.2 to 15 nmol/L (54 to 4086 ng/L). Some commercial suppliers indicate a different assay protocol with a shorter incubation period for IVF samples.

In saliva, levels are about 5 to 40 pmol/L (1 to 12 ng/L) and an assay with a detection limit of at least 200 fg per well or tube (<1 fmol per well) is necessary for 100 μL samples (De Boever, et al., 1990).

Estrone

During the menstrual cycle, estrone is present at similar concentration to that of estradiol-17β and changes in concentration are also similar. Determination of estrone levels has been suggested as useful in the diagnosis of polycystic ovarian syndrome (McKenna, 1988) and a number of commercial radioimmunoassays (RIAs) with preliminary extraction are available, in some cases with a column chromatographic purification step (Wheeler, 1993). However, these are mainly for research purposes.

Estriol

Estriol concentration increases during the second and third trimesters of pregnancy due to the combined metabolic processes of the fetoplacental unit. Measurement of estriol has been used extensively to monitor fetal well-being and a wide range of assays are commercially available, but this has been largely rendered unnecessary by ultrasonographic procedures. It is, however, routinely measured in some laboratories as part of a triple screening test (estriol, hCG, alpha-fetoprotein) for the prenatal diagnosis of Down's syndrome (Cheng, et al., 1993), although the value of three measurements over the measurement of HCG-β and alpha-fetoprotein alone is being questioned (Spencer, 1993; see also later discussion under Pregnancy.)

Androgens

The level of testosterone in men decreases with age and it is measured in investigations of hypogonadism, infertility, and lack of libido. In women it is measured most often in hirsutism. RIAs for the direct measurement of free testosterone are also available. These are used for men with suspected altered levels of sex hormone binding globulin and for women with hirsutism.

In many tissues concerned with external sexual characteristics, testosterone acts as a prohormone and must be converted in situ to 5α-dihydrotestosterone, and in cases of suspected 5α-reductase deficiency this is determined in serum, plasma, or tissue. The commercial assays available are mostly RIA with ^{3}H labels and an initial extraction step, often accompanied by chromatographic purification. Other androgens of clinical interest and measured by commercially available immunoassays include androstenedione, 3α-androstanediol glucuronide, and epitestosterone (Wheeler, 1993). The first two are measured in investigations of hirsutism and the last as a measure of exogenous testosterone administration.

Sex Hormone Binding Globulin

Sex hormone binding globulin (SHBG), which has a high binding affinity for testosterone, dihydrotestosterone, and estradiol-17β, is a β-globulin of 95,000 mol wt synthesized in the liver. Commercial immunoassays for SHBG, either reagent excess or reagent-limited in format, are occasionally used in investigations of hirsutism, because in some instances this may be due to high free testosterone concentration as a result of lowered SHBG levels (Wheeler, 1993). Simultaneously, the total testosterone concentration may be normal.

Protein and Peptide Hormones

The pituitary gonadotropins luteinizing hormone (LH, lutropin), follicle-stimulating hormone (FSH, follitropin), and human chorionic gonadotropin (hCG) resemble thyroid-stimulating hormone (TSH) and have similar mechanisms of action. Each has a molecular weight of about 30,000, consists of 15% to 30% carbohydrate and is composed of two subunits, the α subunit which is the same in all of these hormones and the β subunit which determines biologic specificity, but is completely inactive when dissociated. The β subunit of hCG has a heavily glycosylated, 30 amino acid extension at the carboxyl terminus and has many other differences in sequence from that of the subunit of LH.

The lower detection limits (Garibaldi, et al., 1991; Salameh, et al., 1992) and better specificity (Huhtaniemi, et al., 1992; Ditkoff, et al., 1993) of immunometric assays have led to a steady change from RIAs for the measurement of gonadotropins, often with nonisotopic labeling substances such as enzymes, or fluorimetric or luminometric molecules. Immunometric assays with enzyme labels are especially versatile because they can be formulated as high performance assays for use in sophisticated laboratories or as self-contained kits sold over-the-counter for home use.

There are three main strategies for the use of antibodies in sandwich assays: matched pair of monoclonal antibodies; monoclonal (usually on solid phase) and polyclonal antibodies; or monoclonal label with a mixture of monoclonal antibodies on the solid phase. These strategies, together with the choices of antibodies used, offer the possibilities of extremely narrow or relatively broad specificity with respect to the multiple isoforms in which many protein hormones exist.

The possibility that immunoassays for gonadotropins and other protein hormones might underestimate biologic activity and/or measure biologically inactive peptides has long been discussed. In vitro microbioassays, based on monitoring a biochemical change in isolated target cells exposed to the hormone to be determined, are often as sensitive as equivalent immunoassays and can be used in the determination of ratios of immunologic to biological activity in normal serum samples. For example, Leydig cells incubated with increasing concentrations of LH secrete testosterone in a dose-dependent manner. In general, bioassays and radioreceptor assays (with specific receptors as binding proteins) tend to support the biologic relevance of most modern immunometric assays (Urban, et al., 1991; Huhtaniemi, et al., 1992; see next section, Luteinizing Hormone).

As with other immunoassays, assays for gonadotropins can be susceptible to interference from heterophilic antibodies and human anti-mouse antibodies (see Chap. 1 and 8). One published account described eight cases of false hypergonadotropinemia where both LH and FSH were found to be elevated when determined by RIA but not when determined by immunoradiometric assay (IRMA) and enzyme-linked immunosorbent assay (ELISA) systems (Padova, et al., 1991). The need for greatly improved assay standardization is also apparent as shown by a recent study which prompted the conclusion that "FSH and [estradiol-17β] levels used to predict chances for achieving a viable pregnancy through in vitro fertilization should be interpreted with caution across institutions" (Hershlag, et al., 1992; see also Chap. 4).

Luteinizing Hormone

Immunometric assays for LH dominate the commercial market because they are faster and have lower detection limits, as compared with RIAs (Ditkoff, et al., 1993). High sensitivity is particularly useful for the diagnosis of conditions leading to an abnormal tempo of sexual maturation (Garibaldi, et al., 1991) and for the accurate assessment of LH pulse characteristics when LH levels are low or suppressed (Salameh, et al., 1992).

The great majority of kits presently employ two different monoclonal antibodies, but some use more than one immobilized monoclonal antibody and are referred to as multiple-site, as opposed to two-site assays. The remainder have one monoclonal and one polyclonal antibody, most often with the monoclonal antibody linked to the solid phase (Seth, 1992). In addition, the individual antibodies may bind to the β subunit only, α subunit only or intact LH only, although many manufacturers do not disclose such information. The standardization of LH immunoassay kits is relatively poor (Seth, et al., 1992; Seth, et al., 1991), partially because of this variety of antibodies and their combinations, and the consequent variety of degree of specificity. While some are highly specific for LH, others are susceptible to interference from free β subunit and/or hCG. (The latter are even preferred in some laboratories because they will detect unsuspected pregnancy in investigations of amenorrhoea.) However, highly specific assays may be so selective that they do not measure some genetically determined isoforms of LH. These immunologically distinct variants are not bound by some monoclonal antibodies recognizing epitopes located on intact "normal" LH. Therefore such isoforms, which apparently make up a portion of the LH in about 25% of individuals and are the predominant form in some people, are not detected by some two-site monoclonal antibody assays (Pettersson, et al., 1991; Pettersson, et al., 1992).

Further research is needed to immunologically map the surface of LH, choose sets of appropriate epitopes (e.g., Bidart, et al., 1993), identify minor isoforms, and design assays with appropriately high levels of specificity. In the meantime, the best assays may be those that use a pair of monoclonal antibodies (one against the α and one against the β subunit), are specific, and have consistently performed well in external quality assessment schemes.

Follicle-Stimulating Hormone

The most important applications of FSH determination are for investigations of pubertal disorders, menstrual irregularities, male and female infertility and the onset of the menopause. Many of the considerations discussed above with respect to LH apply, or may apply in the future, to FSH also. In addition, the standardization of FSH assays is complicated by the general use of a crude pituitary extract as calibration material (IRP 78/549). Another International Standard (IS 83/575) that is much more pure has recently become available and the changeover to this will be desirable in the long term. However, there may be some confusion with respect to appropriate diagnostic reference ranges, as the new standard would give lower patient results with more specific assays and higher results for assays with polyclonal antisera (Seth, et al., 1992). However, the practice of using inappropriate reference ranges for FSH diagnoses already exists, with some users apparently ignoring, for no good reason, ranges appropriate to the method they use (Seth, et al., 1991).

A radioligand receptor assay for FSH with calf testes receptors was recently described for investigations of premature ovarian failure and was recommended for use in conjunction with immunoassay to better define the relative contributions of FSH isohormones and FSH-receptor binding competitors (Schneyer et al., 1991).

Human Chorionic Gonadotropin

HCG is measured for the diagnosis of varied conditions, from pregnancy to cancer. However, like other glycoprotein hormones, it exists as subforms that are of possible diagnostic significance and that can differ greatly between serum and urine. The techniques used for the determination of hCG (Norman, et al., 1990) and the applications, chemistry, and standardization of hCG measurements (Stenman, et al., 1993) have recently been reviewed.

There are a wide range of quick urine pregnancy-detection kits for use by medical or paramedical personnel outside the laboratory, or by women themselves at home. Longer established tests are often based on latex agglutination, while the most modern are mainly formulations of two-site immunometric assays with enzymes or brightly colored latex particles for labeling (Daviaud, et al., 1993). Many are extremely easy to use and interpret, and some have built-in controls. Most detect pregnancy soon after the first missed period. More sensitive assays for hCG in serum can be used to diagnose pregnancy close to the time of implantation and have been used in investigations of hormonal parameters associated with early pregnancy loss (Baird, et al., 1991).

The best known forms of hCG of diagnostic interest are intact, whole hCG, free hCG β subunit (hCG-β) and the core fragment of hCG-β (hCG-βcf) (a two-peptide assembly held together by disulfide bonds consisting of residues 6–40 and 55–92 of hCG-β), which is found in large quantities in pregnancy urine (Stenman, et al., 1993). Construction of epitope maps of hCG and the other heterodimeric glycoprotein hormones is an important prerequisite to the informed choice of monoclonal antibodies for use in immunometric assays for detection of the intact hormone or the individual subunits (Fig. 9–2).

Measurement of hCG-β is used to screen for Down's syndrome (Spencer, 1993) and to diagnose persistent trophoblastic disease (invasive mole and choriocarcinoma). However, hCG and hCG-β also exist in "nicked" forms (hCGn and hCG-βn), in which the peptide chain of the β subunit is cleaved in the region of residues 43–49. These nicked forms are detected by some but not all immunoassays, resulting in large scale, assay-dependent variations in the levels of hCG and hCG-β detected (Kardana and Cole, 1992; Stenman, et al., 1993; Cole, et al., 1993). (See also below under Pregnancy and Prenatal Diagnosis.)

Inhibin

Inhibin may be termed a gonadal hormone that selectively suppresses secretion of pituitary FSH. There are at least two biologically active inhibin molecules, inhibin A ($\alpha\beta_A$) and inhibin B ($\alpha\beta_B$), both of which belong to a large family of proteins with similar sequences, including transforming growth factor-β (TGF-β) and müllerian inhibiting substance (Josso, et al., 1991). The β subunits of the inhibins also form homo- and heterodimers named activins, which stimulate the release of pituitary FSH

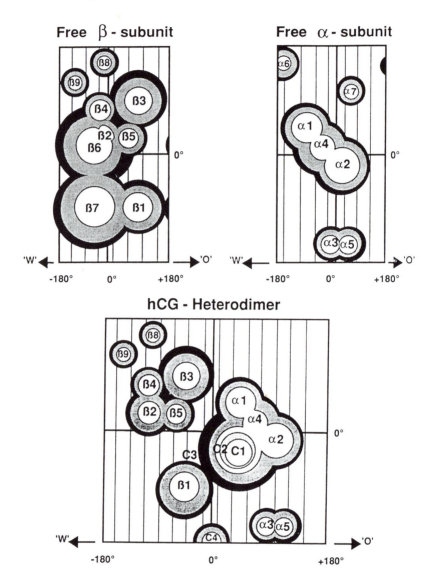

Figure 9–2.   Schematic epitope maps of free hCG-β, free hCG-α, and hCG heterodimer, with the three molecules being depicted as globules in cylindric Mercator projections. Epitopes (α1 to α7, β1 to β9, and C1 to C4) are represented by concentric circles which can merge to form larger antigenic domains with common outer boundaries. On free hCG-β a large domain comprising epitopes β1 to β7, all of which are shared by hCG-βcf, is flanked by two spatially distinct epitopes on the carboxyl terminal peptide extension (β8 and β9). (This extension peptide is not found in the other glycoprotein hormones.) Four spatially distinct antigenic domains on free hCG-α can be defined (α1, α2 and α4; α3 and α5; α6; and α7). Upon assembly of the subunits to give the hCG dimer, epitopes α6, α7, β6, and β7 disappear and the C-epitopes emerge. Three of the C-epitopes overlap with the central domain (α1, α2, and α4) of the free α subunit.

(Shintani, et al., 1991). Follistatin is a glycosylated, single-chain polypeptide, also found in human follicular fluid, that also suppresses FSH release.

An RIA based on synthetic human inhibin α-chain peptide, suitable for the measurement of inhibins in follicular fluid, seminal plasma or amniotic fluid, has recently been described (Sinosich, et al., 1991). The measurement of inhibin (Matson, et al., 1991) or follistatin (Sugawara, et al., 1990) has been proposed as an aid in monitoring superovulation treatment for in vitro fertilization procedures.

Prolactin and Placental Lactogen

Prolactin and placental lactogen have similar structures and resemble growth hormone closely in size and sequence. They have 170 or 191 amino acid residues, respectively, and occur as monomers, dimers, aggregates, and in glycoslyated forms.

Prolactin (mol wt 25,000) is secreted by the anterior pituitary due to stimulation by one or more prolactin releasing factors (PRF). Putative PRFs include thyrotropin releasing hormone (TRH), vasoactive intestinal peptide (VIP), gonadotropin releasing hormone (GnRH), neurotensin, and cholecystokinin. Prolactin is measured in patients suspected of having a prolactinoma or other prolactin secreting tumor, in whom galactorrea may be an associated symptom. Medications are common causes of hyperprolactinemia, including dopamine-depleting agents (e.g., reserpine) and dopamine receptor-blocking agents (e.g., phenothiazines). Elevated concentrations of prolactin can cause hypogonadism resulting in menstrual disorders and infertility in women, and decreased libido and impotence in men. Almost all commercial assays are immunometric and most employ two monoclonal antibodies.

Placental lactogen (mol wt 22,000) is secreted by the syncytiotrophoblasts from about the 10th week of pregnancy with its concentration increasing steadily until about 5 weeks before parturition, when it levels off (Handwerger, 1991). Its concentration in blood is proportional to placental weight and is determined in the assessment of placental function. Many available assays are competitive immunoassays but two-site immunometric assays are becoming increasingly available (Seth, 1992).

SEXUAL DIFFERENTIATION AND DEVELOPMENT

In girls, sexual maturation usually begins with breast development (thelarche) and pubic hair growth (pubarche) followed by menarche at about 13 years (range 10 to 16 years). In boys, testicular development begins at about age 11.5 with pubic hair and penile enlargement at about 14.5 years (range 13 to 16 years). The criteria for precocious and delayed puberty plus their diagnosis and treatment are discussed in

---

Epitopes were defined by monoclonal antibodies and their topographic arrangement resolved by two-site immunoassays. Modified from Bidart J-M, et al. Immunochemical mapping of hCG and hCG-related molecules. Scand J Clin Lab Invest 1993;53(suppl 216):118–136. Reproduced with permission.

standard texts (e.g., Kelch, 1990). Precocious puberty may be isosexual (much more common in girls than boys) due to hormone secreting tumors or adrenal disorders, or contrasexual due to congenital adrenal hyperplasia (CAH) or steroid secreting tumors. In contrast, delayed puberty is much more common in boys.

The majority of cases of early puberty in girls are idiopathic (Rosenfield, 1991). Advanced bone age should prompt a search for a gonadal or adrenal tumor, or CAH. In true precocious puberty, there is a pubertal gonadotropin response to GnRH; for girls this would mean an increase of LH greater than 12 mIU/mL and FSH greater than 3 mIU/mL. A gonadal tumor is suggested when serum estradiol-17β exceeds 275 pmol/L (75 ng/L). A masculinizing disorder is implied by plasma testosterone exceeding 1.5 nmol/L (45 ng/dL) or dehydroepiandrosterone sulfate exceeding 11 μmol/L (3500 μg/L).

In boys if puberty does not start, or if pubertal development plateaus, endocrine or nonendocrine causes are possible, including psychosocial factors. Endocrine evaluation, if necessary, should include the measurement of gonadotropin and steroid concentrations. GnRH stimulation testing to evaluate the level at which the deficiency occurs is only necessary if both gonadotropins and testosterone levels are low (Roth, 1972). Blood samples are obtained before, and 30 and 60 minutes after intravenous injection of 100 μg of GnRH. A normal (pubertal) response varies among laboratories, with LH usually increasing greater than 3 mIU/mL and FSH greater than 3mIU/mL in males. Hypothalamic disease can be separated from pituitary disease by priming with GnRH treatment for 3 to 7 days, then repeating the stimulation test (Frohman, 1987).

In boys the majority of cases of precocious pubertal development are a consequence of a central nervous system lesion (Styne, 1991).

FEMALE REPRODUCTIVE FUNCTION

The Normal Menstrual Cycle

Throughout the menstrual cycle the secretion of the reproductive hormones is dynamic (Fig. 9–3). GnRH and, consequently, gonadotropin secretion occur in bursts that differ in amplitude and frequency, and are modulated by steroid and peptide hormones acting as feedback regulators at the levels of the pituitary and hypothalamus. LH and FSH can change dramatically in blood samples taken at 10 minutes or shorter intervals, and the levels of estradiol-17β and progesterone vary from day to day.

In the early follicular phase, FSH secretion stimulates follicular development with gradually increasing secretion of estrogens by maturing follicles. Toward the late follicular phase there is increased secretion of estradiol-17β yielding serum levels of about 1.45 nmol/L (400 ng/L). The resulting LH surge, possibly triggered by preovulatory estradiol-17β and progesterone secretion (Batista, et al., 1992) from basal pulsing levels of 0 to 30 to 100 to 150 IU/L (0 to 30 to 60 to 150 mIU/mL), stimulates release of chemical mediators including plasmin, which in turn facilitate ejection of the egg from the follicle. As the nondominant follicles regress, estrogen levels fall. Progesterone levels gradually increase with maturation of the corpus luteum, which ultimately secretes more estradiol than preovulatory follicles. Secretory

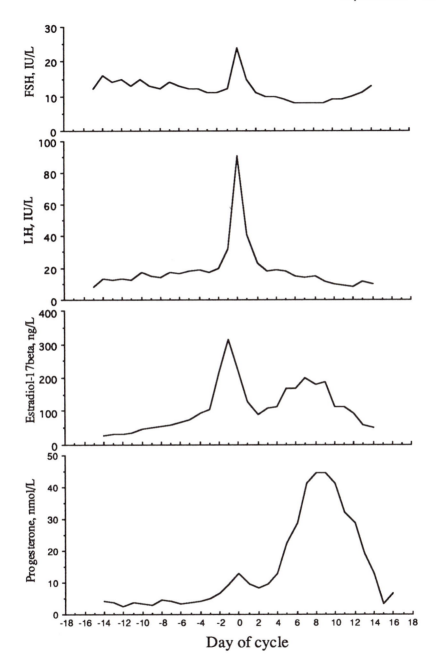

Figure 9–3.   Average variations in the concentrations of four hormones during the menstrual cycle in healthy women of childbearing age. The hormone relevant to each plot is indicated in the label of the y-axis; from top to bottom they are FSH, LH, estradiol-17β and progesterone, respectively. Data from Rebar RW, et al. The normal menstrual cycle and the control of ovulation. In: Becker KL, ed. Principles and Practice of Endocrinology and Metabolism. Philadelphia: JB Lippincott, 1990;788–797.

changes and enhanced vascularity are induced in the endometrium. The ovary also secretes a number of active peptides, including inhibin, that selectively inhibit FSH secretion and thereby contribute to the differential regulation of gonadotropin secretion (Jaffe, et al., 1990).

If pregnancy occurs, the corpus luteum continues its functions until the placenta takes over the production of steroid hormone secretion at about 7 weeks' gestation. If the corpus luteum is not exposed to hCG from a conceptus it regresses and circulating concentrations of inhibin, estradiol-17β, and progesterone levels begin falling in the late luteal phase, several days before menstruation begins. An increase in FSH production heralds the onset of the next cycle.

Female Androgens

With gonadarche, plasma testosterone in healthy females can reach 1.4 to 1.7 nmol/L (40 to 50 ng/dL) and vellous hair is transformed to coarser terminal hair. Total production of testosterone in the female is 0.2 to 0.3 mg (0.6 to 1 μmol) per day. About 50% is secreted by the ovaries and adrenals, chiefly the former, and the other 50% comes from peripheral conversion of androstenedione, also secreted by the ovaries and adrenals. Testosterone is largely bound to SHBG and only 1% to 2% is free, but free testosterone may be increased to 4% or higher in some hirsute women.

Dehydroepiandrosterone (DHEA) and DHEA sulfate (DHEAS) constitute about 80% of urinary 17-ketosteroids. DHEAS is the preferable steroid to measure because of its relatively long half-life and because it better reflects adrenal androgen activity. Although a weak androgen, DHEA is converted in the pilosebaceous unit to testosterone and 5α-dihydrotestosterone, which is about three times more potent than testosterone in terms of hair growth stimulation. Both these androgens are ultimately metabolized to 3α-androstandediol glucuronide, which, because it has been claimed to provide an index of peripheral androgen action (Horton, et al., 1982), is measured in plasma in investigations of hirsutism. However, the clinical utility of 3α-androstanediol glucuronide measurements in cases of hirsutism has been questioned (Rittmaster, 1993).

Menstrual Disturbances

Menarche or established menstruation can be suppressed (primary or secondary amenorrhea, respectively) by physical activity such as intensive ballet training, by maintaining low body weight, or by significant physical or mental stress, and such conditions are best treated by change of lifestyle or diet.

Hypergonadotropic hypogonadism with primary amenorrhea generally indicates Turner's syndrome, with the rare patient not developing clinical ovarian failure until her thirties. Some individuals with a variant form of Turner's syndrome may transiently menstruate in early adolescence. The causes of amenorrhea are many and many be suggested by other symptoms (Table 9–1). It should be noted that patients

Table 9–1 Secondary Symptoms Suggesting Causes for Secondary Amenorrhea That Can be Tested and Proved

Symptom	Cause of Amenorrhea
Galactorrhea	Hyperprolactinemia
Hirsutism and acne	Syndrome of androgen excess
Significant weight loss or heavy physical training	Suppression of the reproductive axis
Postpartum hemorrhage	Hypopituitarism (Sheehan's syndrome)
Dilatation and curettage following abortion or delivery	Uterine synechiae with end-organ failure (Asherman's syndrome)
General	Autoimmune oophoritis

with prolactinoma often do not have galactorrhea, and therefore a plasma prolactin level should be measured in every woman with unexplained amenorrhea (Vance, 1991). Hyperprolactinemia is excluded by a level of serum prolactin less than 888 pmol/L (20 μg/L) despite time of day or menstrual cycle. Mean levels are 222 pmol/L (5 μg/L) and 355 pmol/L (8 μg/L) in healthy men and women, respectively.

Oligomenorrhea implies irregular, infrequent menstrual bleeding often representing anovulation with estrogen deficiency, while dysfunctional uterine bleeding signifies irregular, frequent bleeding, often indicating anovulation with adequate estrogen. However, the causes of these conditions are similar, and vary from subtle abnormalities in GnRH production, to thyroid disease, to disorders of androgen secretion or metabolism.

Polycystic ovary syndrome (PCO) is a common heterogeneous disorder in which menstrual disturbances (amenorrhea, oligomenorrhea, or dysfunctional uterine bleeding) and infertility may be associated with hirsutism and obesity. It occurs in association with CAH, Cushing's syndrome, hyperprolactinemia, and hyperinsulinemia with insulin insensitivity, and may be thought of as a condition of chronic anovulation with an excess synthesis of androgens.

There are probably a number of mechanisms by which PCO can ultimately occur (Nestler, et al., 1989; McKenna, 1988). Dale, et al. (1992) suggest that there are two subgroups of cases: those with obesity, insulin resistance, hyperinsulinemia, and normal/minimally elevated LH levels; and those with normal body weight, elevated LH levels, and normal insulin levels. Because of advances in ovarian imaging techniques PCO is now often detected in patients with more subtle clinical and endocrinologic abnormalities and in girls during puberty. Increased insulin and insulin-like growth factor-I(IGF-I) concentrations have been suggested as inducing factors in pubertal PCO (Nobels and Dewailly, 1992), and chronic hypersecretion of androgen precursors due to an inborn enzyme defect has been suggested as causing a reduction in insulin sensitivity (Speiser, et al., 1992).

Premature menopause is suspected when gonadotropin levels are elevated to the menopausal range and amenorrhea is associated with hot flushes. Rarely, such patients have "resistant ovary syndrome" when ovarian biopsy shows primordial rather

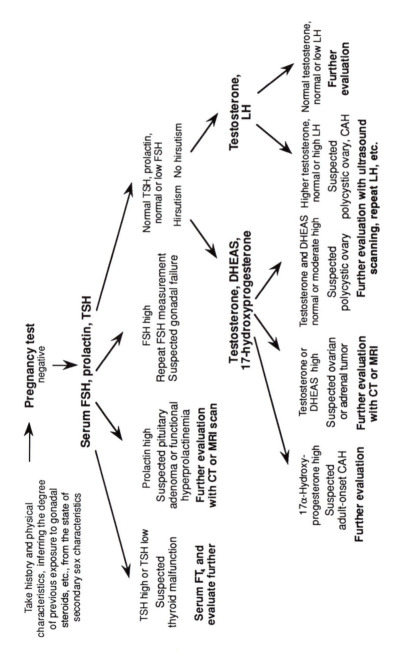

Figure 9–4.   General guide to the laboratory based evaluation of amenorrhea.

than atretic follicles, or their biopsy shows no follicles. They may also spontaneously ovulate and conceive (Rebar and Cedars, 1992).

A general guide to the laboratory based evaluation of amenorrhea is given in Figure 9–4.

Hirsutism

Causes of hirsutism include ovarian pathology (PCO syndrome, hyperthecosis, and ovarian tumors), adrenal pathology (CAH, Cushing's syndrome, or androgen secreting tumor), and target organ sensitivity (increased 5α-reductase activity). In attempts to characterize androgen production in hirsute women, investigators assess production rates, plasma or saliva levels, concentrations in adrenal versus ovarian veins, as well as carrying out adrenocorticotropic hormone (ACTH) stimulation tests and dexamethasone and GnRH agonist suppression tests (Lanzone, et al., 1990). However, much of this testing is expensive and unhelpful (Rittmaster, 1992) and most patients can be screened for serious pathology by measuring only serum testosterone and DHEAS. Carmina, et al. (1992) proposed the ratio of androstenedione:11β-hydroxyandrostenedione serum concentrations as an indicator of excess adrenal androgen secretion.

When marked hirsutism is accompanied by acne, temporal balding, deep voice, increased musculature and clitoromegaly, this is known as virilization. This infrequent condition is caused by a high blood level of an androgen, usually testosterone exceeding 200 ng/dL (7 nmol/L), and generally results from an ovarian tumor (McLachlan, et al., 1987).

Infertility

Reproductive hormonal assays comprise a surprisingly minor portion of the evaluation of female infertility when menses occur regularly and there is no clinical hyperandrogenism. FSH and progesterone are used to assess follicular and endometrial maturation. The concentration of FSH on cycle day 3 is predictive of poor egg viability and in vitro fertilization outcome (Scott, et al. 1989). Estradiol-17β levels are followed on a daily basis during ovulation induction with gonadotropins (Blacker, 1992).

Ovarian function must be normal in two general respects for successful conception and pregnancy. Ovulation must occur and there must be luteal sufficiency. Ovulation can be assumed if the cycles are regular, 1 month apart, and can be confirmed inexpensively by basal body temperature monitoring. Urine ovulation-prediction immunoassay kits measure the augmented preovulatory urinary LH excretion and provide prospective timing of ovulation. Luteal phase deficiency is suggested by an interval of less than 11 days between ovulation and menstruation (Crosignani, 1990). More commonly, inadequate secretory endometrial maturation is assumed when there is normal luteal phase length but midluteal progesterone levels less than 10 μg/L (32 nmol/L). Salivary analysis with frequent sampling may be used for the fine diagnosis of recurrent luteal phase defects (Finn, et al., 1988, 1990, 1992).

Pregnancy

Corpus luteum function is necessary for the first 7 weeks of pregnancy but is probably unnecessary after 8 weeks. Progesterone and 17α-hydroxyprogesterone levels increase sharply to 80 nmol/L (25 μg/L) and 13 nmol/L (4μg/L) respectively by 4 weeks, the latter then declining as luteal steroid production wanes. Progesterone continues to increase, although at a slower rate, as a combination of luteal and placental contributions.

HGC is detectable in serum by day 9 or 10, and its measurement forms the basis for pregnancy testing. Levels double each 1.7 to 2.0 days, with serum values rising precipitously from weeks 5 to 10 and peaking at 10,000 to 100,000 IU/L by the end of the first trimester. Levels then decline, falling by 90% by the end of the second trimester. HCG functions to maintain the early corpus luteum, to promote fetoplacental steroidogenesis, and to stimulate fetal testicular testosterone secretion. Clinically, hCG levels can be low or can anomalously decline in some (but not all) patients with ectopic pregnancy.

The placenta uses maternal and fetal circulating DHEAS to synthesize estradiol and estrone which return to the maternal circulation, with small amounts going to the fetus. In the fetus DHEAS is transformed in the liver to 16α-hydroxydehydroeplandrosterone sulfate which is then converted by the placenta to estriol, and its concentration in the maternal circulation starts to slowly increase at the 9th to 10th week of gestation. Clinically, urinary and plasma estriol levels are observed to fall with fetal deterioration or death, but a low estriol level is not pathognomonic and it should be correlated with other tests of fetoplacental integrity.

Pregnancy-associated plasma protein A (PAPP-A), a tetrameric glycoprotein of mol wt 720,000 can be detected in maternal serum from the sixth week of gestation. Its concentration, as measured by immunoenzymometric assay (IEMA), is reduced in ectopic pregnancies and impending fetal loss, and is raised in preeclamptic toxemia (Ward, 1993).

Prenatal Diagnosis

While scanning by means of ultrasound has greatly facilitated the early detection of a wide range of physical defects in the developing fetus, many abnormalities (including the most common chromosomal abnormality, Down's syndrome) are usually diagnosed by amniocentesis and investigations of the fetal cells thereby obtained, including karyotyping. However, because of an associated risk of spontaneous miscarriage of between 0.3% and 1% with amniocentesis, the measurement of biochemical markers in the maternal bloodstream has received much attention.

Markers for Down's syndrome that have been considered include alpha-fetoprotein (a 63,000 mol wt glycoprotein synthesized in the fetal liver and yolk sac from the 10th week), unconjugated estriol, pregnancy-specific Beta 1 glycoprotein, CA-125, urea-resistant neutrophil alkaline phosphatase, hCG, and hCG-β. The combined use of alpha-fetoprotein, hCG, and estriol as a second-trimester screening test for Down's syndrome has been reviewed by Cheng, et al. (1993). A good method may be a combination of maternal age and measurement of alpha-fetoprotein and hCG-β, which gave a detection rate of 66% for a 5.9% false positive rate (Spencer, 1993). There was no increase in detection rate with the further addition of unconjugated estriol, although estriol may be preferable to alpha-fetoprotein under some circumstances (Cuckle, 1992). A further advantage is that the detection rate was found to be higher earlier, that is, 77% at 14 to 16 weeks. A simultaneous dual immunoassay for alpha-fetoprotein and hCG-β has been developed and applied to routine screening for Down's syndrome (Macri, et al., 1992). The above-mentioned high detection rates were obtained with monoclonal antibodies that could bind to hCG-βn as well as hCG-β (e.g., antibody FBT11) as opposed to another commonly used antibody, 1E5 (Kardana and Cole, 1992; Spencer, 1993).

Elevated maternal serum alpha-fetoprotein concentrations are also found in association with neural tube defects and major ventral wall abnormalities.

Menopause

Approximately 96% of women experience menopause between the ages of 42 and 56. With the start of the menopause, FSH rises earlier than LH (as occurs acutely after oophorectomy) and a concentration of FSH in excess of 25 IU/L on day 3 of the menstrual cycle prognosticates little chance for future pregnancy (Toner, et al., 1991). Plasma concentrations of FSH, LH and α subunit peak 2 to 3 years after the onset of the menopause, and then gradually and minimally decline over many years (Kwekkeboom, et al., 1990).

MALE REPRODUCTIVE FUNCTION

The intertubular Leydig cells of the testis are the major source of testosterone. While there is also testicular secretion of dihydrotestosterone and estradiol, 70% to 80% of these hormones arise from their conversion from the prohormone testosterone in sexually responsive tissues. In adults 5α-dihydrotestesterone is the final hormone in the reproductive tract, skin and bone tissue, 5β-dihydrotestesterone is the final hormone in bone marrow tissue, while in brain tissue estradiol is formed from testosterone, where it controls male cerebral sexual differentiation. Androstendione (a preandrogen in the female), testosterone, and 5α-dihydrotestosterone are metabolized to 3α-androstanediol.

Hypogonadism

Male hypogonadism is caused by reduced testosterone secretion or diminished end-organ responsiveness. Reduced secretion can be caused by a hypothalamic, pituitary, or testicular lesion. In general, severe disorders result in reduced testosterone levels and elevated gonadotropins, but patients with GnRH deficiency present with a failure to undergo puberty and low gonadotropin levels (Crowley and Jameson, 1992). A congenital lesion may be apparent at birth, become evident during adolescence, or appear in adult life. Acquired lesions peak in men at about 50 years of age.

The disorders that lead to primary hypogonadism include congenital anorchia, gonadal dysgenesis, Klinefelter's syndrome, "Sertoli cell only" syndrome and myotonic dystrophy. Lesions of the hypothalamus or pituitary (arising because of a destructive tumor or as the result of surgery or pituitary irradiation) can lead to secondary hypogonadism.

Gynecomastia (enlargement of the male breast) is often the presenting complaint in men with hypogonadism, yet most men with gynecomastia have a normal reproductive axis. Gynecomastia may be a reflection of persistent physiologic changes of adolescence; exogenous, possibly environmental estrogen exposure; disease of the liver, kidneys, or thyroid gland; a drug effect (e.g., marijuana); a clue to an hCG secreting neoplasm, usually testicular; or the result of abnormal adrenal or testicular metabolism or function. Evaluation may continue to include tests of liver and kidney function, serum testosterone, gonadotropins, hCG-β, prolactin, TSH, and estradiol-17β.

Impotence is infrequently attributable to hypogonadism. More commonly it is a consequence of a vascular lesion, particularly in older or diabetic men with cardiac risk factors, or a psychological problem. Serum testosterone, which may fall by as much as one third with advancing age (Bardin, 1991), and may to some extent be a consequence of reduced mass of GnRH released at a normal pulse frequency (Kaufman, 1991), should be measured in conjunction with LH and prolactin. Hypogonadism should be considered if libido is depressed in addition to potency.

Infertility

In most men with a persistently abnormal semen analysis, an identifying cause cannot be found. Potential etiologies include diethylstilbestrol exposure in utero, congenital hernia, cryptorchidism, CAH, severe genital trauma, mumps orchitis, varicocele, a variety of medications or drugs, and environmental exposures.

When the semen analysis is consistently abnormal, serum FSH and LH are most accurately checked by pooling three samples drawn at 30-minute intervals to allow for inherent variation due to pulsatile secretion. Plasma testosterone should also be measured. In general, four patterns of hormone levels are observed (Clarke and Sherins, 1990):

- Normal testosterone, LH and FSH, leading perhaps to a diagnosis of unexplained infertility
- Low testosterone and elevated gonadotropins indicating primary testicular failure
- Low testosterone and low or normal gonadotropins indicating secondary testicular failure due to gonadotropin or GnRH deficiency
- High FSH but normal LH and testosterone due to a mild form of germ cell depletion or seminiferous tubular damage with reduced inhibin secretion

In some cases of initially inexplicable infertility the cause may be immunologic, due to the formation of antibodies to functionally important sperm antigens in the male or female partner (Snow and Ball, 1992).

REFERENCES

Baird DD, Weinberg CR, Wilcox AJ, McConnaughy DR, Musey PI, Collins DC. Hormonal profiles of natural conception cycles ending in early, unrecognized pregnancy loss. J Clin Endocrinol Metab 1991;72:793–800.

Bardin CW, Swerdloff RS, Santen RJ. Androgens: risks and benefits. J Clin Endocrinol Metab 1991;73:4–7.

Batista MC, Cartledge TP, Zellmer AW, Nieman LK, Merriam GR, Loriaux DL. Evidence for a critical role of progesterone in the regulation of the midcycle gonadotropin surge and ovulation. J Clin Endocrinol Metab 1992;74:565–570.

Bidart J-M, Birken S, Berger P, Krichevsky A. Immunochemical mapping of hCG and hCG-related molecules. Scand J Clin Lab Invest 1993;53 (suppl 216):118–136.

Blacker CM. Ovulation stimulation and induction. Endocrinol Metabol Clin North Am 1992;21:57–84.

Carmina E, Stanczyk FZ, Chang L, Miles RA, Lobo RA. The ratio of androstenedione: 11β-hydroxyandrostenedione is an important marker of adrenal androgen excess in women. Fertil Steril 1992;58:148–152.

Cheng EY, Luthy DA, Zebelman AM, Williams MA, Lieppman RE, Hickok DE. A prospective evaluation of a 2nd-trimester screening test for fetal Down syndrome using maternal serum alpha-fetoprotein, hCG, and unconjugated estriol. Obstet Gynecol 1993: 81;72–77.

Clarke RV, Sherins RJ. Male infertility. In: Becker KL, ed. Principles and Practice of Endocrinology and Metabolism. Philadelphia: JB Lippincott, 1990;985–991.

Cole LA, Kardana A, Park S-Y, Braunstein GD. The deactivation of hCG by nicking and dissociation. J Clin Endocrinol Metab 1993;76:704–710.

Crosignani PG. Luteal defect: a rational approach to diagnosis and treatment. In: Adashi EY, Mancuso S, eds. Major Advances in Human Female Reproduction. New York: Raven Press, 1990;73:199–204.

Crowley WF Jr, Jameson JL. Clinical Counterpoint: Gonadotropin-releasing hormone deficiency: perspectives from clinical investigation. Endocr Rev 1992;13:635–640.

Cuckle HS. Measuring unconjugated estriol in serum to screen for fetal Down syndrome (editorial). Clin Chem 1992;38:1687–1689.

Dale PO, Tanbo T, Vaaler S, Åbyholm T. Body weight, hyperinsulinemia, and gonadotropin levels in the polycystic ovarian syndrome: evidence of two distinct populations. Fertil Steril 1992;58:487–491.

Daviaud J, Fournet D, Ballongue C, Guillem GP, Leblanc A, Casellas C, Pau B. Reliability and feasibility of pregnancy Home-Use tests-laboratory validation and diagnostic evaluation by 638 volunteers. Clin Chem 1993;39;53–59.

De Boever J, Kohen F, Bouve J, Leyseele D, Vandekerckhove D. Direct chemiluminescence immunoassay of estradiol in saliva. Clin Chem 1990;36:2036–2041.

Ditkoff EC, Levin JH, Paul WL, Lobo RA. Time-resolved fluroimmunoassay compared with radioimmunoassay of luteinizing hormone. Fertil Steril 1993:59;305–310.

Finn MM, Gosling JP, Tallon DF, Madden ATS, Meehan FP, Fottrell PF. Normal salivary progesterone levels throughout the ovarian cycle as determined by a direct enzyme immunoassay. Fertil Steril 1988;50:882–887.

Dale PO, Tanbo T, Vaaler S, Åbyholm T. Body weight, hyperinsulinemia, and gonadotropin levels in the polycystic ovarian syndrome: evidence of two distinct populations. Fertil Steril 1992;58:487–491.

Daviaud J, Fournet D, Ballongue C, Guillem GP, Leblanc A, Casellas C, Pau B. Reliability and feasibility of pregnancy Home-Use tests-laboratory validation and diagnostic evaluation by 638 volunteers. Clin Chem 1993:39;53–59.

De Boever J, Kohen F, Bouve J, Leyseele D, Vandekerckhove D. Direct chemiluminescence immunoassay of estradiol in saliva. Clin Chem 1990;36:2036–2041.

Ditkoff EC, Levin JH, Paul WL, Lobo RA. Time-resolved fluroimmunoassay compared with radioimmunoassay of luteinizing hormone. Fertil Steril 1993;59;305–310.

Finn MM, Gosling JP, Tallon DF, Madden ATS, Meehan FP, Fottrell PF. Normal salivary progesterone levels throughout the ovarian cycle as determined by a direct enzyme immunoassay. Fertil Steril 1988;50:882–887.

Finn MM, Gosling JP, Tallon DF, Joyce LA, Meehan FP, Fottrell PF. Follicular growth and corpus luteum function in women with unexplained infertility, monitored by ultrasonagraphy and measurement of daily salivary progesterone. Gynecol Endocrinol 1990;3:297–308.

Finn MM, Gosling JP, Tallon DF, Meehan FP, Fottrell PF. Sampling frequency and the diagnosis of luteal phase defects by salivary sampling and progesterone analysis. Gynecol Endocrinol 1992;6:127–134.

Frohman LA. Diseases of the anterior pituitary. In: Felig P, Baxter JD, Broadus AE, Frohman LA eds. Endocrinology and Metabolism. New York: McGraw-Hill, 1987;2:247–337.

Garibaldi LR, Picco P, Magier S, Chevli R, Aceto T Jr. Serum luteinizing hormone concentrations, as measured by a sensitive immunoradiometric assay, in children with normal, precocious or delayed pubertal development. J Clin Endocrinol Metab 1991; 72:888–898.

Handwerger S. Clinical counterpoint: The physiology of placental lactogen in human pregnancy. Endocr Rev 1991;12:329–336.

Hershlag A, Lesser M, Montefusco D, et al. Interinstitutional variability of follicle-stimulating hormone and estradiol levels. Fert Steril 1992;58:1123–1126.

Horton R, Hawks D, Lobo R. 32,17β-androstanediol glucuronide in plasma: a marker of androgen action in idiopathic hirsutism. J Clin Invest 1982;69:1202–1206.

Huhtaniemi I, Ding YQ, Tahtela R, Valimaki M. The bio/immunoratio of plasma luteinizing hormone does not change during the endogenous secretion pulse: reanalysis of the concept using improved immunometric techniques. J Clin Endocrinol Metab 1992; 75:1442–1445.

Jaffe RB, Rabinovici J, Spencer SJ. Inhibin and activin: functional and developmental aspects. In: Adashi EY, Mancuso S, eds. Major Advances in Human Female Reproduction. New York: Raven Press, 1990;73:117–122.

Josso N, Boussin L, Knebelmann B, Nihoul-Fékété C, Picard J-Y. Anti-Müllerian hormone and intersex states. Trends Endocrinol Metab 1991;2:227–233.

Kardana A, Cole LA. Polypeptide nicks cause erroneous results in assays of human chorionic gonadotropin free β-subunit. Clin Chem 1992;38:26–33.

Kaufman JM, Giri M, Deslypere JM, Thomas G, Vermeulen A. Influence of age on the gonadotrophs to luteinizing hormone-releasing hormone in males. J Clin Endocrinol Metab 1991;72:1255–1260.

Kelch RP. Sexual precocity and retardation. In: Becker KL, ed. Principles and Practice of Endocrinology and Metabolism. Philadelphia: JB Lippincott, 1990;747–759.

Kwekkeboom DJ, de Jong FH, van Hemert AM, et al. Serum gonadotropins and α-subunit decline in aging normal postmenopausal women. J Clin Endocrinol Metab 1990; 70:944–950.

Lanzone A, Fulghesu AM, Guido M, et al. The evaluation of ovarian and adrenal compartments in hyperandrogenized women. In: Adashi EY, Mancuso S, eds. Major Advances in Human Female Reproduction. New York: Raven Press, 1990;73:317–325.

Macri JN, Spencer K, Anderson R. Dual analyte immunoassay in neural tube defect and Down's syndrome screening. Ann Clin Biochem 1992;29:390–396.

Matson PL, Morris ID, Sun JG, Ibrahim ZHZ, Liebermann BA. Serum inhibin as an index of ovarian function in women undergoing pituitary suppression and ovarian stimulation in an in vitro fertilization program. Horm Res 1991;35:173–177.

McKenna TJ. Current concepts: pathogenesis and treatment of polycystic ovary syndrome. N Engl J Med 1988;318:558–562.

McLachlan RI, Healy DL, Burger HG. The ovary: clinical. In: Felig P, Baxter JD, Broadus AE, Frohman LA, eds. Endocrinology and Metabolism. New York: McGraw-Hill, 1987;2:951–983.

Nestler JE, Clore JN, Blackward WG. The central role of obesity (hyperinsulinemia) in the pathogenesis of the polycystic ovary syndrome. Am J Obstet Gynecol 1989; 161:1095–1097.

Nobels F, Dewailly D. Puberty and polycystic ovarian syndrome: the insulin/insulin-like growth factor I hypothesis. Fertil Steril 1992;58:655–666.

Norman RJ, Buck RH, De Medeiros SF. Measurement of human chorionic gonadotrophin (hCG): indications and techniques for the clinical laboratory. Ann Clin Biochem 1990;27:183–194.

Padova G, Briguglia G, Tita P, Munguira ME, Arpi ML, Pezzina V. Hypergonadotropinemia not associated with ovarian failure and induced by factors interfering in radioimmunoassay. Fertil Steril, 1991;55:637–639.

Pettersson K, Ding YQ, Huhtaniemi I. Monoclonal antibody-based discrepancies between two-site immunometric tests for lutropin. Clin Chem 1991;37:1745–1748.

Pettersson K, Ding YQ, Huhtaniemi I. An immunologically anomalous luteinizing hormone variant in a healthy woman. J Clin Endocrinol Metab 1992;74:164–171.

Rebar RW, Kenigsberg D, Hodgen GD. The normal menstrual cycle and the control of ovulation. In: Becker KL, ed. Principles and Practice of Endocrinology and Metabolism. Philadelphia: JB Lippincott, 1990;788–797.

Rebar RW, Cedars MI, Hypergonadotropic forms of amenorrhea in young women. Endocrinol Metab Clin North Am 1992;21:173–191.

Rittmaster RS. Hyperandrogenism—what is normal? N Engl J Med 1992;327:194–195.

Rittmaster RS. Androgen conjugates:physiology and clinical significance. Endocr Rev 1993;14:121–132.

Rosenfield RL. Puberty and its disorders in girls. Endocrinol Metab Clin North Am 1991;20:15–42.

Roth JC, Kelch RP, Kaplan SL, Grumbach MM. FSH and LH response to luteinizing hormone-releasing factor in prepubertal and pubertal children, adult males and patients with hypogonadotropic and hypergonadotropic hypogonadism. J Clin Endocrinol Metab 1972;35:926–930.

Salameh W, Bhasin S, Steiner BS, Peterson M, Swerdloff RS. Effect of improved assay sensitivity on luteinizing hormone pulse detection after gonadotropin-releasing hormone antagonist treatment in man. J Clin Endocrinol Metab 1992;75:1479–1483.

Schneyer AL, Sluss PM, Whitcomb RW, Hall JE, Crowley WF Jr, Freeman RG. Development of a radioligand receptor assay for measuring follitropin in serum: application to premature ovarian failure. Clin Chem 1991;37:508–514.

Scott RT, Toner JP, Muasher SJ, et al. Follicle stimulating hormone levels on cycle day 3 one predictive of in vitro fertilization outcome. Fertil Steril 1989;51:651–654.

Seth J, ed. Peptide Hormones, vol 2, part 1. In: Seth J, ed. The Immunoassay Kit Directory, Series A: Clinical Chemistry. Norwell MA: Kluwer Academic Publishers, 1992.

Seth J, Ellis AR, Al-Sadie R. Causes of method bias in assays for pituitary gonadotrophins in serum. Communications in Laboratory Medicine 1992;3:25–28.

Seth J, Sturgeon CM, Al-Sadie R, Hanning I, Ellis AR. External quality assessment of immunoassays of peptide hormones and tumour markers: principles and practice. Ann Ist Super Sanitá 1991;27:443–452.

Shintani Y, Takada Y, Yamasaki R, Saito S. Radioimmunoassay for activin A/EDF: method and measurement of immunoreactive actinin A/EDF levels in various biological materials. J Immunol Methods 1991;137:267–274.

Sinosich MJ, Sieg S, Zakher A, et al. Rosenwaks Z, Hodgen GD. Radioimmunoassay of inhibin based on synthetic human inhibin α-chain peptide. Clin Chem 1991;37:40–46.

Snow K, Ball GD. Characterization of human sperm antigens and antisperm antibodies in infertile patients. Fertil Steril 1992;58:1011–1019.

Speiser PW, Serrat J, New MI, Gertner JM. Insulin insensitivity in adrenal hyperplasia due to nonclassical steroid 21-hydroxylase deficiency. J Clin Endocrinol Metab 1992;75: 1421–1424.

Spencer K. Screening for Down syndrome: the role of intact hCG and free subunit measurement. Scand J Clin Lab Invest 1993;53 suppl 216:79–97.

Stenman U-H, Bidart J-M, Birkin S, Mann K, Nisula B, O'Connor J. Standardization of protein immunoprocedures. Choriogonadotropin (CG). Scand J Clin Lab Invest 1993;53 suppl 216:42–78.

Styne DM. Puberty and its disorders in boys. Endocrinol Metab Clin North Am 1991;20:43–69.

Sugawara M, Depaolo L, Nakatani A, Dimarzo SJ, Ling N. Radioimmunoassay of follistatin: application for in vitro fertilization procedures. J Clin Endocrinol Metab 1990;71: 1672–1674.

Tallon DF, Gosling JP, Buckley PM, et al. Direct solid-phase enzyme immunoassay of progesterone in saliva. Clin Chem 1984;30:1507–1511.

Toner JP, Philput CB, Jones GS, Muasher SJ. Basal follicle stimulating hormone level is a better predictor of in vitro fertilization performance than age. Fertil Steril 1991;55:786–791.

Urban RJ, Padmanabhan V, Beitins I, Veldhuis D. Metabolic clearance of human follicle-stimulating hormone assessed by radioimmunoassay, immunoradiometric assay, and *in vitro* sertoli cell bioassay. J Clin Endocrinol Metab 1991;73:818–823.

Vance ML. When bromocriptine fails. Endocrinologist 1991;1:119–124.

Ward, TM, ed. Proteins and Tumour Markers, vol 2, part 3. In: Seth J, ed. The Immunoassay Kit Directory, Series A: Clinical Chemistry. Norwell MA: Kluwer Academic Publishers, 1993.

Wheeler MJ, ed. Steroid and Thyroid Hormones, vol 2, part 2. In: Seth J, ed. The Immunoassay Kit Directory, Series A: Clinical Chemistry. Norwell MA: Kluwer Academic Publishers, 1993.

Zacur HA, Linkins S, Chang V, Smith B, Kimball AW, Burkman R. Ethinyl estradiol and norethindrone radioimmunoassay following Sephadex LH-20 column chromatography. Clin Chim Acta 1991;204:209–215.

CHAPTER 10

Bone and Mineral Metabolism

Michael Power and
Patrick F. Fottrell

In 1987 an international Consensus Development Conference on osteoporosis high-lighted the requirement for research into methods for the prevention, diagnosis, and treatment of osteoporosis. About 20 million women are affected by osteoporosis in the United States alone, at an annual cost of $10 billion in health care and lost pro-ductivity, and by the year 2000 this is set to increase to $20 billion. In the United States also osteoporosis is responsible for, or contributes to, 1,500,000 broken bones per annum including 250,000 hip fractures (Riggs and Melton, 1992). In fact, in de-veloped countries about 75% of all fractures in women older than 45 years are related to osteoporosis. These fractures are a significant cause of morbidity and mortality, but with early detection of bone deterioration, many may be prevented.

The recent development of specific and sensitive immunoassay procedures for measuring bone proteins has increased the possibility of monitoring even small changes in bone metabolism. These developments and their clinical applications are the major focus of this chapter.

BONE METABOLISM

Bone matrix is composed of two phases: (1) the organic phase, composed mainly of type I collagen (90%), with smaller amounts of the noncollagenous proteins, and (2) the inorganic phase, composed of hydroxyapatite crystals (90%), with bicarbon-ate, citrate, and fluoride. The noncollagenous proteins include growth factors for the control and regulation of the activity of osteoblasts and osteoclasts (Canalis and Lian, 1988; Mundy, 1992), matrix gla protein, and osteocalcin. These last two proteins con-tain γ-carboxyglutamic acid, and are involved in the attraction of osteoclasts to the site of bone resorption and the subsequent differentiation of these cells (Glowacki, et al., 1991; Loesser and Wallin, 1992).

173

Even in adults, bone is very active metabolically, but formation and resorption are coordinated and coupled, so that over a period of time the amount of bone formed closely approximates the amount removed. Resorption is carried out by the osteoclasts which break down matrix components, and release into the bloodstream both inorganic (calcium, phosphate, and other mineral salts) and organic constituents (collagenous proteins, and noncollagenous proteins and their fragments). Osteoblasts synthesize collagen, alkaline phosphatase, osteocalcin, and other noncollagenous proteins.

Measurements of serum and urinary concentrations of organic bone components and their breakdown products are used to monitor rates of bone formation and resorption, although they vary in their sensitivity and specificity as indices of bone metabolism (Table 10–1). The control of bone metabolism involves the interplay of many regulatory systems both systemically and in the local environment (Canalis and Lian, 1988; Kennedy and Jones, 1991; Mundy, 1992).

Many diseases that affect bone metabolism, such as Paget's disease, renal failure, hyperparathyroidism, and osteoporosis, increase the rate of bone resorption relative to the rate of bone formation. Even very subtle alterations in the relative metabolic activities of the osteoblasts and osteoclasts that have little initial effect, can result in significant losses over time.

REGULATION OF BONE METABOLISM

Growth factors formed by osteoblasts (autocrine control) and related or nearby cells (paracrine control) regulate the activity of osteoblasts, and these in turn may be controlled by hormones (endocrine control). The growth factors include the insulin-like growth factors (IGF-I and IGF-II), transforming growth factor-β (TGF-β), and interleukin-6 (IL-6) (Canalis and Lian, 1988; Jilka, et al., 1992). The control of their for-

Table 10–1   Biochemical Markers of Bone Turnover

Sample Type	Bone Formation	Bone Resorption
Serum	Total alkaline phosphatese	Total hydroxyproline
	Bone-specific alkaline phosphatase	Tartrate-resistant acid phosphatase
	Osteocalcin	
	Procollagen 1 carboxy terminal	
	Extension peptide	
Urine	Nondialyzable hydroxyproline	Total and dialyzable hydroxyproline
		Hydroxylysine glycosides
		Collagen crosslinks

Modified from Delmas PD. Biochemical markers of bone turnover in osteoporosis. In: Riggs BL, Melton LJ, eds. Osteoporosis: Etiology, Diagnosis and Management. New York: Raven Press, 1988;297–316; and from Epstein S. Serum and urinary markers of bone remodeling: assessment of bone turnover. Endocr Rev 1988;9:437–449.

mation and secretion is being investigated in several centers, including the effects of the calcitrophic hormones such as parathyroid hormone (PTH), calcitonin (Ct), and vitamin D metabolites. The thyroid hormones (triiodothyronine [T_3] and thyroxine [T_4]), steroids such as estradiol-17β, progesterone (Komm, et al., 1988), and testosterone (Kasperk, et al., 1989) also affect bone metabolism. Receptors for these steroid hormones have been detected in osteoblasts (Komm, et al., 1988) and osteoclasts (Pensler, et al., 1990). In osteoblasts, estradiol-17β, progesterone, and testosterone stimulate the formation of IGF-I, IGF binding proteins, TGFβ (Komm, et al., 1988), type I collagen, and bone alkaline phosphatase (Prior, 1990). Osteoblasts also have receptors for thyroid (Rizzoli, et al., 1986) and glucocorticoid hormones (Chen, et al., 1986).

The influence of steroid hormones on osteoblasts and of IGFs, TGF-β, IL-6 on osteoblasts and osteoclasts has been reviewed (Kennedy and Jones, 1991). The IGFs and TGF-β promote the anabolic activity of osteoblasts, whereas IL-6 promotes the differentiation of osteoclasts. Other hormones that may influence the metabolism of osteoblasts include growth hormone (Johansen, et al., 1990) and insulin (Verhaeghe, et al., 1989, 1992).

MEASUREMENT OF BONE MASS

Techniques related to two basic radiographic approaches are generally used to measure noninvasively bone mass: gamma (or x-ray) photon absorptiometry and quantitative computed tomography. Current versions of bone densitometers use dual energies to cancel out the effects of variable soft tissue contributions, as in dual photon absorptiometry with ^{125}I and ^{153}Gd sources, dual energy x-ray absorptiometry (DEXA), and dual energy quantitative computed tomography (DEQCT). DEXA is now widely used, but because DEQCT also takes protein conformation into account, it promises to be more valuable.

A recent study has indicated that standard bone mass measurements (DEXA) combined with relatively cheap biochemical assessments (urinary hydroxyproline and total alkaline phosphatase) are better than bone mass measurements alone (Hansen, et al., 1991). This also clearly implies that the use of newer, more specific markers of bone metabolism will be even more efficient at early prediction of bone disease. Biochemical markers of bone metabolism may reflect the tensile strength of bone as well as bone mass (Screening for Osteoporosis, 1992).

MARKERS OF BONE TURNOVER

Bone Formation

Osteocalcin

Osteocalcin (bone Gla protein), the most abundant noncollagenous protein in mature human bone (1% to 2% total protein), is a relatively small (mol wt 5800) bone-specific protein, synthesized by osteoblasts and incorporated into the bone matrix (Fig. 10–1). Its precise function is not known but the three γ-carboxyglutamic acid (Gla) residues confer on it the ability to bind free calcium and the hydroxyapatite of bone matrix. It may play a role in the movement of osteoclasts to a site of bone resorption and promote their activity at this area. 1,25-Dihydroxyvitamin D_3 (calcitriol) stimulates the biosynthesis of osteocalcin, and vitamin K_1 is a cofactor for carboxylation of its glutamic acid residues. Part of the newly synthesized osteocalcin that is not adsorbed to hydroxyapatite escapes into the plasma, and therefore the measurement of intact osteocalcin in plasma has received considerable attention as a possible marker for bone formation. Its concentration is raised in patients with metabolic bone disease characterized by increased bone turnover (Epstein, 1988).

Most commercial immunoassay kits for serum osteocalcin use ^{125}I-iodinated or enzyme-labeled osteocalcin in competitive assays. Because of the close homology between bovine and human osteocalcin (they differ by only 5 amino acids out of 50), antisera raised against bovine osteocalcin cross-react strongly with the human protein, and most commercial immunoassays have antisera raised against bovine osteocalcin. However, some immunoassays are available with antibodies against intact human osteocalcin, or against peptides with amino acid sequences homologous with human osteocalcin, but these latter assays are likely to detect similar peptides as well as intact osteocalcin. Two-site immunometric assays have also been developed (e.g.,

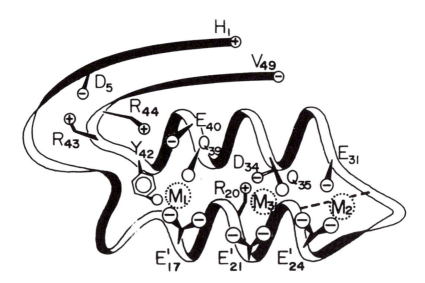

Figure 10–1. Structure of human osteocalcin which, as in most species, has 49 amino acid residues. Common structural features found in osteocalcins include the strongly conserved central portion consisting of two antiparallel α-helical domains, and the Gla residues (E') at positions 17, 21, and 24. These together with glutamate (E), aspartate (D), and other residues in the midregion give osteocalcin its Ca^{2+} indicated by M^1, M^2 and M^3) binding properties. (From the cover of *The Anatomical Record* 1989, 224, issue 2. Reproduced with permission.)

Monaghan, et al., 1993) and these may offer advantages because of their greater intrinsic specificity and sensitivity.

The pronounced differences between published serum osteocalcin concentration ranges for healthy persons is probably due to differences in the specificities of the different antisera used (Power and Fottrell, 1991). Some antisera of all types detect peptides derived from osteocalcin as well as the intact molecule, and these peptieds may reflect the rate of bone resorption rather than the rate of bone formation, which is the objective of measuring the intact molecule.

In the selection of a suitable immunoassay kit for the measurement of osteocalcin, attention should be paid to several criteria, including cross-reactivity of the antibody with osteocalcin-related peptides and the extent to which the assay has been analytically and clinically validated. In this regard, particular attention should be given to the degree to which the assay measures osteocalcin in human serum independently of the volume of the sample being measured.

Serum osteocalcin concentrations are measured to monitor bone formation in osteoporosis, renal failure, Paget's disease, hyperthyroidosis, skeletal metastases, and diseases related to excess glucocorticoids (Epstein, 1988; Lian and Gundberg, 1988). Osteocalcin measurements provide a more specific index of bone metabolism than indices such as total serum alkaline phosphatase or urinary hydroxyproline. Its level in serum correlates with two of the most reliable methods for measuring bone density: DEXA and dual photon absorbtiometry (Lee et al., 1990). Its measurement may, therefore, be a useful adjunct to the latter technology in the management of patients at risk for osteoporosis. However, the variety of analytic and physiologic factors that probably contribute to the wide range of published values must first be addressed (Azria, 1989; Power and Fottrell, 1991). Normal concentration ranges should be established in men and women by means of fully validated and standardized immunoassays, and these studies must also take into account ethnic factors, age, circadian, menstrual and seasonal variations, as well as levels of exercise and the use of drugs (Delmas, et al., 1990; Power and Fottrell, 1991).

Bone Isoenzyme of Alkaline Phosphatase

The function of the bone isoenzyme may include hydrolysis of pyrophosphate, inhibition of mineralization, release of phosphate from bone for the mineralization process, localization of phosphate for the initiation of mineralization, and as a nucleator for the mineralization process (Beertsen and VandenBos, 1992). Because of its relatively large molecular weight (140,000), alkaline phosphatase is not excreted by the kidney, and has a half life of 1 to 2 days in the circulation (Posen and Gruntstein, 1982). Its levels in plasma are therefore not influenced significantly by decreases in the glomular filtration rate which, in contrast, influences the serum concentrations of many other bone biomarkers such as serum osteocalcin and the pyridinoline crosslinks (Delmas, et al., 1983).

Total serum alkaline phosphatase measurements have been used for at least 60 years in the management of patients with various bone disorders. However, its specificity is limited because it represents the combined activities of at least *five* isoenzymes from liver, bone (also found in liver and early placenta), placenta, intestine, and germ cells (Fishman, 1990).

The amino acid sequences of the placental, germ cell, and intestinal enzymes closely resemble each other, but are different from the tissue-unspecific isoenzymes from bone, kidney, and liver. In all tissues the isoenzymes are attached to the plasma membrane and enter the circulation when the membranes are damaged. It appears that most of the enzyme activity is releasable from the membrane by phosphatidylinositol-specific phospholipase C (Incerpi, et al., 1992) and that it is anchored to the cell membrane via a phosphoinositide linked to the hydrophobic carboxy terminal of the peptide backbone (Fishman, 1990).

Several methods have been devised to differentiate the isoenzymes of alkaline phosphatase in serum including electrophoresis, heat- and urea-based selective denaturatin, kinetic methods, and chromatograhic procedures with wheat-germ lectin or ion-exchange resins. Although these methods do not totally discriminate between the isoenzymes, relatively good correlations have been obtained with histologic parameters of bone formation in some studies (Brixen, et al., 1989). Antisera have been developed against the bone isoenzyme, which differs in cross-reactivity with other isoenzymes of alkaline phosphatase; one antiserum has only 3% cross-reactivity with the liver isoenzyme (Duda, et al., 1988). Immunoassays for bone alkaline phosphatase are available commercially, but have not yet undergone thorough clinical evaluation.

Type I Collagen Extension Peptide (pColl-1-C)

The collagens found most extensively in bone are types I and III, although the latter is not specific to bone matrix. Carboxy- and amino-terminal fragments released after collagen biosynthesis are excreted in the urine, and their concentrations are indicative of the rate of collagen formation (Simon, et al., 1984). An immunoassay for the measurement of C-terminal peptide (pColl-1-C) in urine has been developed. In Paget's disease the concentrations of pColl-1-C are increased (Taubman, et al., 1976), and during treatment with antiresorptive agents, such as calcitonin and the bisphosphonates, levels decrease significantly (Hassager, et al., 1991). The concentration of pColl-1-C is higher in postmenopausal than in premenopausal women. Treatment with antiresorptive agents and regimens, such as estrogen-progestagen hormone replacement therapy and anabolic steroids, results in a relatively rapid decrease in the levels of urinary pColl-1-C (Hassager, et al., 1991).

The main problem with measurement of pColl-1-C is the interference of peptides from the less specific type III collagen, which are also present in urine. This should be eliminated by the use of more specific antisera. Another factor that must be considered is interindividual variation in the clearance rates of pColl-1-C (Parfitt and Kleerekopper, 1984). The development of more specific, fully validated immunoassays and their clinical evaluation will contribute to the elucidation of the role of pColl-1-C measurements in the investigation of bone disorders.

Bone Resorption

Collagen Crosslinks

Collagen conformation is stabilized by the nonreducible pyridinoline crosslinks, hydroxylysylpyridinoline and lysylpyridinoline (Fig. 10–2). The lysylpyridinoline crosslinks are primarily found in the type I collagen of bone, whereas the hydroxylysylpyridinoline derivative is present in collagen from several tissues (Eyre, 1984). During bone resorption by osteoclasts the lysylpyridinoline links are released and are excreted in urine. They are relatively stable and their urinary concentration reflects the rate of bone resorption (Uebelhart, et al., 1990, 1991). Interestingly, lysylpyridinoline concentrations decrease on administration of inhibitors of osteoclastic activity such as the bisphosphonates, calcitonin, and anabolic steroids, after hormone replacement therapy (Uebelhart, et al., 1991; Robins, et al., 1991a), and after parathyroidectomy (Seibel, et al., 1992). Levels have been measured in patients with increased rates of bone resorption, for example, in Paget's disease, primary hyperparathyroidism, osteoporosis, and osteomalacia (Table 10–2). Lysylpyridinoline concentrations are decreased in collagen from the femoral head of osteoporotic patients, and may therefore be associated with the increase in bone fragility associated with osteoporosis (Bailey, et al, 1992).

The most commonly used procedure to measure lysylpyridinoline or hydroxylysylpyridinoline crosslinks is high performance liquid chromatography (HPLC) (Robins, et al., 1991a), but the published methods have a low throughput of samples. In addition, the validation of many of these methods as published may not have been sufficiently rigorous. There is also the possibility of interference from glycosylated

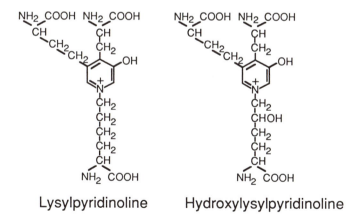

Lysylpyridinoline   Hydroxylysylpyridinoline

Figure 10–2. Structures of the nonreducible pyridinoline crosslinks of collagen, hydroxylysylpyridinoline, and lysylpyridinoline.

Table 10–2   Concentrations of Lysylpyridinoline in Metabolic Bone Diseases

Reference	Control	Lysylpyridinoline (pmol/μmol creatinine in urine)			
		Paget's disease	*Hyperpara-thyroidism*	*Osteo-malacia*	*Osteo-porosis*
Robins, et al., 1991	1–14*	80 ± 57[†]	52 ± 26	45 ± 19	—
Black, et al., 1988	3–11	494	—	—	—
Uebelhart, et al., 1991					
Pre HRT[‡]	—	—	—	—	2–18
Post HRT	—	—	—	—	2–7.5
Uebelhart, et al., 1990	6.3 ± 3.4	75 ± 80	15.8 ± 9.9	—	—

*Range of concentrations found.
[†]Mean ± SD.
[‡]HRT, hormone replacement therapy.

forms of the pyridinolines, which may coelute with the analyte if elution conditions are not optimized.

Immunoassays have been developed for free hydroxylysylpyridinoline derivative in urine (Robins, 1982) and, more recently, for the pyridinoline crosslinked carboxy-terminal telopeptide of type I collagen, without the need for preliminary hydrolysis and extraction steps (Ristelli, et al., 1993). Preliminary hydrolysis steps may alter the chemical structure of collagen crosslinks, and promote the formation of diastereoisomers. Free crosslinks cross-react only about 5% with antisera raised against the acid treated pyridinolines (Robins, et al., 1991b). Generally, all three hydrolysis steps are better omitted at all stages for the preparation of immunogen, standard and for the pretreatment of samples.

A monoclonal antibody against type I collagen crosslinked N-telopeptides has been obtained and used to develop a labeled second-antibody, limited-reagent assay for urine samples (Hanson, et al., 1992). The authors claim that in a study of early postmenopausal women this assay was able to distinguish high bone-resorbing subjects with greater consistency than analysis of urinary pryridinolines or hydroxyproline.

The measurement of urinary collagen crosslinks has considerable potential for monitoring bone resorption. The extent to which this potential will be realized must await comprehensive studies with fully validated immunoassays on samples from both controls and patients with metabolic bone diseases.

Tartrate-Resistant Acid Phosphatase

Bone tartrate-resistant acid phosphatase (TRAP) (isoenzyme type 5b) is a lysosomal enzyme found mainly in osteoclasts, platelets, spleen, and erythrocytes whose function in bone is not understood (Minkin, 1982). It is resistant to tartrate, unlike the prostate isoenzyme, and it has been used clinically as a marker of bone resorption. Levels fivefold higher than controls have been found in patients with Paget's disease and primary hyperparathyroidism, which have relatively high rates of bone resorption. Levels of TRAP decrease below control values in postmenopausal women on hormone replacement therapy or anabolic steroids (Stepan, et al., 1989). There is some doubt, however, whether TRAP activity is confined to osteoclasts because macrophages in tissue culture also express the enzyme (Modderman, et al., 1991).

An immunoassay for TRAP has been developed with an antibody raised against enzyme from human leukemic spleen (Kraenzlin et al., 1990) and increased levels were detected in patients with Paget's disease and primary hyperparathyroidism, which are characterised by increased rates of bone resorption. While there is good correlation between serum levels of TRAP, osteocalcin, and serum levels of bone-specific alkaline phosphatase, further studies are required to assess its clinical potential.

Hormones Controlling Calcium Metabolism

In general, parathyroid hormone (PTH) acts to maintain a normal level of calcium in extracellular fluids by promoting renal calcium reabsorption and phosphate excretion, and by promoting the conversion of 25-hydroxyvitamin D to 1,25-dihydroxy-vitamin D. PTH release is mainly stimulated by low ambient calcium levels. 1,25-Dihydroxyvitamin D increases intestinal absorption of calcium, in part by inducing the synthesis of intestinal calcium-binding protein. Calcitonin inhibits the function of osteoclasts reducing bone resorption, and decreases the renal reabsorption of calcium.

Parathyroid Hormone

The measurement of serum PTH has been used in the management of bone and related diseases for many years. Its major present applications are in the investigation of hypocalcemia and hypercalcemia, and in the management of patients with renal bone disease.

PTH has 84 amino acid residues and is released in the intact form from the parathyroid gland. It is subsequently cleaved by the Kupffer cells of the liver and by other tissues to give various fragments, classed as C-terminal, midregion, and N-terminal. Most biologic activity in the circulation is due to intact PTH, but some N-terminal fragments have PTH activity (Armitage, 1986). PTH is also being used therapeutically to increase the rate of bone turnover.

Immunoassays for PTH may be divided into three types (Mallette, 1991): (1) two-site immunometric assays for intact PTH, which are now the most common; (2) competitive immunoassays which detect intact PTH and midregion peptides, intact PTH and N-terminal peptides, or intact PTH and C-terminal peptides; and (3) competitive immunoassays which detect C-terminal peptides (65–84), midregion peptides (34–68), or N-terminal peptides (1–34) only. Because they are cleared more slowly, midregion and C-terminal fragments may represent an index of integrated PTH secretion. The measurement of N-terminal peptides may facilitate the monitoring of acute changes in PTH secretion. Measurements of intact PTH correlate best with biologically active hormone.

Some PTH radioimmunoassays (RIAs) take from 36 to 136 hours, while immunometric assays with nonisotopic label take as little as 2 hours. PTH assays are among the most widely used immunoassays in the clinical laboratory (Bilezikian, 1992; Mallette, 1991). Midregion and intact PTH assays are generally accepted as being more useful, although all assays can distinguish between PTH levels due to hyperparathyroidism and malignancy-associated hypercalcemia (Goltzman and Hendy, 1990), where PTH levels are often below the sensitivity of most immunoassays.

Some fragments from the C-terminal region of PTH-related peptide (PTHrP is a 139 residue protein secreted by a variety of cancers) inhibit bone resorption and may be responsible for hypercalcemia of malignancy (Fenton, et al., 1991). An immunometric assay for PTHrP is now commercially available and has recently been evaluated in the diagnosis of hypercalcemia of malignancy (Fraser, et al., 1993).

See Tables 10–3 and 10–4 for information on the differential diagnosis of hypocalcemia and hypercalcemia, respectively.

Vitamin D and Its Metabolites

While recent research has confirmed the action of vitamin D as a hormone essential for the efficient absorption and utilization of calcium metabolism, its roles have been greatly extended and its action shown to be nongenomic as well as genomic (Walters, 1992).

Immunoassays and protein binding assays (with animal vitamin D binding protein) for 25-hydroxyvitamin D in plasma having similar cross-reactivity with vitamins D_2 and D_3 are used to determine vitamin D nutritional status (Hollis, et al., 1993). The development of assays for the detection of biologically active vitamin D (1,25 dihydroxyvitamin D_2 or D_3) in serum is difficult because of interference from structurally related metabolites such as 25-hydroxyvitamin D (Fig. 10–3), present at 1000-fold higher concentrations (Christakos, et al., 1989). Therefore, a purification/concentration step is required prior to immunoassay (Clemens, 1990). The development of highly specific and high off limits antisera leading to assays not requiring a preassay purification step would be a major advantage.

Calcitonin

Calcitonin is a 32 amino acid peptide produced by the C cells in the thyroid gland in response to increased plasma calcium concentrations. Most of the circulating calcitonin is present as aggregates of unknown biologic activity (Eastell, et al., 1988) that may include a carrier protein.

The development of immunoassays for calcitonin has suffered many of the problems already discussed with reference to the measurement of PTH and 1,25-dihydroxyvitamin D. Some immunoassays require an extraction step with silica gel to separate monomeric calcitonin from larger complexes before assay, but they detect only 15% to 20% of the total immunoreactive calcitonin in the circulation (Body and Heath, 1983). In addition, levels determined after extraction do not agree well with total levels (Eastell, et al., 1988). Other assays require an initial immunoextraction procedure (Shamonki, et al., 1988). Calcitonin is now also determined by means of two-site immunometric assays with monoclonal antibodies and without an extrac-

Table 10–3   Differential Diagnosis of Hypocalcemia

	PTH	Phosphate	25-Hydroxy-vitamin D	1,25 Dihydroxy-vitamin D	Other Indications
25-Hydroxyvitamin D deficiency (dietary deficiency or malabsorption)	High	Low	Low	Low to normal	Blood alkaline phosphatase elevated
1,25 Dihydroxyvitamin D deficiency (renal failure)	High	Low to high	Normal	Very low	Blood phosphate usually high in renal failure
Resistance to 1,25-dihydroxy vitamin D	High	Low	Normal	Very high	Urinary cAMP* secretion usually normal to high
PTH deficiency (hypoparathyroidism)	Very low	High	Normal	Low	Low blood Mg^{2+}, TRP† is reduced after exogenous PTH
PTH resistance (pseudo-hypoparathyroidism) types 1 and 2	High	High	Normal	Normal to low	Type 1: no cAMP or TRP response to exogenous PTH. Type 2: normal cAMP but no TRP response to PTH.

*cAMP, 3′,5′-Cyclic adenosine monophosphate. A range of enzyme, radioimmunoassay, and competitive protein binding assays with tritiated labels, mostly validated for the analysis of urine samples, are commercially available.

†TRP, Tubular response of phosphate. The TRP is reduced after the administration of exogenous PTH in healthy persons.

Table 10–4   Differential Diagnosis of Hypercalcemia

	PTH	Phosphate	1,25 Dihydroxy-vitamin D	Urine Ca^{2+}	Urine cAMP*	Other Indications
Primary hyper-parathyroidism	Very high	Low	High	High	High	
Humoral hyper-parathyroidism of malignancy	Very low	Normal or low	Normal or low	High	High	PTHrP may be elevated (60% of cases)
Familial hypocalciuric hypercalcemia	Normal, low or high	Normal or low	Normal	Very low	Normal	Ratio of (Ca^{2+} clearance)/(creatinine clearance) < 0.01
Granulomatous disease	Low	Normal	High or normal	Normal or high	Low	
Vitamin D intoxication	Low	High	Very high	High	Low	25-Hydroxy-vitamin D very high
Immobilization	Normal to low	Normal or low	Low	High	Low or normal	Seen in Paget's disease
Milk-alkali syndrome	Low	High	Low	Normal or low	Low	Renal function diminished

*cAMP, 3′,5′-Cyclic adenosine monophosphate; see also note to Table 10–3.

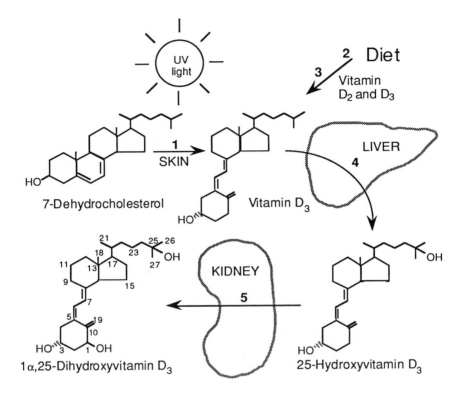

Figure 10–3. The main reactions of vitamin D production and activation, and their locations. In addition, the keratinocytes, which produce vitamin D, can also hydroxylate 25-hydroxyvitamin D to 1,25 dihydroxyvitamin D_3, and this regulates their proliferation and differentiation (Bickle and Pillai, 1993). The term vitamin D includes vitamin D_3 (shown above) and vitamin D_2 (which has an extra methyl group at C24 and an extra double bond between C22 and C23). Either may be added to foods and both are metabolized by the same pathways giving the corresponding vitamin D_2 metabolites. The points where blocks can occur are numbered. *1.* Very low exposure to sunlight and/or heavy pigmentation. 2. Nutritional inadequacy. *3.* Malabsorption syndromes or surgery of the gastrointestinal tract. *4.* Liver disease or anticonvulsant drugs. *5.* Renal failure, 1α-hydroxylase deficiency, nephrectomy, and hypoparathyroidism. In addition, functional defects in the intracellular receptor binding of 1,25-dihydroxyvitamin D can also result in symptoms corresponding to vitamin D deficiency.

tions step, and these may give much higher levels than some previous RIAs (Yatscoff and Dube, 1988; Kempter and Ritter, 1991).

Calcitonin assays are used in the management of patients with medullary thyroid carcinoma and as part of the pentagastrin stimulation test for the early discovery of relevant multiple endocrine neoplasia syndromes (Chap. 16). Calcitonin has not received much attention as a bone biomarker, because its levels are apparently not decreased in osteoporosis or other bone related conditions (Saggese, et al., 1992).

Synthetic salmon calcitonin is used to inhibit osteoclast activity in patients with metabolic bone disease and its level in the circulation may be monitored by means of a specific immunoradiometric assay (Deftos, 1992).

The measurement of specific bone markers such as osteocalcin, lysylpyridinoline, and the bone isoenzyme of alkaline phosphatase is supplanting the less specific markers such as urinary hydroxyproline and total serum acid- and alkaline-phosphatases. However, extensive studies with fully validated assays are essential to properly assess their full clinical potential.

The only cost-effective approach to osteoporosis is prevention. Intervention can be initiated in post- or perimenopausal women who are at risk for osteoporosis because of low bone density. A combination of the measurement of bone density, and the measurement of specific bone biomarkers may identify "rapid bone losers" and predict the risk of fractures better than bone density measurements alone (Riggs and Melton, 1992; Dixon, 1992).

The measurement of PTH remains exceedingly important in the evaluation of the patient with hypercalcemia.

REFERENCES

Armitage EK. Parathyrin (parathyroid hormone) metabolism and methods for assay. Clin Chem 1986;32:418–424.

Azria M. The value of biomarkers in detecting alterations in bone metabolism. Calcif Tiss Int 1989;45:7–11.

Bailey AJ, Wotton SF, Sims TJ, Thompson PW. Post-translational modifications of the collagen of human osteoporotic femoral head. Biochem Biophys Res Commun 1992; 185:801–805.

Beertsen W, VandenBos T. Alkaline phosphatase induces the mineralization of sheets of collagen implanted subcutaneously in the rat. J Clin Invest 1992;89:1874–1980.

Bickle DD, Pillai S. Vitamin D, Calcium and epidermal differentiation. Endocr Rev. 1993;14:3–19.

Bilezikian JP. Clinical utility of assays for parathyroid hormone-related protein. Clin Chem 1992;38:179–181.

Black D, Duncan A, Robins SP. Quantitative analysis of the pyridinium crosslinks of collagen in urine using ion-paired reverse-phase high-performance liquid chromatography. Analyt Biochem 1988;169:197–302.

Body JJ, Heath H III. Estimates of circulating calcitonin: physiological studies in normal and thyroidectomized men. J Clin Endocrinol Metab 1983;57:897–903.

Brixen K, Nielsen HK, Eriksen EF, Charles P, Mosekilde L. Efficacy of wheat germ lectin-precipitited alkaline phosphatase in serum as an estimator of bone mineralization rate. Calcif Tiss Int 1989;44:93–98.

Canalis E, Lian JB. Effects of bone associated growth factors on DNA, collagen, and osteocalcin synthesis, in cultured rat fetal calvariae. Bone 1988;9:243–246.

Chen TL, Hauschka PV, Feldman D. Dexamethasone increases 1,25 dihydroxyvitamin D receptor levels and augments responses in rat osteoblast-like cells. Endocrinology 1986;118:1119–1126.

Christakos S. Gabrielidis C, Rhoten WB. Vitamin D-dependant calcium binding proteins: chemistry, distribution, functional considerations, and molecular biology. Endocr Rev 1989;10:3–26.

Clemens TL. Useful clinical assays for vitamin D metabolites. Trends Endocrinol Metab 1990; Jan/Feb:129–133.

Consensus development conference: prophylaxis and treatment of osteoporosis. Br Med J 1987;295:914–915.

Deftos LJ. Two-site immunoradiometric assay of intact salmon calcitonin. Clin Chem 1992;38:2284–2286.

Delmas PD. Biochemical markers of bone turnover in osteoporosis. In: Riggs BL, Melton LJ, eds. Osteoporosis: Etiology, Diagnosis and Management. New York: Raven Press, 1988;297–316.

Delmas PD, Christiansen C, Mann KG, Price PA. Bone gla protein (osteocalcin) assay: standardization report. J Bone Miner Res 1990;5:5–11.

Delmas PD, Wilson DM, Mann KG, Riggs BL. Effect of renal function on plasma levels of bone Gla-protein. J Clin Endocrinol Metab 1983;57:1028–1030.

Dixon A St.-J. Health of the nation and osteoporosis. Ann Rheum Dis 1992;51:914–918.

Duda RJ, O'Brien JF, Katzmann JA, Peterson JM, Mann KG, Riggs BL. Concurrent assays of circulating bone Gla protein and bone alkaline phosphatase: effects of age, sex and metabolic bone disease. J Clin Endocrinol Metab 1988;66:951–957.

Eastell R, Heath H III, Kumar R, Riggs BL. Hormonal factors: PTH, vitamin D, and calcitonin. In: Riggs BL, Melton LJ, eds. Osteoporosis: Etiology, Diagnosis, and Management. New York: Raven Press, 1988;373–388.

Epstein S. Serum and urinary markers of bone remodeling: assessment of bone turnover. Endocr Rev 1988;9:437–449.

Eyre DR. Cross-linking in collagen and elastin. Annu Rev Biochem 1984;53:717–748.

Fenton AJ, Kemp BE, Hammonds RG Jr, et al. A potent inhibitor of osteoclastic bone resorption within a highly conserved pentapeptide region of parathyroid hormone-related protein, PTHrP [107–111]. Endocrinology 1991;129:3424–3426.

Fishman WH. Alkaline phosphatase isozymes: recent progress. Clin Biochem 1990;23:99–104.

Fraser WD, Robinson J, Lawton R, et al. Clinical and laboratory studies of a new immunoradiometric assay of parathyroid hormone-related protein. Clin Chem 1993;39:414–419.

Glowacki J, Rey C, Glimcher MJ, Cox KA, Lian J. A role for osteocalcin in osteoclast differentiation. J Cell Biochem 1991;45:292–302.

Goltzman D, Hendy GN. Parathyroid hormone. In: Becker KL, ed. Principles and Practice of Endocrinology and Metabolism. Philadelphia: JB Lippincott, 1990;402–412.

Hansen M, Overgaard K, Riis B, Christiansen C. Role of peak bone mass and bone loss in postmenopausal osteoporosis. Br Med J 1991;303:961–964.

Hanson DA, Weis MAE, Bollen AM, Maslan SL, Singer FR, Eyre DR. A specific immunoassay for monitoring human bone resorption: quantitation of type I collagen cross-linked N-telopeptides inurine. J Bone Miner Res 1992;7:1251–1258.

Hassager C, Jensen L T, Johansen JS, et al. The carboxy-terminal propeptide of type I procollagen in serum as a marker of bone formation: the effect of nandrolene decanoate and female sex hormones. Metabolism 1991;40:205–208.

Hollis BW, Kamerud JQ, Selvaag SR, Lorenz JD, Napoli JL. Determination of vitamin D status by radioimmunoassay with an ^{125}I-labeled tracer. Clin Chem 1993;39:529–533.

Incerpi S, Baldini P, Belo M, Luly P. Insulin-dependent release of 5'-nucleotidase and alkaline phosphatase from liver plasma membranes. Biosci Rep 1992;12:101–108.

Jilka RL, Hangoc G, Girasole G, et al. Increased osteoclast development after estrogen loss; mediation by interleukin -6. Science 1992;257:88–91.

Johansen J, Pedersen S, Jorgensen S, et al. Effects of growth hormone (GH) on plasma bone Gla protein in GH-deficient adults. J Clin Endocrinol Metab 1990;70:916–919.

Kasperk C, Wergedal JE, Farley JR, Linkhart TA, Turner RT, Baylink DJ. Androgens directly stimulate proliferation of bone cells in vitro. Endocrinology 1989;124:1576–1578.

Kempter B, Ritter MM. Unexpected high calcitonin concentrations after pentagastrin stimulation. Clin Chem 1991;37:473–474.

Kennedy RL, Jones TH. Cytokines in endocrinology: their effects in health and in disease. J Endocrinol 1991;129:167–178.

Komm B S, Terpening CM, Brnz DJ, et al. Estrogen binding, receptor mRNA, and biological response in osteoblast-like osteosarcoma cells. Science 1988;241:81–83.

Kraenzlin M, Lau KHW, Liang L, et al. Development of an immunoassay for human serum osteoclastic tartrate-resistant acid phosphatase. J Clin Endocrinol Metab 1990; 71:442–451.

Lee MS, Kim SY, Lee MC, et al. Negative correlation between the change in bone mineral density and serum osteocalcin in patients with hyperthyroidism. J Clin Endocrinol Metab 1990;70:766–770.

Lian JB, Gundberg CM. Osteocalcin, biochemical considerations and clinical applications. Clin Orthop Relat Res 1988;226:267–291.

Loesser RF, Wallin R. Cell adhession to matrix Gla protein and its inhibition by the Arg-Gly-Asp-containing peptide. J Biol Chem 1992;267:9459–9462.

Mallette LE. Immunologic assays for parathyroid hormone: principles and utilization in disease states. Adv Endocrinol Metab 1991;2:183–204.

Minkin C. Bone acid phosphatase: tartrate-resistant acid phosphatase as a marker of osteoclast function. Calcif Tiss Int 1982;34:285–290.

Modderman WE, Tuinenburg-Bol Raap AC, Nijweide PJ. Tartrate-resistant acid phosphatase is not an exclusive marker for mouse osteoclasts in cell culture. Bone 1991;12:81–87.

Monaghan DA, Power MJ, Fottrell PF. Sandwich enzyme immunoassay of osteocalcin in serum with use of an antibody against human osteocalcin. Clin Chem 1993;39:942–947.

Mundy GR. Cytokines and local factors which affect osteoclast function. Int J Cell Cloning 1992;10:215–222.

Parfitt AM, Kleerekopper M. Diagnostic value of bone histomorphometry and comparison of histological measurements and biochemical indices of bone remodeling. In: Christiansen C, Arnaud CD, Nordin BEC, Parfitt AM, Peck WA, Riggs BL, eds. Osteoporosis. Glostrup, Denmark: Aalborg Stiftsbogtrykeri, 1984;111–120.

Pensler JM, Radosevich JA, Higbee R, Langman CB. Osteoclasts isolated from membranous bone in children exhibit nuclear estrogen and progesterone receptors. J Bone Miner Res 1990;5:797–802.

Posen S, Gruntstein HS. Turnover rate of skeletal alkaline phosphatase in humans. Clin Chem 1982;28:153–154.

Power MJ, Fottrell PF. Osteocalcin: diagnostic methods and clinical applications. Crit Rev Clin Lab Sci 1991;28:287–335.

Prior G. Progesterone as a bone-trophic hormone. Endocr Rev 1990;11:386–398.

Riggs BL, Melton LJ. The prevention and treatment of osteoporosis. New Engl J Med 1992;327:620–627.

Ristelli J, Elomaa I, Niemi S, Novamo A, Ristelli L. Radioimmunoassay for the pyridinoline cross-linked carboxy-terminal telopeptide of Type I collagen: a new serum marker of bone collagen degradation. Clin Chem 1993;39:635–640.

Rizzoli R, Poser J, Burgi U. Nuclear thyroid hormone receptors in cultured bone cells. Metabolism 1986;35:71–74.

Robins SP, Black D, Paterson CR, Reid DM, Duncan A, Seibel MJ. Evaluation of urinary hydroxypyridium crosslink measurement as resorption markers in metabolic bone diseases. Eur J Clin Invest 1991a;21:310–315.

Robins SP, Duncan A, McLaren AM. Structural specificity of an ELISA for the collagen cross links, pyridinoline: implications for the measurement of free pyridinium cross links as indices of resorption in metabolic bone diseases. J Bone Miner Res 1991b; (suppl 6):S244.

Robins SP. An enzyme-linked immunoassay for the collagen crosslink, pyridinoline. Biochem J 1982;207:617–620.

Saggese G, Berteloni S, Bareoncelli GOI, Federico G. Assessment of thyroidal "C" cell secretion in osteoporotic girls with Turner's syndrome. Acta Paediatr 1992;81:532–535.

Screening for Osteoporosis to Prevent Fractures. Effective Health Care. Leeds: University of Leeds, 1992; 1–11.

Seibel MJ, Robins SP, Bilizekian JP. Urinary pyridinium cross links of collagen: specific markers of bone resorption in metabolic bone disease. Trends Endocrinol Metab 1992;3:263–270.

Shamonki IM, Frumar AM, Tatanya IV, et al. Age related changes in calcitonin secretion in females. J Clin Endocrinol Metab 1980;50:437–439.

Simon LS, Parfitt AM, Villanueva AR, Krane SM. Procollagen type 1 C-terminal extension peptide (p Coll-1-C) in serum as a marker of collagen syntheseis: correlation with iliac trabecular bone formation rate. Calcif Tiss Int 1984;36:498.

Stepan JJ, Pospichal J, Schreiber V, Kanka J, Presl J, Pacovsky V. The application of plasma tartrate-resistant acid phosphatase to assess changes in bone resorption in response to artificial menopause and its treatment with estrogen or norethisterone. Calcif Tiss Int 1989;45:273–280.

Taubman MB, Kammerman S, Goldberg B. Radioimmunoassay of procollagen in serum of patients with Paget's disease. Proc Soc Exp Biol Med 1976;152:284–290.

Uebelhart D, Gineyts E, Chapuy M-C, Delmas PD. Urinary excretion of the pyridinium crosslinks: a new marker of bone resorption in metabolic bone disease. Bone Miner 1990;8:87–96.

Uebelhart D, Schlemmer A, Johansen JS, Gineyts E, Christiansen C, Delmas PD. Effect of menopause and hormone replacement therapy on urinary excretion of pyridinium excretion of pyridinium cross-links. J Clin Endocrinol Metab 1991;72:367–373.

Verhaeghe J, Suiker AMH, Nyomba BL, et al. Bone mineral homeostasis in spontaneously diabetic rats. II. Impaired bone turnover and decreased osteocalcin synthesis. Endocrinology 1989;124:573–582.

Verhaeghe J, Suiker AHM, Visser VJ, van Herck E, van Bree R, Bouillon R. The effects of systemic insulin, insulin-like growth factor-1, and growth hormone on bone growth and turnover in spontaneously diabetic BB rats. J Endocrinol 1992;134:485–492.

Walters MR. Newly identified actions of the vitamin D endocrine system. Endocr Rev 1992;13:719–764.

Yatscoff RW, Dube WJ. Reference interval for basal calcitonin and calcitonin concentrations after pentagastrin infusion. Clin Chem 1988;34:1931–1932.

CHAPTER 11

Gastrointestinal Tract Hormones and Lipoproteins

Penelope M. Clarke

The gastrointestinal tract (GIT) is a large and complex organ with many functions, most of which are directly related to the digestion and absorption of food. Although the GIT has long been known to have an endocrine role (secretin was discovered in 1902 and was the first substance to be named a hormone), an understanding of the complexity of the GIT's endocrine functions has developed only recently. This is mainly because many of its endocrine functions are associated with specialized cells that are scattered throughout the gastrointestinal mucosa rather than gathered together as glands.

The absorption of lipids from the small intestine, their transport to the liver and adipose and other tissues, and the mobilization of lipid stores are all dependent on the participation of the apolipoproteins. Although many apolipoproteins are synthesized in non-GIT tissues, immunoassays for both the apolipoproteins and the GIT hormones, and their clinical applications, are discussed in this chapter.

GASTROINTESTINAL HORMONES

There have been over 40 peptides identified in the GIT and pancreas that may have regulatory functions and, as such, act as endocrine or paracrine agents or as neurotransmitters. Table 11–1 lists some of the most important and their locations. Many have a broad distribution throughout the GIT, for example, vasoactive intestinal peptide (VIP); and others are more localized to a particular cell type, for example, insulin in the cells of the islets of Langerhans (Said, 1980; Ballesta, et al., 1985). Much of the clinical interest in measuring many of these hormones is because they are associated with GIT tumors.

The pancreatic endocrine tumors (Table 11–2) may contain different cell types; the predominant cell type and its secreted hormone usually define the clinical syn-

Table 11–1   Some Hormonally Active Peptides Found in the
Gastrointestinal Tract

Peptide	Location
Cholecystokinin (CKK)	Small intestine
Enteroglucagon (GLI)	Small and large intestine
Gastrin	Stomach and small intestine
Glucagon	Pancreas
Glucose-dependent insulinotropic hormone (GIP)	Small intestine
Insulin	Pancreas
Motilin	Small intestine
Neurotensin	Small intestine
Pancreatic polypeptide (PP)	Pancreas
Peptide histidine methionine (PHM)	Whole GIT
Peptide tyrosine tyrosine (PYY)	Small and large intestine
Secretin	Small intestine
Somatostatin	Whole GIT
Vasoactive intestinal paptide (VIP)	Whole GIT

drome. However, a significant number (20% to 40%) are nonfunctioning. It is also possible that co-occurring peptide release may modify the clinical expression of the tumor. A significant number of patients with such tumors are found on long-term follow-up examination to have significant elevations in other GIT hormones.

Assay Methods

While many of these hormones can and were first measured by bioassay, the expense and technical difficulties of bioassays limit their use and thus immunoassay is the method of choice. Radioimmunoassays (RIAs) have been most widely used (Yalow and Straus, 1980). Two-site immunometric assays have not been widely applied to these peptides, because of the small size of the hormones and the consequent restrictions on antigen-antibody binding sites. The advantages of enzymes as labels, such as longer reagent shelf-life and safety, have been recognized and they are used in assays for gastrin and insulin (von Grünigen, et al., 1991; Alpha, et al., 1992).

Sample Collection and Storage

Many of these hormones are unstable in samples of peripheral blood. Therefore, blood should be collected into lithium heparin tubes (maximum 20 U/mL) containing aprotinin (Trasylol), a protease inhibitor, and the tubes transported on ice to the laboratory for immediate centrifugation and separation of the plasma. Suitable collection conditions may vary depending on which assay is used, so these conditions should always be checked with the laboratory beforehand. Hemolysis and lipemia should be avoided.

Table 11–2 Islet Cell Tumors and Their Hormones

Tumor Syndrome	Clinical Features	Upper Limit of Reference Range[*,†]
Insulinoma	Hypoglycemia	25 mU/L
Glucagonoma	Necrolytic migratory erythema, diabetes, diarrhea, venous thrombosis	91 pmol/L
Somatostatinoma	Dyspepsia, diabetes, gallstones, steatorrhea, hypochlorhydria	42 pmol/L
PPoma[‡]	None generally recognized	90–100 pmol/L (age related)
Gastrinoma	Peptic ulcer disease, diarrhea	40 pmol/L
VIPoma	Secretory diarrhea, hypokalemia, hypochlorhydria, metabolic acidosis	30 pmol/L
Calcitoninoma	Diarrhea	0.08 µg/L
Neurotensinoma	None generally recognized	68 pmol/L

[*]Approximate reference range. These will be assay dependent and should be checked with the service laboratory or assay manufacturer.

[†]Chiang,et al. Multiple hormone elevations in Zollinger-Ellison syndrome. Gastroenterology 1990;99:1565–1575.

[‡]Pancreatic polypeptide-oma.

Standardization

The ideal standard will show immunochemical identity with the unknown samples, which is indicated, but this is not proven by parallel dilution curves over a wide concentration range. With GIT hormones this may be difficult to achieve because: (1) the hormone may be heterogeneous; (2) nonhuman sources of standards are often used and species differences may be important; or (3) when both plasma samples and tissue extracts must be assayed, each may present special characteristics. Similar difficulties are encountered with control materials. Commercially available synthetic peptides and preparations from specialized institutes, such as the National Institute for Biological Standards and Control (Potters Bar, Herts, EN6 3QG, UK) are used as standards.

Assay Constraints

Labeled Antigen

For RIA the peptide itself is usually labeled with ^{125}I. For assays with extended incubation times, which are not uncommon, special care must be taken to avoid iodination damage to the labeled peptide. This may be aided by chromatographic purification of the iodinated peptide and by optimizing storage conditions (Raggatt and Hales, 1982). In the case of secretin, which contains no tyrosyl residues, an analog containing tyrosine is used.

Matrix Effects

There may be particular problems when tissue extracts must be assayed. Assay buffers (ionic strength, pH, additives such as proteins and detergents) should be optimized to minimize differences between standards and samples, and the effects of sample dilution carefully monitored.

Sensitivity

For some GIT hormones, the lowest concentration that can be detected by RIA may not be sufficient to reach the lower limit of a "normal" reference range, for example, fasting gastrin, glucagon, and pancreatic polypeptide; and in some cases in vivo stimulation tests are used, for example, the secretin test for gastrinomas.

Specificity

RIAs using polyclonal antisera may have particular problems of specificity, first being the need to distinguish structurally related but different hormones, such as secretin, VIP, glucagon and gastric inhibitory polypeptide (GIP) and, second the heterogeneity of some hormones, often a size heterogeneity. This may necessitate a preliminary chromatographic separation step, for example, cholecystokinin (CCK) elutes as CCK-58, CCK-33, CCK-22, and CCK-8 (Cantor and Rehfeld, 1987), the suffixes indicating the number of amino acid residues.

The Major Analytes

Glucagon

Mammalian pancreatic glucagon is a single-chain polypeptide of 29 amino acid residues which is structurally similar to secretin, GIP, and VIP. Glucagon is synthesized as a preprohormone which also contains a signal peptide (20 residues), enteroglucagon related polypeptide (30 residues), and glucagon-like peptides-1 and -2 (GLP-1, GLP-2) (37 and 34 residues, respectively). The amino acid sequences of GLP-1 and GLP-2 are similar to that of glucagon. Glucagon stimulates hepatic glucose release and the conversion of amino acids to glucose in the liver. It has important roles in preventing hypoglycemia in the neonate and during prolonged exercise.

Glucagon is not very immunogenic and coupling of the antigen to albumin leaving the C-terminal free is thought to improve immunogenicity (Holst and Aasted, 1974; Heding, 1971). One major limitation of RIA for glucagon may be cross-reactivity with enteroglucagon, GLP-1, and GLP-2. Interestingly, GLP-1 has been demonstrated in the plasma of three patients with glucagonomas, although the diagnostic significance is not established (Uttenthal, et al., 1985). Low concentrations of

GLP-1 relative to glucagon are found in pancreatic tissue, suggesting that normally the majority of proglucagon is cleaved such that GLP-1 is not produced.

Gastrin

Gastrin has been identified in several molecular weight forms (G-17, G-34, and G-14) which may have different tissue distributions. In turn, each of these forms may or may not be sulfated. Initial proteolytic cleavage of progastrin gives a glycine-extended form which is relatively inactive but acts as a substrate for the formation of active peptide (DelValle, et al.,1989). Gastrin stimulates hydrochloric acid and pepsinogen secretion.

The specificity of gastrin immunoassays is generally limited. In particular there is often cross-reactivity with CCK, and different antisera detect the various forms of gastrin differently. Some Zollinger-Ellison syndrome patients who do not have elevated plasma gastrin concentrations have been found to have glycine-extended gastrin in the plasma, although the significance of this is not clear (DelValle, et al., 1987).

In the investigation of gastrinomas it is important to exclude other causes of hypergastrinemia such as renal failure, pernicious anemia, retained antrum, antral gastral cell hyperplasia, atrophic gastritis, and prior vagotomy. While dynamic function tests may be used (e.g., the secretin test [Billingham, et al., 1987] in the case of gastrinomas), plasma gastrin concentrations greater than 476 pmol/L (1000 pg/mL) are usually diagnostic.

Insulin, Proinsulin, Split Proinsulins, and C-Peptide

Proinsulin is synthesized as preproinsulin in the beta cell and undergoes limited proteolysis, at sites where there are pairs of basic amino acids, to yield partially processed forms and, finally insulin and C-peptide (Fig. 11–1) (Guest and Hutton, 1992). Only insulin is thought to have any significant biologic activity. Insulin and C-peptide are secreted directly into the portal circulation in equimolar amounts, and the liver variably extracts 40% to 60% of the insulin delivered to it. C-peptide is excreted in the urine.

The introduction of RIA for insulin (it was the first RIA) made it possible to measure plasma insulin concentrations in large numbers of samples and subsequently RIAs for proinsulin were developed. It is now appreciated that there were significant problems of cross-reactivity in these early assays (Temple, et al., 1990), which may explain some of the differences in reported plasma concentrations.

Attempts to improve the specificity of, for example, proinsulin assays have included the use of chromatographic separation or prior extraction with immunoadsorbent (Heding, 1977). The availability of biosynthetic proinsulin and split proinsulins allowed development of monoclonal antibodies to those peptides and the better standardization of assays. In particular, specificity can be improved by the use in sandwich immunometric assays of pairs of monoclonal antibodies to two different epitopes on the analyte of interest. This technique has been applied to insulin, proinsulin, and split proinsulins (Sobey, et al., 1989; Temple, et al., 1992). Of interest too

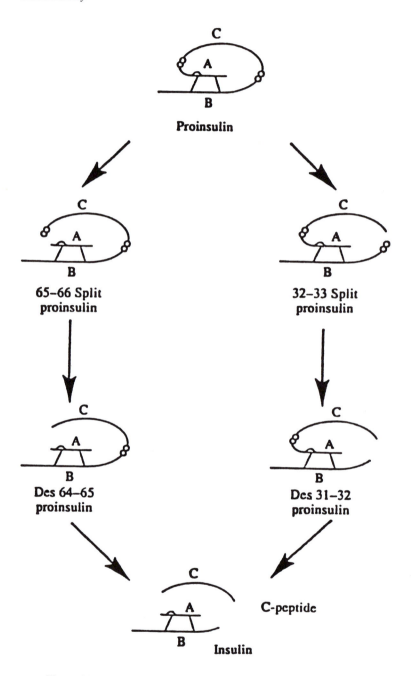

Figure 11–1. Processing of proinsulin to C-peptide and insulin.

is the development of nonisotopic immunometric assays for these peptides, for example enzyme-amplification and time-resolved fluorescence assays (Alpha, et al. 1992; Dhahir, et al., 1992; Storch, et al., 1993).

Measurement of C-peptide in place of insulin may be preferred in the investigation of hypoglycemia, due to the longer in vivo half-life of C-peptide, and because of possible interferences in insulin assays from exogenous insulin and antibodies to insulin in the patient's plasma. Generally, RIAs are used for the measurement of C-peptide with the main analytic challenges being the need to improve the antigenicity of the peptide for immunization and the need to introduce tyrosine residues into the peptide for ease of iodination (Heding, 1987).

The measurement of plasma (pro)insulins and C-peptide concentrations is central to the investigation of hypoglycemia, and elevated plasma concentrations should raise the possibility of an endocrine tumor (Marks and Teale, 1991). Adult fasting reference ranges increase with obesity. The approximate normal ranges for nonobese, fasting concentrations are insulin 33 to 170 pmol/L (5 to 25 mU/L); proinsulin less than 7 pmol/L; and C-peptide 0.3 to 1.16 nmol/L.

Other Analytes

Immunoassays, mostly RIAs, are commercially available for the determination of other peptides that are secreted by the GIT. These include CCK, octapeptide, neurotensin, somatostatin, and VIP. VIP is measured in the diagnosis of Verner-Morrison syndrome.

APOLIPOPROTEINS

The metabolism of lipids and the apolipoproteins, involving the small intestine, liver and muscle-adipose tissue, is complex and dynamic. The apolipoproteins act as lipid transporters. They bind cellular receptors and activate lipolytic enzymes. The lipoproteins are classified on the basis of their densities as defined by ultracentrifugation and have different compositions (Table 11–3). The reader is referred to a review of their physiology and pathology by Bhatnagar and Durrington (1991). Disorders of lipid metabolism can be considered as either genetic (primary) or due to acquired disease (secondary), although clinically the two can occur together, for example, familial and alcohol related hypertriglyceridemia. Diagnosis is based on family history, physical examination, and lipid analyses. More specialized tests such as ultracentrifugation, apolipoprotein analyses, and receptor studies are used in a minority of cases (Study Group, European Atherosclerosis Society, 1988). Thus the measurement of, for example, apolipoprotein B in familial combined hyperlipidemia, apolipoprotein C-II in hyperchylomicronemia, and apolipoprotein E genotyping in remnant hyperlipidemia may be useful. More generally, the measurements of apolipoproteins A-I and B in the assessment of risk of coronary heart disease, and possibly as alternatives to measurement of high density lipoprotein (HDL) and low density lipoprotein (LDL), have been advocated but are not widely accepted as rou-

Table 11–3   Composition and Function of the Lipids and Apolipoproteins

	Chylo-microns	VLDL[†]	IDL	LDL	HDL
Density (g/mL)	< 0.93	0.93–1.006	1.006–1.019	1.019–1.063	1.063–1.210
Composition (%)					
Triglycerides	90	65	35	10	5
Cholesterol	5	20	40	50	35
Phospholipid	4	10	15	20	35
Protein	1	5	10	20	25
Principal apoli-poproteins*	A-I	B-100	B-100	B-100	A-I A-II
	B-48	E			C
	C	C			E
	E				

*Key to apolipoprotein functions:

Protein	Function
A-I	Structural protein in HDL, LCAT activator, receptor ligand
A-II	Structural protein in HDL
B-48	Chylomicron structural protein
B-100	VLDL-LDL structural protein
C-I	LCAT activator
C-II	LpL cofactor
C-III	LpL modulator
E	Receptor ligand

[†]IDL, intermediate density lipoprotein; LDL, low density lipoprotein; VLDL, very low density lipoprotein; LCAT, lecithin-cholesterol acyltransferase; LpL, lipoprotein lipase.

tine. Clinical use has been limited by lack of comparability of results between laboratories (Cooper, et al., 1991a). It is clear that a number of analytic problems are common to the analyses of the apolipoproteins, particularly the lack of adequate standardization and reference methodologies (Labeur, et al., 1990).

Assay Methods

All the major immunoassay formats have been used for the analysis of the apolipoproteins, each with its advantages and disadvantages (Labeur, et al., 1990). Consideration of the workload, turnaround time, and facilities required may influence the choice of assay. Some of the limitations may be peculiar to apolipoprotein assays, as follows.

1. *Radial Immunodiffusion/Immunoelectrophoresis.* These techniques, which rely on the migration of lipid particles through an agarose gel, are limited in terms of speed of assay and the number of samples that can easily be assayed. In addition there may be problems of accuracy because different lipoprotein fractions

migrate through the gel at different rates. Lyophilized preparations may also behave differently to fresh serum as shown by assays for apolipoprotein B (Smith, et al., 1990).

2. *Radioimmunoassays.* Isolation of pure apolipoprotein for iodination may result in aggregation of the labeled protein and differences in the reactivity of standard compared with sample.

3. *Nephelometric/Turbidimetric Assays.* These techniques have been widely used for the assay of apolipoproteins and are easily automated, fast, and precise. However, they are very sensitive to sample turbidity and the optimization of sample pretreatment with enzyme or detergent is critical (Brustolin, et al., 1991).

4. *Immunometric Assays.* Two-site assays with two antibodies (either polyclonal or monoclonal) have been used for the apolipoproteins, with the possibility of improved specificity, for example, for the determination of lipoprotein (a) (Labeur, et al., 1989). However, two-site assays may be particularly susceptible to epitope masking (Gries, et al., 1988) and this may vary between sample and standard and between samples. Therefore, thorough validation of these assays in terms of accuracy is essential.

In general, accurate quantitation by any of the above methods may be difficult because (1) antigenic sites may be masked by lipid; (2) a given apolipoprotein may be distributed variably between different lipoprotein fractions; and (3) there may be differences between the relative concentrations and the compositions of lipoprotein fractions between individual samples and standards.

Sample Collection, Storage, and Pretreatment

It is generally recommended that the patient should be fasting (12 hours or overnight) when a blood sample is collected. This minimizes problems of sample turbidity in nephelometric/turbidimetric assays. Serum is preferred to plasma to avoid interference by fibrin. Samples may be stored at 4°C for a few days, or at −70°C for longer times, with a minimum delay before freezing, a minimum number of freeze-thaw cycles, and with thawing at 37°C. Possible storage effects may be method dependent, and hence collection and storage conditions should be validated for each assay (Cooper, et al., 1985; Marcovina and Albers, 1989). In particular, freezing of samples for apolipoprotein A-I is not recommended, as this may result in disruption of lipid particles and consequent variability of measured protein. Sample storage tubes should also be standardized.

The antigenic sites of the apolipoproteins may be completely or partially masked by the lipid moiety. Sample pretreatment, either by delipidation or with enzymes and detergents, to unmask the antigenic sites may be necessary for accurate quantitation and to overcome problems of sample turbidity (Brustolin, et al., 1991).

Standardization

Generally, purified apolipoproteins are used as standards. Apolipoprotein A-I may be isolated by chromatography of HDL after delipidation. However, it readily undergoes deamidation, oxidation, proteolytic degradation, and self association; so that care is needed to minimize this in isolation and storage procedures. In addition, post-translational modifications and genetic polymorphisms have been demonstrated and may influence the behavior of preparations as standards. Thus preparation from serum pools made from 'fresh' serum and stored at less than $-50°C$ may be advisable (Steinberg, et al., 1983). Apolipoprotein B may be purified from freshly isolated LDL (Rosseneu, et al., 1983) but it is so hydrophobic that when isolated it is insoluble in aqueous buffers. It may be solubilized with detergents and guanidine hydrochloride. Lyophilization of apolipoproteins may also lead to aggregation and changes in behavior in immunoassays (Marcovina and Albers, 1990; Smith, et al., 1990).

In addition, inconsistencies in standardization may be due to significant variations in the protein measurements and protein standards used to characterize apolipoprotein preparations (Albers, et al., 1989; Henderson, et al., 1990). Efforts are well underway to prepare, validate, and distribute International Reference Materials and primary and secondary standards, particularly for apolipoproteins A1 and B (Cooper, et al., 1991b; Marcovina and Albers, 1989, Albers, et al., 1992; Marcovina et al., 1993).

Selection and Characterization of Antibodies

Polyclonal antisera have been widely used, particularly for assays dependent on precipitation of antigen-antibody complex. Their use may result in loss of specificity and, because of variable epitope expression, there may be nonlinearity of response on dilution of sample, and consequent inaccuracy. Monoclonal antibodies have a number of advantages and their use should improve specificity. However, antibodies must be chosen such that all polymorphisms are detected equally, as should the native and isolated apolipoprotein (Marcovina, et al., 1990).

Apolipoprotein A-I

Apolipoprotein A-I is the major protein of HDL and may be a negative predictor of ischamic heart disease (Cooper, et al., 1991a). It activates the enzyme lecithin-cholesterol acyltransferase (EC 2.3.1.43) (LCAT) which catalyzes the transfer of a C-2 fatty acid from lecithin to cholesterol.

A wide range of immunoassays has been developed for apolipoprotein A-I (Steinberg, et al., 1983) and the common problems of standardization, self association and aggregation, variable masking of antigenic sites, and polymorphism have been described. In order to overcome some of these problems it has been suggested that human serum assayed by isotope dilution for apolipoprotein A-I could be used as a standard (Weech, et al., 1988). (See discussion above under Standardization.)

Apolipoprotein B

High concentrations of serum apolipoprotein B may show a relationship with the development of coronary heart disease even in individuals with normal serum concentrations of cholesterol. Several forms of apolipoprotein B have been described, most notably B-100 and B-48 which differ in molecular weight. B-48 is synthesized in the adult intestine and consists of 2152 amino acids that are homologous with the first 2152 residues of B-100. B-48 is a constituent of chylomicrons and chylomicron remnants. B-100 is synthesized primarily by the liver and is a constituent of low, intermediate, and very low density lipoproteins. In addition, acetylation and glycosylation have been demonstrated.

Several immunoassays have been described for apolipoprotein B but they tend to show discrepancies (Bury and Rosseneu, 1988). For normal sera this may be due, in the main, to differences in the standards used and in the lack of comparability between specimen antigen and standard. This becomes compounded in dyslipoproteinemic sera by sample turbidity, different lipoprotein distribution between the fractions, and by the presence of "abnormal" fractions (Rosseneu, et al., 1983).

A number of assays for apolipoprotein B have been described that have monoclonal antibodies in both competitive (Waterson, et al., 1987) and noncompetitive (Albers, et al. 1989) formats. The latter approach may have the advantage of increased specificity and avoids the possibility of epitope changes on binding the antigen to a solid phase, as used in some competitive assays. Using two monoclonal antibodies, one to B-100 and B-48 and one specific for B-100, it has been possible to develop an assay specific for B-100 (Albers, et al., 1989) and, by also measuring total apolipoprotein B, it may be possible to estimate B-48. However, the large amount of lipid in chylomicrons is likely to mask some of the epitopes, making accurate quantitation of B-48 difficult.

Lipoprotein (a)

Lipoprotein (a) or Lp (a), consists of a glycoprotein apo (a) linked through disulfide bonds to apolipoprotein B-100 in the lipoprotein particle. Lp (a) has been shown to have a high degree of homology with plasminogen and to consist of a serine protease-like domain, a kringle-5-like domain, and a large number of kringle-4-like repeats. It shows size polymorphism with an inverse relationship between Lp (a) size and plasma concentration (Gaubatz, et al., 1990). Plasma concentrations of Lp (a) in the population show a highly skewed distribution and are independent of diet and age, although showing ethnic variation. High plasma concentrations have been associated with premature coronary heart disease, stroke, and atherosclerosis (Editorial, 1991). In view of its possible importance as an independent risk factor for coronary heart disease, immunoassays of most types have been developed and used for its measurement (Molinari, et al., 1983; Gillery et al., 1993), including rapid, noninstrumented, screening methods (Lou et al., 1993).

The two-site immunoassay principle has been applied to Lp (a) with all the types of antibody combinations being used: polyclonal antibody both as solid phase and as label (Abe, et al., 1988); polyclonal on solid phase and monoclonal label (Doetsch, et al, 1991), and matched monoclonal antibodies used for solid phase and label (Wong, et al., 1990). The last approach has the advantage of being able to define specificity. Thus monoclonal antibodies used in combination might be expected to minimize cross-reactivity with plasminogen and free Lp (a) (Fless, et al., 1989).

Mixtures of monoclonal antibodies have been used in some assays in order to minimize the effects of variable epitope expression on different individual plasma samples (Vu-Dac, et al., 1989). It has been suggested that monoclonal antibodies directed to epitopes on kringle-5 or the protease domain of Lp (a) should be selected to avoid differences in immunoreactivity due to the number of epitopes depending on the number of kringle-4 repeats (Albers, et al., 1990).

As with the other lipoproteins, there are common analytic problems such as variable epitope expression due to masking by lipid moieties and lack of a primary reference material. Delipidated Lp (a) will self associate and form irreversible aggregates and is not suitable as a primary standard. Lp (a) has been suggested as a primary standard, although there have been reports of monoclonal antibodies showing different reactivity to isolated Lp (a) and Lp (a) with intact disulfide bonds. Additionally, there are discrepancies in determining by independent chemical means the absolute mass of the primary standard. Traditionally this has been expressed as total lipoprotein mass (lipid, protein, and carbohydrate), but because of the technical difficulty of this and the variability in Lp (a) particles this should be discouraged. Alternatively, calibration in terms of absolute protein mass has been used. Lp (a) synthetic peptide could be used if its immunologic activity is identical to that of naturally occurring Lp (a) and its mass can be determined from its amino acid sequence, which is constant. However, such a standard cannot be used for assays using anti-apolipoprotein B antibodies. Last, the problems of calibration are further complicated by the variation in mass of the various Lp (a) isoforms, differences in the ratios of apolipoprotein a to apoliproprotein B, matrix effects, and the possible detrimental effects of lyophilization.

There have been a number of reference ranges reported for the apolipoproteins, all of which are assay dependent. Most show a skewed distribution and the following are given for guidance only: serum apolipoprotein A-I, 1.08 to 1.89 g/L; apolipoprotein B, 0.6 to 1.94 g/L; Lp (a) less than 30 mg/dL (Zunic, et al., 1992).

REFERENCES

Abe A, Maeda S, Makizo K, et al. Enzyme-linked immunosorbent assay of lipoprotein (a) in serum and cord blood. Clin Chim Acta 1988;177:31–40.

Albers JJ, Lodge MS, Curtiss LK. Evaluation of a monoclonal antibody-based enzyme-linked immunosorbent assay as a candidate reference method for the measurement of apolipoprotein B-100. J Lipid Res 1989;30:1445–1458.

Albers JJ, Marcovina SM, Lodge MS. The unique lipoprotein (a), properties and immunochemical measurement. Clin Chem 1990;36:2019–2026.

Albers JJ, Marcovina SM, Kennedy H. International Federation of Clinical Chemistry standardization project for measurements of apolipoproteins A-1 and BII. Evaluation and selection of candidate reference materials. Clin Chem 1992;38:658–662.

Alpha B, Cox L, Crowther N, Clark PMS, Hales CN. Sensitive amplified immunoenzymometric assays (IEMA) for human insulin and intact proinsulin. Eur J Clin Chem Clin Biochem 1992;30:27–32.

Ballesta J, Bloom SR, Polak JM. Distribution and localization of regulatory peptides. CRC Crit Rev Clin Lab Sci 1985;22:185–218.

Bhatnagar D, Durrington PN. Clinical value of apolipoprotein measurement. Ann Clin Biochem 1991;28:427–437.

Billingham MS, Wheeler MJ, Hall RA. Biochemical function tests. Oxford: Blackwell Scientific Publications, 1987.

Brustolin D, Maierna M, Aguzzi F, Zoppi F, Tarenghi G, Berti G. Immunoturbidimetric method for routine determinations of Apolipoproteins A-1 and B. Clin Chem 1991;37:742–747.

Bury JB, Rosseneu MY. Apolipoprotein quantitation by ELISA: Technical aspects and clinical applications. Rev Immunoassay Tech 1988;1:1–30.

Cantor P, Rehfeld JF. The molecular nature of cholecystokinin in human plasma. Clin Chim Acta 1987;168:153–158.

Chiang H-CV, O'Dorisio TM, Huang SC, Maton PN, Gardner JD, Jensen RT. Multiple hormone elevations in Zollinger-Ellison syndrome. Gastroenterology 1990;99: 1565–1575.

Cooper GR, Smith SJ, Wiebe DA, Kuchmak M, Hannon WH. International survey of apolipoprotein A1 and B measurements (1983–1984). Clin Chem 1985;31:223–228.

Cooper GR, Henderson LO, Smith SJ, Hannon WH. Clinical applications and standardization of apolipoprotein measurements in the diagnostic workup of lipid disorders. Clin Chem 1991a;37:619–620.

Cooper GR, Myers GL, Henderson LO. Establishment of reference methods for lipids, lipoproteins and apolipoproteins. Eur J Clin Chem Clin Biochem 1991b;29:269–275.

Dhahir FJ, Cook DB, Self CH. Amplified enzyme-linked immunoassay of human proinsulin in serum (Detection limit = 0.1 pmol/L). Clin Chem 1992;38:227–232.

DelValle J, Sugano K, Yamada T. Progastrin and its glycine-extended posttranslational processing intermediates in human gastrointestinal tissues. Gastroenterology 1987;92: 1908–1912.

DelValle J, Sugano K, Yamada T. Glycine-extended processing intermediates of gastrin and cholecystokinin in human plasma. Gastroenterology 1989;97:1159–1163.

Doetsch K, Roheim PS. Thompson JJ. Human lipoprotein (a) quantified by 'capture' ELISA. Ann Clin Lab Sci 1991;21:216–224.

Editorial. Lipoprotein (a). Lancet 1991;337:397–398.

Fless GM, Snyder ML, Scanu AM. Enzyme-linked immunoassay for LP (a). J Lipid Res 1989;30:651–662.

Gaubatz JW, Ghanem KI, Guevera J, Nava M L Patsch W, Morrisett JD. Polymorphic forms of human apolipoprotein (a): inheritance and relationship of their molecular weights to plasma levels of lipoprotein (a). J Lipid Res 1990;31:603–613.

Gillery P, Arthuis P, Cuperlier C, Circaud R. Rate nephelometric assay of serum lipoprotein (a). Clin Chem 1993;39:503–508.

Gries A, Fievet C, Marcovina S, et al. Interaction of LDL, Lp (a) and reduced Lp (a) with monoclonal antibodies against apo B. J Lipid Res 1988;29:1–9.

Guest PC, Hutton JC. Biosynthesis of insulin secretory granule proteins. In: Flatt PR, ed., Nutrient Regulation of Insulin Secretion. London: Portland Press, 1992;59–82.

Heding LG. Radioimmunological determination of pancreatic and gut glucagon in plasma. Diabetologia 1971;71:10–19.

Heding LG. Specific and direct immunoassay for human proinsulin in serum. Diabetologia 1977;13:467–474.

Heding LG. Radioimmunoassays for insulin, C-peptide and proinsulin. Lancaster, PA: MTP Press, 1987.

Henderson LO, Powell MK, Smith SJ, Hannon WH, Cooper GR, Marcovina SM. Impact of protein measurements on standardization of assays of apolipoproteins A-1 and B. Clin Chem 1990;36:1911–1917.

Holst JJ, Aasted B. Production and evaluation of glucagon antibodies for radioimmunoassay. Acta Endocrinol 1974;77:715–726.

Labeur C, Michiels G, Bury J, Usher DC, Rosseneu M. Lipoprotein (a) quantified by an enzyme-linked immunosorbent assay with monoclonal antibodies. Clin Chem 1989; 35:1380–1384.

Labeur C, Shepherd J, Rosseneu M. Immunological assays of apolipoproteins in plasma: methods and instrumentation. Clin Chem 1990;36:591–597.

Lou SC, Patel C, Ching SF, Gordon J. One-step competitive immunochromatographic assay for semiquantitative determination of lipoprotein(a) in plasma. Clin Chem 1993;39: 619–624.

Marcovina S M, Albers J J. Standardization of the immunochemical determination of apolipoproteins A-1 and B: A report on the International Federation of Clinical Chemistry meeting on standardization of apolipoproteins A-1 and B measurements (basis for future consensus), Vienna, Austria, 18–19 April, 1989. Clin Chem 1989; 35:2009–2015.

Marcovina SM, Albers JJ. Apolipoprotein assays: standardization and quality control. Scand J Clin Lab Invest 1990;198 (suppl 50):58–65.

Marcovina SM, Albers JJ, Henderson LO, Hannon WH. International Federation of Clinical Chemistry Standardization Project for measurements of apolipoproteins A-I and B. III. Comparability of apolipoprotein A-I values by use of International Reference Material. Clin Chem 1993;39:773–781.

Marcovina SM, Curtiss LK, Milne R, Albers JJ. Selection and characterization of monoclonal antibodies for measuring plasma levels of apolipoproteins A-1 and B. J Int Fed Clin Chem 1990;2:138–144.

Marks V, Teale JD. Tumours producing hypoglycaemia. Diabetes Metab Rev 1991;7:79–91.

Molinari E, Pichler P, Krempler F, Kostner GM. A rapid screening method for pathological lipoprotein Lp(a) concentrations. Clin Chim Acta 1983;128:373–378.

Raggatt PR, Hales CN. Immunoassays using labeled antigens or antibodies. In: Lachmann PJ, Peters DK, eds. Clinical Aspects of Immunology. Oxford: Blackwell Scientific Publications, 1982;309–342.

Rosseneu M, Vercaemst R, Steinberg KK, Cooper GR. Some considerations of methodology and standardization of apolipoprotein B immunoassays. Clin Chem 1983;29:427–433.

Said SI. Peptides common to the nervous system and the gastrointestinal tract. In Frontiers in Neuroendocrinology, vol 6. New York: Raven Press, 1980;293–331.

Smith SJ, Henderson LO, Hannon WH, Cooper GR. Effects of analytical method and lyophilized sera on measurements of apolipoproteins A-1 and B, an international survey. Clin Chem 1990;36:290–296.

Sobey WJ, Beer SF, Carrington CA, et al. Sensitive and specific two-site immunoradiometric assays for human insulin, proinsulin, 65–66 split and 32–33 split proinsulins. Biochem J 1989;260:535–541.

Steinberg KK, Cooper GR, Graiser SR, Rosseneu M. Some considerations of methodology and standardization of apolipoprotein A-1 immunoassays. Clin Chem 1983;29:415–426.

Storch M-J, Morbach P, Kerp L. A time-resolved fluoroimmunoassay for human insulin based on two monoclonal antibodies. J Immunol Methods 1993;157:197–201.

Study Group, European Atherosclerosis Society. The recognition and management of hyperlipidaemia in adults: a policy statement of the European Atherosclerosis Society. Eur Heart J 1988;9:571–600.

Temple R, Clark PMS, Hales CN. Measurement of insulin secretion in type 2 diabetes: problems and pitfalls. Diabe Med 1992;9:503–512.

Temple RC, Clark PMS, Nagi DK, Schneider AE, Yudkin JS, Hales CN. Radioimmunoassay may overestimate insulin in non-insulin dependent diabetes. Clin Endocrinol 1990;32: 689–693.

Uttenthal LO, Ghiglione M, George SK, Bishop AE, Polak JM, Bloom SR. Molecular forms of glucagon-like peptide-1 in human pancreas and glucagonomas. J Clin Endocrinol Metab 1985;61:472–479.

Von Grünigen R, Siglmüller G, Papini A, et al. Enzyme immunoassay with captured hapten: a sensitive gastrin assay with biotinyl-gastrin derivatives. Biol Chem Hoppe-Seyler 1991;372;163–172.

Vu-Dac N, Mezdour H, Parra HJ, Luc G, Luyeye I, Fruchart JC. A selective bi-site immunoenzymatic procedure for human Lp(a) lipoprotein quantification using monoclonal antibodies against apo(a) and apo B. J Lipid Res 1989;30:1437–1443.

Waterson M, Samuel L, Norman M. The production and use of monoclonal antibodies to measure apolipoprotein B by a competitive enzyme-linked immunoassay. Ann Clin Biochem 1987;24:301–308.

Weech PK, Jewer D, Marcel YL. Apolipoprotein A1 assayed in human serum by isotope dilution as a potential standard for immunoassay. J Lipid Res 1988;29:85–93.

Wong WLT, Eaton DL, Berlaul A, Fendly B, Hass PE. A monoclonal-antibody-based enzyme-linked immunosorbent assay of lipoprotein (a). Clin Chem 1990;36:192–197.

Yalow RS, Straus E. Problems and pitfalls in the radioimmunoassay of gastrointestinal hormones. In: Jerzy-Glass GB, ed. Gastrointestinal Hormones. New York: Raven Press, 1980;751–767.

Zunic G, Jelic-Ivanovic Z, Spasic S, Stojiljkovic A, Majkic-Singh N. Reference values for apolipoproteins A-1 and B in healthy subjects by age. Clin Chem 1992;38:566–569.

CHAPTER 12

Disorders of Blood

Sheldon Davidson

This chapter starts with a brief review of the hematopoietic system followed by a discussion of immunoassays and related methods in the diagnosis of disorders of erythrocytes, white blood cells, plasma cells, and the hemostatic system.

THE HEMATOPOIETIC SYSTEM

The pluripotential stem cells of the bone marrow give rise to the precursor cells that differentiate to form erythrocytes, platelets, and leukocytes (Fig. 12–1). Hematopoiesis is maintained and controlled by specific cell-cell interactions in the microenvironment provided by the stromal matrix of the bone marrow and by a wide range of synergistically interacting, glycoprotein growth factors, each of which is usually produced by many cell types and affects more than one lineage (Table 12–1) (Hoffbrand and Pettit, 1993). Immunoassays for the measurement of individual interleukins and other growth factors have been developed (e.g., IL-1a, IL-1b, and IL-2 [Grassi, et al., 1991]; granulocyte-macrophage colony-stimulating factor [Zenke, et al., 1991]) but are not in routine clinical use (see also Chap. 15).

Erythropoiesis, that portion of hematopoiesis concerned with the formation of erythrocytes (red blood cells), is regulated by erythropoietin, which is synthesized in the kidney and liver and is stimulated by low arterial oxygen tension.

Leukocytes (white blood cells) are of two types: phagocytes and immunocytes. Phagocytes include granulocytes (subclassified as neutrophils [polymorphs], eosinophils, and basophils) and monocytes. Immunocytes, the cells of the immune system, include B and T lymphocytes, their precursor cells, and plasma cells. Plasma cells, derived from B lymphocytes, produce and secrete immunoglobulins.

Granulocytes and monocytes (monocytes become macrophages in the tissues) function primarily as cells of defense against microorganisms and directly attack such organisms, although their function is highly interdependent on the immune system. Monocytes and neutrophils can phagocytize microorganisms, antibody-coated erythrocytes and tumor cells, as well as unsensitized tumor cells. They display surface antigens and receptors that allow their identification, including Fc, C3b and Mac-1

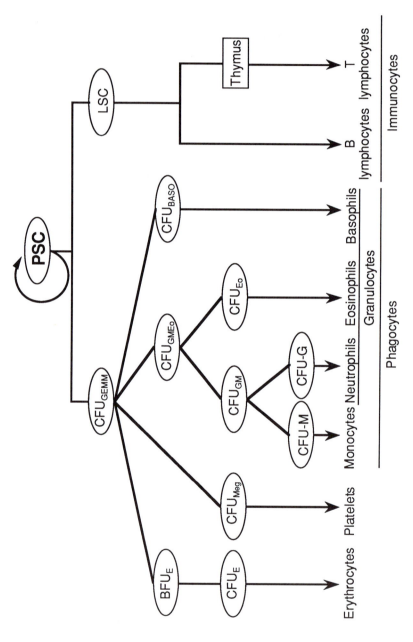

Figure 12-1.   Blood cell formation from a common pluripotential stem cell (PSC), which can renew itself. After a number of divisions and differentiation steps a series of separate progenitor cells are formed, which continue to form further specialized progenitor cells and/or differentiate, and migrate to the bloodstream. Other abbreviations: baso, basophil; BFU, burst forming unit; CFU, colony forming unit; Eo, erythroid; GEMM, mixed granulocyte, erythroid, monocyte, megakaryocyte; GM, granulocyte, monocyte; LSC, lymphoid stem cell; Meg, megakaryocyte.

Table 12–1   Growth Factors Regulating Hematopoiesis

Endogenous Factors

Stimulate stromal cells* to secrete GM-, G-, M-CSF, IL-6:
  Interleukin-1 (IL-1)
  Tumor necrosis factor

Acts on pluripotential cells:
  Stem cell factor (SCF)

Act on early multipotential cells:
  Interleukin-3 (IL-3)
  Interleukin-4 (IL-4)
  Interleukin-6 (IL-6)
  Granulocyte-macrophage colony-stimulating factor (GM-CSF)

Act on cells committed to a specific lineage or two:
  Granulocyte colony stimulating factor (G-CSF)
  Macrophage colony stimulating factor (M-CSF)
  Interleukin-5 (IL-5)
  Erythropoietin

Inhibits the growth of many types of hematopoietic cells:
  Transforming growth factor-β (TGF-β)

Other factors that may also be important:
  Interleukin-8 (IL-8)
  Interleukin-9 (IL-9)
  Interleukin-10 (IL-10)
  Interleukin-11 (IL-11)

Exogenous Factors

Stimulate T lymphocytes to secrete IL-3, IL-5:
  Antigens

Stimulate monocytes to secrete TNF, IL-1, IL-6, GM-, G-, C-CSF:
  Endotoxins

Inhibits erythropoietin synthesis in kidney and liver:
  Oxygen tension

---

*The stromal matrix cells of the hematopoietic bone marrow include endothelial cells, fibroblasts, fat cells, and macrophages.

receptors. Leukocytes are also classified according to the antigens they display, such as human leukocyte antigen (HLA) class I and class II antigens, cluster differentiation (CD) antigens, or neutrophil antigens (NA, NB, etc). (Hoffbrand and Pettit, 1993).

Platelets, which are incomplete cells, are derived from megakaryocytes in the bone marrow and have a major role in hemostasis.

ERYTHROCYTES

The nucleus-containing normoblasts of bone marrow are committed to develop into erythrocytes. Losing their nuclei, they become hemoglobin-synthesizing reticulocytes which move into the blood. Mature erythrocytes are fully charged with hemoglobin and other proteins and lack even RNA. The complex process of red cell regeneration requires a wide range of competent genes and good nutrition, including adequate intakes of iron, magnesium, cobalt, folate, vitamins B_{12}, C, and E, pyridoxine, thiamine, riboflavin, and pantothenic acid; and the stimulatory effects of many growth factors and hormones, including stem cell factor (SCF), interleukin-3 (IL-3) and granulocyte-macrophage colony-stimulating factor (GM-CSF), erythropoietin, androgens, and thyroxine. Too few, or incompetent, red cells, as well as red cells with a short half-life, lead to anemia, while excess red cells are associated with polycythemia (erythrocytosis).

Iron Deficiency and Related Anemias

The differential diagnosis of iron deficiency anemia, the most common of all anemias, from the anemia of chronic disease and sideroblastic anemia (a form of myelodysplastic syndrome) is aided by measurement of serum ferritin concentrations (Table 12–2). In sideroblastic anemia a bone-marrow iron-stain shows an increase in red cell precursors containing iron in the mitochondria, frequently forming a ring around the nucleus (ringed sideroblasts).

Table 12–2   Diagnostic Indicators of Iron Deficiency and Related Anemias

	Parameters measured			
Type of Anemia	*Serum iron*	*Serum iron binding capacity*	*Serum ferritin*	*Bone marrow iron*
Iron deficiency	Low	High	Low	Very low
Chronic disease	Low	Low	High	High
Sideroblastic	High	Normal	High	High
Iron overload	High	Normal	Very high	High

Ferritin

Ferritin is the iron storage protein, and each molecule (apoprotein mol wt 450,000) binds iron as a crystalline ferric hydroxide-phosphate complex. It is mainly intracellular but is also found in the bloodstream, and blood ferritin concentrations depend upon the total iron reserves in the body.

A wide range of immunoassays are commercially available for the measurement of ferritin in serum or plasma (Ward, 1992). Most are two-site immunometric assays, most employing enzymes (usually horseradish peroxidase) or ^{125}I as labeling substance. Less than 10% of assays are liquid phase and a very wide variety of solid phase materials are used in the others, the most popular being microtiter wells, tubes, magnetizable particles, and large beads.

Ferritin is also determined by nephelometric immunoassay which can be automated by means of suitable equipment (Flowers, et al., 1986; Borque, et al., 1992). One fully automated system for nephelometric immunoassay is supplied by Behringwerk AG (Marberg, Germany), and ferritin reagents are available from Boehringer Mannheim (Mannheim, Germany). These include latex particles covalently coated with rabbit antibodies against human placental ferritin, which aggregate in the presence of ferritin forming large light-scattering particles.

Megaloblastic Anemia

Megaloblastic anemia is caused by defects in DNA synthesis. The most common causes are deficiencies in vitamin B_{12} (cyanocobalamin) and folic acid, both of which are essential for DNA synthesis. Affected erythopoietic cells are characterized by a nucleus which is immature compared with the level of maturation of the cytoplasm.

When vitamin B_{12} is ingested it combines with intrinsic factor, a protein secreted by parietal cells in the stomach. The resulting complex is then carried through the small intestine to the ileum, where the vitamin B_{12} is absorbed by combining with receptors in the ileoepithelium. The vitamin B_{12} then separates and combines with three primary transport proteins in the blood, TC-1, TC-2, and TC-3. In the absence of intrinsic factor, vitamin B_{12} cannot be absorbed and vitamin B_{12} deficiency, with consequent megaloblastic anemia, ultimately results. Pernicious anemia is etiologically an autoimmune disorder with autoantibodies that destroy the gastric parietal cells and bind intrinsic factor, leading to a deficiency of intrinsic factor and consequent malabsorption of vitamin B_{12}.

The most specific test for pernicious anemia is the Schilling test in which absorbed ^{57}Co-labeled vitamin B_{12} is flushed into a 24-hour urine sample by a large dose of nonradioactive vitamin B_{12} given simultaneously. If the radioactive vitamin B_{12} is absorbed adequately, it is excreted in the urine, but in the absence of absorption the amount of radioactivity in the urine is very small. If vitamin B_{12} excretion becomes normal when intrinsic factor is administered simultaneously with labeled vitamin$_{12}$, a diagnosis of pernicious anemia is confirmed. Absorption is not improved in general malabsorption states. Either way, the treatment is by injecting vitamin B_{12} parenterally.

Another common cause of megaloblastic anemia is folic acid (pteroylmono-glutamic acid) deficiency. Folic acid is a water-soluble vitamin which is stored in the body in only limited quantities. Deficiency can be due to decreased intake, taking drugs that block folic acid absorption or metabolism and, as with vitamin B_{12} deficiency, intestinal disorders that disturb absorption. Alternatively, deficiency may arise from an increased requirement, as in pregnancy.

Vitamin B_{12} is necessary for activation of the reduced form of folic acid and, in its absence, inactive forms of folate accumulate. Consequently, vitamin B_{12} cannot reverse folate deficiency but, on the other hand, large quantities of folic acid may reverse the anemia caused by vitamin B_{12} deficiency. Neurologic damage caused by vitamin B_{12} deficiency does not involve folic acid, and therefore it is essential to determine which of the two vitamins is truly deficient, as administration of folic acid alone to a patient deficient in vitamin B_{12} may precipitate neurologic damage.

Vitamin B_{12} Assay

To measure vitamin B_{12}, it must first be liberated from binding proteins and converted to stable cyanocobalamin. This may be done by heating the serum in the presence of cyanide ions at an acid pH, or by treatment with a pH greater than 12.5. Then, according to a competitive format equivalent to a radioimmunoassay (RIA), labeled vitamin B_{12} (e.g., ^{57}Co-vitamin B_{12}) and intrinsic factor reagent are added and unknown or standard vitamin B_{12} and radioactive vitamin B_{12} compete for binding sites, after which the free fraction is separated by centrifugation and the label counted. Vitamin B_{12} concentrations in the patient serum samples are then determined by comparison with standard readings (Dacie and Lewis, 1991).

In the past such assays were often unreliable because the preparations of intrinsic factor used contained R-binders which are forms of transcobalamin, primarily transcobalamin-1, which can bind cobalamins other than vitamin B_{12} itself. Therefore, the vitamin B_{12} serum levels tended to be overestimated. The use of intrinsic factor that has been characterized by microbiologic assay is now recommended (National Committee for Clinical Laboratory Standards, 1980).

Folate Assay

Folate deficiency is best diagnosed by the determination of serum folic acid. ^{125}I-folic acid is mixed with the serum sample and the mixture heated to destroy indigenous binders, before β-lactoglobulin, the binding agent, is added. After incubation, the bound and free label are separated and the radioactivity in the supernatant counted. Alternatively, folate can be determined in the red cells rather than in the serum. The red cells are separated and hemolyzed and the hemolysate analyzed in the same way as the serum (Dacie and Lewis, 1991).

Autoantibodies

Intrinsic factor antibodies can be detected by a radiometric assay procedure using ^{57}Co-vitamin B_{12}, (Dacie and Lewis, 1991). The intrinsic antibodies are of two types, blocking and binding (types I and II) and immunoassays with [125]I (Conn, 1986) or enzyme labels (Waters, et al., 1989) can be used to detect both simultaneously.

The test for antibodies against parietal cells employs stomach sections as the substrate for the assay. Diluted serum is assayed by incubation with tissue segments of mouse or rat stomach. A positive reaction can be identified with immunofluorescent staining of the parietal cells with labeled anti-human antibodies (Bigazzi, et al., 1992).

Hemolytic Anemia

Erythrocytes have a mean lifespan of 120 days before they are destroyed and their basic components, such as amino acids and iron, are recycled. A low red cell count due to an increase in the rate of erythrocyte destruction is defined as hemolytic anemia, and may be acquired or hereditary. Acquired hemolytic anemia can be autoimmune, alloimmune (following blood transfusion or marrow transplantation), drug induced, or chemically induced. Autoimmune hemolytic anemias are due to antibodies that bind to red cells, and are divided into "warm" and "cold" types according to whether the antibody reacts better at 37°C or 4°C.

To confirm abnormal hemolysis a range of indirect tests, documenting increased red cell production (which results in reticulocytosis and bone marrow erythroid hyperplasia), and direct tests, which confirm decreased red cell survival, are used. Direct tests include measurements of urinary urinobilinogen, fecal stercobilinogen, and serum haptoglobin. Coombs' test is used to identify autoimmune disease by detecting anti–red cell antibodies.

Haptoglobin

Haptoglobin binds free hemoglobin released from hemolyzed red cells to form stable complexes which are removed from the circulation by the reticuloendothelial system. It is composed of two nonidentical pairs of polypeptide chains, α and β, with 19% carbohydrate on the β-chain, and occurs in three genetically determined forms based on differences in the α-chain. Reduced levels of haptoglobin indicate increased release of free hemoglobin resulting from hemolysis. Haptoglobin is measured mainly by turbidometric or nephelometric immunoassays or by radial immunodiffusion and a range of commercial kits are available (Ward, 1993).

Coombs' Test

This is also called the antiglobulin test and exists in two forms. In the direct test, the patient's red cells are mixed with Coombs' reagent (antiserum containing antibodies directed against human immunoglobulins and/or complement components, e.g., IgM, IgA, C3, and C4). The anti-human antibodies attach to any immunoglobulin molecules on the red cell surfaces resulting in agglutination of the red cells. In the indirect test, patient plasma is incubated with normal red cells and, after washing, anti–red cell immunoglobulins are detected after the addition of Coombs' reagent (Dacie and Lewis, 1991).

Two kinds of Coombs reagent are available. Broad spectrum Coombs reagent contains antibodies against both immunoglobulins and complement factors, and therefore will pick up both immunoglobulin and complement molecules on the red cell surface. Specific Coombs reagents are antisera against a mixture of immunoglobulin heavy chains (γ, μ and α chains), individual class or subclass heavy chains (μ chain or IgM Fc, or $\gamma1$), or mixed or individual complement components (e.g., C4 or C3)(see Chap. 14). Patients who have only complement components on the red cell surface, as is seen in cold agglutinin hemolytic anemias and IgM mediated hemolytic anemias, are positive with broad spectrum but not with many more specific antisera. Improved reagents with broad specificity but reduced tendency to give false positives can be made from cocktails of specific antibodies (Dacie and Lewis, 1991).

In patients with high titers of anti–red cell antibodies, free anti–red cell antibodies may be found in the plasma. These can be identified with the indirect Coombs' test, since test red cells with different antigen components (e.g., with different blood group antigens) can be used, which also allows the specificity of the "auto"-antibodies to be characterized. In a patient who has received a blood transfusion, if the direct test is negative and an indirect test with donor-type red cells is positive, then allo- rather than autoantibodies are probably responsible for the anemia.

Polycythemia

Polycythemia is a condition in which the number of red cells is abnormally high. Patients who have elevated hemoglobin and hematocrit levels with a normal red cell mass are defined as having pseudopolycythemia and this is usually associated with a reduced plasma volume. In true polycythemia there is an increase in red cell mass which can be divided into primary and secondary forms. Secondary polycythemia, in turn, is divided into appropriate and inappropriate. Conditions defined as appropriate are those in which there is reduced oxygen supply, such as severe pulmonary disease with hypoxia. Conditions defined as inappropriate are associated with a tumor causing increased but unneeded production of erythropoietin.

Primary polycythemia (polycythemia vera, polycythemia rubra vera) is characterized not just by an elevated red cell mass but also by elevated white cell and platelet counts. The spleen is also enlarged and the serum vitamin B_{12}, vitamin B_{12} binding capacity, and leukocyte alkaline phosphatase levels are elevated.

Erythropoietin

The determination of plasma erythropoietin concentrations is very important for the differential diagnosis of polycythemia syndromes, and for investigations of anemia. Erythropoietin, a 34,000 mol wt glycoprotein (carbohydrate represents 40% of its total mass) with 166 amino acid residues in a single polypeptide chain, stimulates the division of red cell precursors with a subsequent increase in the red cell mass. Erythropoietin blood levels are relatively normal in patients with renal failure, are elevated in secondary polycythemia or hemolytic anemia, but are markedly reduced in true polycythemia.

The performance of early RIAs for erythropoietin was hampered by the use of incompletely purified antigen and standard, but the development of recombinant human erythropoietin expressed in mammalian cells has removed this restriction. The erythropoietin WHO Second International Reference Preparation (no. 67/343) purified from urine is available from the National Institute of Biological Standards (Potters Bar, Herts, UK). All preparations should be calibrated against this standard and the measurements expressed as IU/L. A variety of reliable RIAs have been developed (e.g., Schlageter, et al., 1990) but most are relatively slow (see Tanebe, et al., 1992 for a comprehensive list of references). Many are also relatively insensitive (detection limit >2 IU/L) and incapable of accurately measuring the very low concentrations found in polycythemia, which may be useful for the accurate diagnosis of polycythemia vera. More sensitive immunometric assays have been described. These include an immunoradiometric assay (IRMA) (Andre, et al., 1992) and an immunoenzymometric assay (IEMA) (Tanebe, 1992), both with two monoclonal antibodies, which have detection limits of 0.5 and 0.3 IU/L, and take 3.5 to 2.5 hours to perform, respectively. However, in most cases of polycythemia vera examined, the erythropoietin levels were near or lower than the detection limits of even these assays. In general, measured concentrations were lower than observed with RIA, which is consistent with the improved specificity often observed with immunometric assays.

WHITE CELLS

Neutrophils

Neutropenia is a reduction in the concentration of circulating neutrophils. As with erythrocytes in certain anemias, the cause can be either a decrease in production by the bone marrow or an increased destruction in the peripheral circulation. Usually microscopic examination of a bone marrow aspirate is sufficient to identify decreased granulocyte production. When increased peripheral destruction is the cause, an immune mechanism, perhaps drug precipitated, is the most common etiology, and the detection of antineutrophil antibodies (by immunofluorescence or agglutination assay) would be necessary to confirm a diagnosis of immune neutropenia (Coates, et al., 1992).

Lymphocytes

B cells and T cells have on their surfaces various CD molecules which allow the identification of the different types and degrees of maturation of lymphocytes. Extensive lists of CD molecules with their cellular distributions and properties are included in many manuals and textbooks (e.g., Hoffbrand and Pettit, 1993). The two most important lymphocyte categories are helper T cells (identified by the presence of CD4) and suppressor T cells (CD8). CD5 is typical of B cells of chronic lymphocytic leukemia. CD7 is found in T cells of acute lymphoblastic leukemia. CD10 marks pre-B cells, which are usually found in childhood acute lymphoblastic leukemia and indicate a poor prognosis. Terminal deoxynucleotidyl transferase (TdT), which is present on the surface of cells of thymic origin and in nearly all cases of acute lymphocytic or undifferentiated leukemia, is used to separate a lymphoid from myeloid leukemias. Most malignant lymphomas can be differentiated by morphologic features, but occasionally the determination of specific cell surface antigens is necessary; for example, Ki-67, or CD25 (the IL-2 receptor) surface markers are important adverse prognostic indicators.

Flow Cytometry

Fluorescence activated flow cytometry, with fluorescence-labeled monoclonal antibodies, represents one of the greatest recent advances in diagnostic immunology. It allows the counting of different types of cells in a complex mixture, for example, lymphocytes with distinctive functional activities, lineages, and maturational states. The principle of determination involves the use of fluorescein-conjugated murine monoclonal antibodies against the various CD and other surface markers, with electronic analysis of the fluorescence and other signals originating from single cells as they pass a light source.

The application of flow cytometry in tests for granulocyte, lymphocyte, and monocyte number and function has become routine in the diagnosis of a wide range of neoplastic and other diseases, and in monitoring immunosuppressive and immunorestorative treatments. These are described at length in a recent manual (Giorgi, 1992).

Plasma Cells

Monoclonal proliferations of bone marrow plasma cells can cause neoplastic tumors, many of which are associated with elevated concentrations of a monoclonal protein in serum or urine, or both. The monoclonal protein (paraprotein) may be an immunoglobulin or an immunoglobulin chain, and is fully characterized to exactly diagnose the condition. There are nine types of heavy chains, called $\alpha 1$, $\alpha 2$, ϵ, δ, $\gamma 1$, $\gamma 2$, $\gamma 3$, $\gamma 4$, and μ, and two types of light chains, called λ and κ. Urinary Bence Jones proteins are λ or κ light chains. Serum protein electrophoresis is a simple screening test that can partially identify paraproteins. More exact identification is accomplished by immunofixation or immunoelectrophoresis with antisera specific for each heavy and light chain (Caron and Penn, 1992). (See also under M–protein in Chap. 16.)

β_2-Microglobulin

β_2-Microglobulin, a member of the immunoglobulin superfamily, is a single polypeptide chain of mol wt 11,500, which represents the light chain portion of the major histocompatibility complex found in cell membranes. It is present in plasma and other body fluids and is reabsorbed into the bloodstream when renal tubular function is normal. It is measured in serum and urine samples, but is unstable at low pH, so that levels determined in urine with a pH less than 6.5 are unreliable.

A wide variety of commercial immunoassays for the measurement of β_2-microglobulin are available. Some are competitive (RIA, enzyme immunoassay [EIA], fluoroimmunoassay [FIA]), but many two-site immunometric assays with various labeling substances are also available (Ward, 1993; Kandoussi, et al., 1993). Like ferritin, it may also be automatically determined by means of immunonephelometry (Iguaz, et al., 1992). Elevated plasma β_2-microglobulin distinguishes multiple myeloma from benign monoclonal gammopathy, and can be used to follow the course of the disease. It is also elevated during allograft rejection and chronic renal failure (see also Chap. 16).

PLATELETS AND THE COAGULATION SYSTEM

Platelets are formed in bone marrow by fragmentation of the cytoplasm of very large, multinuclear cells—the megakaryocytes. The two most important features of the platelets are granules (containing adenosine disphosphate [ADP], calcium, serotonin, platelet factors, and coagulation factors) and adhesion proteins on their surface. Hemostasis (coagulation), the mechanism by which bleeding is controlled, is a complex system, defects in any part of which can result in serious abnormalities. Platelet aggregation can directly stimulate the activation of thrombin by means of exposed membrane phospholipid (platelet factor 3).

Platelets

The most common abnormality of platelets is a low platelet count or thrombocytopenia, caused by decreased platelet production (decreased marrow megakaryocytes) or increased platelet destruction (increased megakaryocytes). Immune thrombocytopenic purpura (ITP) is the most common cause of thrombocytopenia. A typical patient with ITP will have a low platelet count, no splenomegaly, and bone marrow with increased megakaryocytes. Measurement of antiplatelet antibodies and platelet membrane associated immunoglobulin may be used to confirm the diagnosis. Their presence has prognostic implications, especially in pregnancy where antiplatelet antibodies may cross the placenta. The antibodies bound to the platelet surface include abnormal autoantibodies, immune complexes bound to Fc receptors, and nonspecific absorbed immunoglobulin. They are detected by immunofluorescent staining or by flow cytometry (Lalezari and Khorshidi, 1992) or with radiolabeled antibodies (Tijhuis, et al., 1991).

Coagulation

The entire clotting process is dedicated to the formation of thrombin, the enzyme which cleaves the fibrinogen molecule to fibrinopeptides A and B, and fibrin monomers. Fibrin monomers spontaneously aggregate to form fibrin polymer, the material of the clot. The coagulation system is tested initially by a prothrombin time, activated partial thromboplastin time, and thrombin time. Fibrinogen is also frequently measured (Dacie and Lewis, 1991), sometimes by radial immunodiffusion, but the calibration of many of the assays used could be improved (Palareti, et al., 1991). Abnormal results for any of these tests mandates further testing.

Degradation Products

One of the most important abnormalities of the fibrinogen system is the syndrome known as disseminated intravascular coagulation. This is associated with a wide range of conditions including sepsis and shock, abnormal late pregnancy, some carcinomas, liver disease, and severe malaria, and results in chronic clotting in small blood vessels or a fulminant hemorrhagic syndrome. The situation is suspected when there is a prolongation of the thrombin time, with decreased platelets and fibrinogen. The diagnosis is confirmed by other test results including high levels of fibrinogen/fibrin degradation products in serum or urine (Dacie and Lewis, 1991; Hillyard, et al., 1987).

Prothrombin fragment 1.2 has been suggested as a biomarker of thrombin formation during coagulation with diagnostic potential for defining the prethrombotic or hypercoagulable state, assessing thrombotic risk, and monitoring anticoagulation therapy (Hursting, et al., 1993a, 1993b). A specific two-site, enzyme-linked immunometric assay, with immobilized monoclonal antibody against the carboxy terminal of fragment 1.2 and horseradish peroxidase conjugated to polyclonal antibody binding the amino terminal region, was recently developed (Hursting, et al., 1993a). The reference interval in healthy persons of fragment 1.2 concentrations has also been determined (Hursting, et al., 1993b).

Antiphospholipid Antibodies

The fibrinolytic system counters excessive clotting, and patients who have defects in this process are termed hypercoagulable. Among the most common causes is the lupus anticoagulant, which is probably an immunoglobulin directed against phospholipids. Quantitation of anticardiolipin and other such antibodies is by immunoassay (Loizou, et al., 1985; Johnstone, et al., 1992) (see also Chap. 13). Patients who are positive for both anticardiolipin antibody and the coagulation test for lupus anticoagulant (Rose and Roberts, 1992) are at particularly high risk for thromboembloic problems.

Coagulation Factors

Most coagulation factors can be determined by means of one-stage coagulation assays in which optimal amounts of all the clotting factors are present except the one to be determined. Of the specific factor deficiencies the most common is X-linked factor VIII deficiency, which is also known as hemophilia A. Factor VIII can be measured with a clot-solubility coagulation assay, but is also determined by immunoelectrophoresis. Hemophilia B, factor IX deficiency, is rare and it can be measured by immunometric assay (Dacie and Lewis, 1991).

Von Willebrand Antigen

Factor VIII, produced in the vascular endothelium, is transported by a complex protein called "factor VIII related antigen" or von Willebrand antigen. Von Willebrand disease is an autosomal dominant disease in which there is an apparent deficiency of factor VIII due to a deficiency of the binding protein. Von Willebrand factor interacts with platelet glycoprotein 1b, and this interaction brings about platelet aggregation. In the absence of von Willebrand factor, the antibiotic ristocetin will not induce platelet aggregation. Von Willebrand's antigen can be measured by immunoelectrophoresis (Dacie and Lewis, 1991), RIA, or IEMA assay (Benson, 1991).

REFERENCES

Andre M, Ferster A, Toppet M, Fondu P, Dratwa M, Bergmann P. Performance of an immunoradiometric assay of erythropoietin and results for specimens from anemic and polycythemic patients. Clin Chem 1992;38:758–763.

Benson RE, Catalfamo JL, Brooks M, Dodds WJ. A sensitive immunoassay for von Willebrand factor. J Immunoassay 1991;12:371–390.

Bigazzi PE, Burek CL, Rose NR. Antibodies to tissue-specific endocrine, gastrointestinal, and surface-receptor antigens. In: Rose NR, deMacario EC, Fahey JL, Friedman H, Penn GM, eds. Manual of Clinical Laboratory Immunology, ed 4. Washington, DC: American Society of Microbiology, 1992;765–774.

Borque L, Rus A, Coro JD, Maside C, Escanero J. Automated quantitative nephelometric latex immunoassay for determining ferritin in human serum. J Clin Lab Analysis 1992;6:239–244.

Caron J, Penn GM. Electroproretic and immunochemical characterization of immunoglobulins. In: Rose NR, deMacario EC, Fahey JL, Friedman H, Penn GM, eds. Manual of Clinical Laboratory Immunology, ed 4. Washington, DC: American Society of Microbiology, 1992;84–95.

Coates TD, Beyer LA, Baehner RL. Laboratory evaluation of neutropenia and neutrophil dysfunction. In: Rose NR, deMacario EC, Fahey JL, Friedman H, Penn GM, eds. Manual of Clinical Laboratory Immunology, ed 4. Washington, DC: American Society of Microbiology, 1992;409–418.

Conn DA. Detection of type I and type II antibodies to intrinsic factor. Med Lab Sci 1986;43:148–151.

Dacie JV, Lewis SM. Practical Haematology, ed 7. Edinburgh: Churchill Livingstone, 1991.

Flowers CA, Kuizon M, Beard JL, Skikene BS, Covell AM, Cook JD. Serum ferritin assay for prevalence studies of iron deficiency. Am J Hematol 1986;23:141–151.

Giorgi JV, ed. Section D. Immune cell phenotyping by flow cytometry. In: Rose NR, deMacario EC, Fahey JL, Friedman H, Penn GM, eds. Manual of Clinical Laboratory Immunology, ed 4. Washington, DC: American Society of Microbiology, 1992;156–235.

Grassi J, Roberge CJ, Frobert Y, Pradelles P, Poubelle PE. Determination of IL1a, IL1b and IL2 in biological media using specific enzyme immunometric assays. Immunol Rev 1991;119:125–145.

Hillyard CJ, Blake AS, Wilson K, et al. A latex aggltination assay for D dimer: evaluation and application to the diagnosis of thrombotic disease. Clin Chem 1987;33:1837–1840.

Hoffbrand AV, Pettit JE. Essential Immunology, ed 3. Oxford: Blackwell Scientific Publications, 1993.

Hursting MJ, Butman BT, Steiner JP, et al. Monoclonal antibodies specific for prothrombin fragment 1.2 and their use in a quantitative enzyme-linked immunosorbent assay. Clin Chem 1993a;39:583–591.

Hursting MJ, Stead AG, Crout FV, Horvath BZ, Moore BM. Effects of age, race, sex and smoking on prothrombin fragment 1.2 in a healthy population. Clin Chem 1993b; 39:683–686.

Iguaz F, Naval J, Borque L. Measurement of serum beta$_2$-microglobulin by a latex nephelometric immunoassay. Clin Biochem 1992;25:245–249.

Johnstone F, Kiltpatrick D, Burns S. Anticardiolipin antibodies and pregnancy: outcome in women with human immunodeficiency virus infection. Obstet Gynecol 1992;80:92–96.

Kandoussi A, Cachera C, Pagniez D, Saile R, Tacquet A. Quantification of β_2-microglobulin and albumin in plasma and peritoneal dialysis fluid by a noncompetitive immunoenzymometric assay. Clin Chem 1993;39:93–96.

Lalezari P, Khorshidi M. Neutrophil and platelet antibodies in immune neutropenia and thrombocytopenia. In: Rose NR, deMacario EC, Fahey JL, Friedman H, Penn GM, eds. Manual of Clinical Laboratory Immunology, ed 4. Washington, DC: American Society of Microbiology, 1992;344–350.

Loizou US, McCrea JD, Rudge AC, Reynolds R, Boyle CC, Harris EN. Measurements of anticardiolipin antibody by ELISA: standardization and quantitation of results. Clin Exp Immunol 1985;62:738–745.

National Committee for Clinical Laboratory Standards. Proposed Standard: PLSA-12 Guideline for Evaluating a B$_{12}$ Assay. NCCLS, 1980.

Palareti G, Maccaferri M, Manotti C, et al. Fibrinogen assays: a collaborative study of six different methods. Clin Chem 1991;37:714–719.

Rose VL, Roberts HR. Immunology of acquired inhibitors to clotting proteins. In: Rose NR, deMacario EC, Fahey JL, Friedman H, Penn GM, eds. Manual of Clinical Laboratory Immunology, ed 4. Washington, DC: American Society of Microbiology, 1992; 351–362.

Schlageter M-H, Toubert M-E, Podgorniak M-P, Najean Y. Radioimmunoassay of erythropoietin: analytical performance and clinical use in hematology. Clin Chem 1990;36: 1731–1735.

Tanebe M, Teshima S, Hanyu T, Hayashi Y. Rapid and sensitive method for erythropoietin determination in serum. Clin Chem 1992;38:1752–1755.

Tijhuis GJ, Klaassen RJL, Modderman PW, Ouwehand WH, Borne AEGK. Quantification of platelet bound immunoglobulins of different class and subclass using radiolabeled monoclonal antibodies: assay conditions and clinical application. Br J Haematol 1991;77:93–101.

Ward TM, ed, Proteins and Tumour Markers, Vol 2, part 3. In: Seth J, ed. The Immunoassay Kit Directory, Series A: Clinical Chemistry. Norwell, MA: Kluwer Academic Publishers, 1993.

Waters HM, Smith C, Howarth JE, Dawson DW, Delamore IW. A new enzyme immunoassay for the detection of total, type I and type II intrinsic factor antibody. J Clin Pathol 1989;42:307–312.

Zenke G, Strittmatter U, Tees R, et al. A cocktail of three monoclonal antibodies significantly increases the sensitivity of an enzyme immunoassay for human granulocyte-macrophage colony-stimulating factor. J Immunoassay 1991;12:185–206.

CHAPTER 13

Rheumatic Disease

Arthur Bobrove

The rheumatic diseases comprise a wide assortment of disorders affecting the musculoskeletal system. They are classified as degenerative, metabolic, infectious, infiltrative or inflammatory, and immunologic. The autoimmune rheumatic diseases include the following:

1. *Rheumatoid arthritis.* A chronic, systemic, inflammatory polyarthritis with the presence of circulating autoantibodies specific for the Fc portion of IgG.
2. *Systemic lupus erythematosus* (SLE). A chronic multisystem disease that may provoke an inflammatory response in many organ systems, and exhibits features of faulty immunoregulation with the development of a wide range of autoantibodies, particularly to antigens found in the cell nucleus.
3. *Systemic sclerosis and overlap syndromes.* Disorders of connective tissue and blood vessels leading to intense fibrosis of the skin and other organs and associated with vasospasm manifested in Raynaud's phenomenon.
4. *Sjögren's syndrome.* A chronic autoimmune disease occurring independently or in association with one of the other diseases described above, and associated with destruction of lacrimal and salivary glands leading to dry eyes and mouth (autoimmune exocrinopathy).
5. *Polymyositis and dermatomyositis.* Idiopathic inflammatory myopathies associated with progressive proximal muscle weakness. A distinct subset is associated with underlying malignancy.

Advances in laboratory diagnosis of the rheumatic diseases have clearly outpaced advances in therapy. Nevertheless, increased knowledge of various immunologic and genetic factors in several of these disorders has also contributed to a greater understanding of their pathophysiology.

AUTOANTIBODIES

Methods of Measurement

The range of methods are described in detail in a recently published manual (Rose, et al., 1992). Tests with immunofluorescence or immunoperoxidase staining and microscope assisted evaluation of the density and pattern of binding by patient antibodies to standardized tissue sections and cultured cells are basic methods for the detection of antibodies binding nuclear and cytoplasmic antigens. Nevertheless, quantitative immunonephelometric and labeled immunoassay methods, designed to measure individual, diagnostically significant antibodies which bind specific antigens, are playing an ever increasing role, which is particularly useful in reducing the rate of false positive results. Already many of the autoantigens are produced in bacteria, etc., by means of recombinant DNA methods (Renz, et al., 1989; Paxton, et al., 1990). Alternative or complementary methods include immunodiffusion assays (Wilson and Sanders, 1992), immunoblot assays (Fonong, et al., 1990), microgel diffusion blotting (DeKeyser, et al., 1990), and enzyme immunoassays for the simultaneous determination of multiple autoantibodies (Paxton, et al., 1990). (See also Chaps. 1, 3, 15, and 17 for further information on assays for specific antibodies.)

Rheumatoid Factors

Rheumatoid factors are IgM, IgG, IgA, and IgE antibodies (see Table 17-1 for their general properties) which bind to the constant region of IgG. They are found in the blood of persons with rheumatoid arthritis or with other rheumatoid or chronic diseases such as mixed essential cryoglobulinemia, Sjögren's syndrome, pulmonary fibrosis, or pulmonary silicosis. They are also found in the joint synovial fluid as large IgM-IgG and IgG complexes which fix complement, and are responsible for complement-mediated tissue damage. Cook and Agnello (1992) describe the range of tests used for rheumatoid factors.

Assays for rheumatoid factors were among the earliest immunoassays. The first were hemagglutination assays with human IgG–coated sheep erythrocytes. In the 1950s IgG coated polystyrene latex particles were introduced, and since then latex slide agglutination tests have been the most popular assays. However, the results from these assays produced in different laboratories or by different companies are only poorly comparable and there has been little pressure to standardize them because the accurate determination of rheumatoid factor concentrations has not been clinically important in most cases. Nevertheless, a reference preparation with defined international units of rheumatoid factor exists (Anderson, et al., 1970), and more quantitative automatic immunonephelometric, immunoturbidimetric, and enzyme linked immunoassays are commercially available. All of the commercial assays detect or measure mainly IgM rheumatoid factors. (See also Chaps. 1, 3, 15, and 17 for further information on assays for specific antibodies.)

Antinuclear Antibodies

Autoantibodies binding to a wide range of constituents of the cellular nucleus are characteristic of a range of autoimmune diseases (Table 13–1). They are described as antinuclear antibodies (ANA) and the antigens include double-stranded and single-stranded DNA, and a range of extractable antigens.

Detection of the presence or absence of ANA in the serum of patients with suspected SLE is clinically useful because they are found in more than 95% of patients with untreated SLE, although they are also found in about 4% of healthy individuals. ANA are detected in serum by means of the indirect fluorescent antibody technique with the antigens supplied as cryostat sections of mouse kidney or liver, or as cultured cells such as human epithelial cell line, HEp-2. The cultured cells are better because they have larger nuclei and some relevant antigens are present in higher concentrations (Fritzler, 1992). ANA may be referred to as FANA (fluorescent ANA) when detected by means of an immunofluorescence test.

Quantitation of ANA in terms of defined units, or in terms of the maximum dilution at which a positive result is obtained in a qualitative assay, helps to distinguish patients with relevant disease from those who give a false positive result. Patterns of FANA staining as obtained with tissue sections or cells are very useful guides to the type of antibody present and correlate with the type of connective tissue disease. For example, a peripheral (or rim) pattern and/or homogeneous pattern correlates with antibodies to DNA and is associated with active SLE, whereas a speckled pattern is caused by antibodies to ribonucleoprotein (RNP) and is seen in patients with scleroderma as well as in some patients with SLE. A nucleolar pattern may be seen in patients with isolated Raynaud's disease (Table 13 –1) (Fritzler, 1992; Mongey, et al., 1991; Tan, 1989).

Antibodies to centromere, a specialized domain at the primary constriction of a eukaryotic chromosome, are found in about 50% of individuals having features of scleroderma. Usually these patients have the limited form, or CREST syndrome (calcinosis cutis, Raynaud's phenomenon, esophageal dysmotility, sclerodactyly, and telangiectasia), and the presence of anticentromere antibodies generally indicates a more favorable prognosis (Steen, et al., 1988).

Anti-DNA Antibodies

The specific detection of antibodies to natural or double-stranded DNA may be performed in a variety of ways. In the modified Farr assay ammonium sulfate is used to precipitate radiolabeled bacterial DNA after addition of patient serum (Isenberg, et al., 1987). Alternatively, *Crithidia luciliae,* a unicellular protozoan with a modified giant mitochondrion (the kinetoplast) containing double-stranded DNA unassociated with RNA or nuclear proteins, is used as the source of DNA and the location of fluorescence examined microscopically after exposure to patient serum and fluorescence-labeled anti-Ig class antibody. The *C. luciliae* test is widely used (Ballou, 1992). However, it has been criticized for poor sensitivity and for not being as accurate as the Farr test (the standard reference method) in monitoring patients with active lupus

Table 13 –1   Antigenic Activity of Antinuclear Antibodies*

Type of Antibody	Disease in Which Antibodies Are Seen	Characteristic of Antigenic Determinants	Pattern Observed by Indirect Immunofluorescence Test	Other Tests Used to Detect Specific Antibody
1. Reacts only double-stranded DNA	Characteristic of SLE; few cases reported	Double-strandedness of DNA essential	Rim and/or homogeneous	RIA, ID, CIE, HA, CF, EIA, special IF
2. Reacts with double- and single-stranded DNA†	High levels in SLE; lower levels in other rheumatic diseases	Related to deoxyribose, purines, and pyrimidines, but not dependent on double helix	Same as no. 1	Same as no. 1
3. Reacts only with single-stranded DNA	Rheumatic and nonrheumatic diseases	Related to purines and pyrimidines with ribose or deoxyribose equally reactive	Not detected on routine screen; special treatment necessary	RIA, ID, CIE, HA, EIA, CF
Deoxynucleoprotein, soluble	LE cell antibody in SLE, drug-induced LE	DNA-histone complex; dissociated components are nonreactive	Rim and/or homogeneous	RIA, ID, EIA, latex, HA, bentonite, LE cell
Histone (H1, H2A, H2B, H3, H4)	SLE, drug-induced SLE, RA	Different classes of histones may have different determinants	Homogeneous and/or rim	CF, IB, RIA, EIA
Histone (H3)	Undifferentiated connective tissue disease	H3	Variable large speckles††	RIA, EIA, IB

Sm†	Highly diagnostic of SLE	Proteins complexed with U1, U2, U4 –U6 snRNA spliceosome component	Speckled	ID, CIE, HA, EIA,IB
Nuclear RNP†	High levels in mixed connective tissue disease and SLE; lower in other diseases	Proteins complexed with U1, U2, snRNA spliceosome component	Speckled	ID, CIE, HA, EIA, IB
Ribosomal RNP†	SLE	Phosphoproteins associated with ribosomes	Nucleolar, cytoplasm	ID, IB
Scl-70	Highly diagnostic of scleroderma	DNA topoiso-merase I	Atypical speckled	ID, IB
Centromere† (kinetochore)	CREST variant scleroderma, less frequently in Raynaud's phenomenon and other diseases	Proteins at inner and outer kinetochore plate	Discrete speckled§	IB

Table 13–1   (*continued*)

Type of Antibody	Disease in Which Anti-bodies Are Seen	Characteristic of Antigenic Determinants	Pattern Observed by Indirect Immuno-Fluorescence Test	Other Tests Used to Detect Specific Antibody
SS-A (Ro)[†]	High prevalence in Sjögren's syndrome sicca complex; sub-acute cutaneous lupus and neonatal lupus syndrome; SLE; lower preva-lence in other rheumatic diseases	Proteins complexed to Y1 –Y5 RNA	Speckled or negative: not consistent on substrates from all sources	ID, EIA, CIE, IB, EIA
SS-B (La, Ha)[†]	High prevalence in Sjögren's syndrome sicca complex; lower prevalence in other diseases	Phosphoprotein complexed with RNA polymerase III transcripts	Speckled	ID, EIA, CIE, EIA, IB
PM-1 (Pm/Scl)	Myositis/sclero-derma overlap	Complex of 11 proteins	Variable, speckled	ID, IB
Jo-1	Polymyositis	Histidyl-tRNA synthetase	?Cytoplasmic	IB
Mi-2	Dermatomyositis	Proteins	Homogeneous	
Ku	SLE	DNA-binding proteins		
PCNA (Ga, LE-4)	SLE	33-kDa protein (cyclin): auxiliary	Variable-size speckles in some cells	ID, IB

NspI	Various rheumatic diseases	80-kDa protein	Speckled interphase cells‡	None
Nucleolar	High prevalence in sclero- derma; SLE	RNA polymerase I; Fibrillarin; nucleolar organizer protein	Nucleolar	IB
Nuclear matrix	SLE, undifferentiated connective tissue disease	HnRNA + matrix proteins	Large speckles‡	None

*Abbreviations: CF, complement fixation; CIE, counterimmunoelectrophoresis in agar gel; EIA, enzyme-linked immunoassay; HA, passive hemagglutination; HnRNA, heterogeneous nuclear RNA; IB, immunoblotting; ID, agar gel double immunodiffusion; IF, immunofluorescence; LE, lupus erythematosus; NSp, nuclear speckled; PCNA, proliferating cell nuclear antigen; PM, polymyositis, RA; rheumatoid arthritis; RANA, rheumatoid arthritis nuclear antigen; RIA, radioimmunoassay; RNP, ribonucleoprotein; Scl, scleroderma; SLE, systemic lupus erythematosus; Sm, Smith; SnRNA, small nuclear RNA; SS, Sjögren's syndrome.

†On acetone-fixed mouse kidney substrate.

‡On HEp-2 and other tissue culture cell substrate.

§Prototype sera available from the Centers for Disease Control (Tan, et al., 1977).

Fritzler M. Immunofluorescent antinuclear antibody test. In: Rose NR, de Macario EC, Fahey JL, et al., eds. Manual of Clinical Laboratory Immunology, ed 4. Washington, DC: American Society for Microbiology, 1992;724–729. Reproduced with permission.

nephritis in which the level of antibodies to double-stranded DNA detected frequently correlates with clinical activity (Monier, et al., 1988). Anti-DNA antibodies may also be quantified by means of enzyme linked assay with natural DNA indirectly absorbed to microtiter plate wells via methylated bovine serum albumin (Rubin, 1992).

Serial measurements for antibodies to natural DNA and concomitant measurements of the complement component C3 and/or C4 (see below under Complement Components) may allow prediction of a flare in lupus activity (an elevation in anti-DNA antibodies with a reduction in serum C3 or C4 [Swaak, et al., 1986]), or may indicate disease remission (a reduction in anti-DNA antibodies and normalization of the C3 or C4 level). Thus, the measurement of antibodies to double-stranded DNA helps in the diagnosis of SLE, prediction of the progress of the disease, and assists in therapeutic decision making (ter Borg, et al., 1990a).

Extractable Nuclear Antigen Antibodies

Extractable nuclear antigen (ENA) antibodies bind a wide range of proteins and nucleoproteins, which were often initially identified simply as disease related antigens but subsequently recognized as known functional entities, for example, the Jo-1 antigen is the amino acid activating enzyme histidyl-tRNA synthetase (Table 13–1). ENA antibodies are detected by methods based on immunofluorescence staining but quantitation of specific antibodies can yield extra diagnostic information. Sm antibodies are highly specific for SLE, whereas antibodies to RNP in high titer are associated with mixed connective tissue disease (Van Venrooy, et al., 1991).

Antihistone Antibodies

While antihistone antibodies are detected in only approximately 20% of patients with SLE, they are found in 100% of patients with procainamide induced lupus, and therefore they are a useful marker in such cases. These samples invariably have FANA which display a diffuse pattern after immunofluorescent staining. Other patterns, such as speckled or nucleolar, essentially exclude the diagnosis of a drug induced lupus (Rubin and Waga, 1987). Antihistone antibodies can also be quantified by means of enzyme-linked assay (Rubin, 1992).

Sjögren's Syndrome (SS) Antibodies

Antibodies to SS-A/Ro antigen (ribonucleoproteins) are detected in about 60% of patients with Sjögren's syndrome and about 35% with SLE. They increase the risk of a woman with lupus having an infant with congenital heart block to about 5%, and they have been shown to bind fetal cardiac tissue (Taylor et al., 1986). Maternal SS-A/Ro antibodies act as a serologic marker for neonatal lupus erythematosus (Lane and Watson, 1984). It has also been demonstrated that many patients with so-called ANA-negative SLE, typified by subacute cutaneous lupus and positive IgM-rheumatoid factor, frequently have antibodies to SS-A/Ro (Maddison, et al., 1981). Thus the non-detection of ANA does not exclude the existence of antibodies to SS-A/Ro.

Antibodies to SS-B/La (phosphoprotein complexes) are found in patients with Sjögren's syndrome with a lower prevalence in other rheumatic diseases. The frequency of these antibodies appears to be less than for SS-A/Ro and it is more common for anti SS-B/La to occur independently (Harley et al., 1986). It has been claimed that the presence of anti SS-B/La also increases the risk of congenital heart block.

Scleroderma (Scl) Antibodies

Scl-70 antibodies are highly specific for diffuse scleroderma, although they are found in only about 30% of patients with this disease (Weiner, et al., 1988). The presence of Scl-70 antibodies in patients with isolated Raynaud's phenomena may have prognostic significance for the development of systemic sclerosis. Scl-70 antibodies are best detected by EIA with immunoblot confirmation (Fonong, et al., 1990).

Myositis-Associated Antibodies

Low titer ANA are found in approximately 50% of patients with idiopathic inflammatory myopathies (e.g., polymyositis or dermatomyositis). On the other hand, homogeneous cytoplasmic staining of HEp-2 cells by sera from patients with inflammatory myositis suggests the presence of myositis-specific antibodies. Jo-1 antibody is the most common of these myositis-specific antibodies and is found in 20% –25% of myositis patients. It is also associated with interstitial lung disease (Love et al., 1991), and the Jo-1 syndrome. This consists of myositis arthritis, Raynaud's phenomenon, interstitial lung disease, and a scaling, cracking rash of fingertips (mechanic's hands) (Miller, 1993). The preferred methods of detection are enzyme-linked immunoassays (Fonong, et al., 1990). Other "myositis-specific" autoantibodies are found in a small percentage of myocitis patients, including anti-Mi2 and anti-SRP. However, these are not routinely measured.

Antiphospholipid Antibodies

Antiphospholipid (cardiolipin) antibodies may be detected by immunoassay, by a clotting assay, or as causing a false positive result in a test for syphilis. They are found in approximately 33% of lupus patients, and are associated with a high incidence of second-trimester fetal wastage in pregnant women, thrombocytopenia, and arterial or venous thrombotic events. Detection of anticardiolipin antibodies is performed by means of enzyme immunoassay (EIA) or radioimmunoassay (RIA) and should include IgG, IgM, and IgA isotypes (Lockshin and Gharavi, 1992; Loizou, et al., 1985). Antiphospholipid antibodies also exist in a clinical disorder separate from SLE, called primary antiphospholipid syndrome. This is characterized by the presence of one or more of the above clinical manifestations but without sufficient clinical criteria to establish a diagnosis of SLE.

A cofactor necessary for the binding of antiphospholipid antibodies to cardiolipin, β_2-glycoprotein 1 (apolipoprotein H), may be important to the thrombotic effects of anticardiolipin antibodies (Lockshin and Gharavi, 1992; McNeil, et al., 1990). The presence of β_2-glycoprotein 1 is also necessary for the detection of antiphospholipid antibodies by immunoassay. It has been traditionally (and unknowingly) supplied by the use of dilute bovine serum in assay buffers, but is now added in controlled amounts in some immunoenzymometric assays (IEMA) (Amiral, 1993).

Anti-Neutrophil Cytoplasmic Antibodies

Anti-neutrophil cytoplasmic antibodies (ANCA) are autoantibodies that bind to specific cytoplasmic proteins of neutrophils and monocytes. ANCA are useful as serologic markers for a number of systemic vasculitides, including Wegener's gran-ulomatosis and subsets of polyarteritis nodosa, leukocytoclastic vasculitis, and cres-centric glomerulonephritis (Jennette, et al., 1992). The most frequently used method for detecting ANCA is indirect immunofluorescence microscopy with alcohol-fixed neutrophils (Roberts and Rubin, 1992). Two patterns of fluorescence are produced by the two major ANCA subtypes, cytoplasmic (C-ANCA) and perinuclear (P-ANCA), and their relative frequencies differ among patients with different vasculitides. Serum ANCA concentrations may also be measured by flow cytometry, and enzyme-linked immunochemical methods are increasingly being used to evaluate and quantitate spe-cific ANCA antibodies. Quantitation of ANCA should help to guide therapy and as-sist in determining the level of disease activity (Van der Woude, et al., 1985).

Anti–Glomerular Basement Membrane Antibodies

Anti-GBM antibodies are found in patients with classical, untreated Goodpasture's syndrome and in a subset of patients with rapidly progressive glomerular nephritis (RP-GN). GBM antibodies react with noncollagenous type IV collagen subunits in human glomerular basement membrane as well as alveolar basement membrane but not membrane from other tissues (e.g., placenta). Because RP-GN may be associated with either GBM antibodies or ANCA and there are differences in the clinical be-havior of the anti-GBM and ANCA related diseases, testing for both is indicated for evaluation of the disease.

PROTEIN MARKERS

C-Reactive Protein

C-reactive protein (CRP) is a sensitive, acute phase reactant and its concentration in serum (normally about 800 μg/L) increases within 6 hours of the onset of inflamma-tion. It is synthesized in the liver and consists of five noncovalently bound subunits forming a 105,000 mol wt complex. Associated with choline-containing complex lipids, it binds to damaged cell membranes and to the capsule of some bacteria. Bound CRP activates the complement cascade. The measurement of CRP offers the added advantage of distinguishing between bacterial infection and a disease flare in SLE and, perhaps, other inflammatory rheumatic diseases (ter Borg, et al., 1990b). Laser nephrolometry, IEMA, fluoroimmunoassay (FIA) and EIA are currently replacing the standard agglutination technique for CRP measurements.

Complement Components

The complement system forms an integral part of the immune system. It is a complex mechanism for the antibody-independent (alternative pathway) or aggregated antibody–antigen complex-assisted (classical pathway, Fig. 13–1) inhibition and lysis of bacterial and other cells recognized as foreign. The total hemolytic complement assay (the CH_{50} assay) tests the ability to lyse 50% of a standard suspension of sheep erythrocytes coated with rabbit antibody. This depends on the activity of the entire classical pathway and the terminal sequence, and is most useful in detecting an isolated hereditary deficiency of one of the complement components (e.g., C2). Nevertheless, because normal serum contains some components in substantial excess, the CH_{50} may be normal when components C3 or C4 are significantly reduced, as in active lupus nephritis (Hebert, et al., 1991). It would appear, therefore, that measuring specific complement components may offer more clinically useful information.

Commercially developed immunoassays are available for individual complement factors, including C1 inhibitor, C1q, C1r, C1s, C2, C3, C3a des Arg, iC3b, C3c, C3d, C4, C4a des Arg, C4c, C4d fragment, C5, C5a, C5 des Arg, C6, C7, C8, and C9 (Ward, 1993). The development and clinical application in cases of rheumatic disease of a time-resolved immunofluorometric assay for C3 in cerebrospinal fluid has recently been described (Gaillard, et al., 1993). A set of two enzyme-linked procedures for the differential diagnosis of defects of the classical pathway (C1, C4, C2), the alternative pathway (C3, factor B, factor D, properdin) and the terminal components (C5–C9) has also been described (Fredrikson, et al., 1993).

REFERENCES

Amiral J. Immunoassays for antiphospholipid antibodies require β2GP1 for a standardized reactivity. Int Biotechnol Lab 1993; July:26.

Anderson SG, Bentzon MW, Houba V, King P. International reference preparation of rheumatoid arthritis serum. Bull WHO 1970;42:311–318.

Ballou S. Crithidia luciliae immunofluorescence test for antibodies to DNA. In: Rose NR, et al., Manual of Clinical Laboratory Immunology, ed 4. Washington, DC: American Society for Microbiology, 1992;730–734.

Cook L, Agnello V. Tests for detection of rheumatoid factors. In: Rose, NR, et al., Manual of Clinical Laboratory Immunology, ed 4. Washington, DC: American Society for Microbiology, 1992;762–764.

DeKeyser F, Verbruggen G, Veys EM, et al. "Microgel diffusion blotting" for sensitive detection of antibodies to extractable nuclear antigens. Clin Chem 1990;36:337–339.

Fonong T, Evans SM, Homburgere HA. Development and comparative evaluation of immunoblot assays for detecting autoantibodies to ScI 70 and Jo 1 antigens in serum. Clin Chem 1990;36:2052–2056.

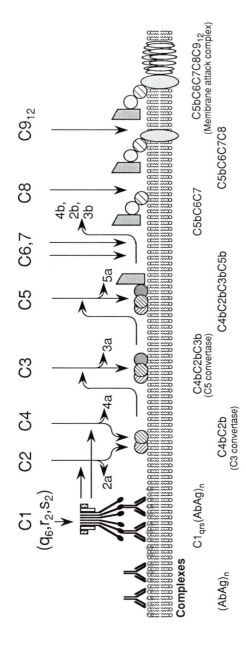

Figure 13-1.   The classical pathway of complement fixation leading to formation of the membrane attack complex. A cluster of foreign antigenic determinants is required to trigger the pathway but, since each activated enzyme (e.g., C3 convertase) cleaves many molecules of the next component, the whole pathway is an amplifying cascade with the formation of many lytic complexes due to the activation of one early component. Many of the activated intermediates bind tightly to membranes, and therefore most of these events take place on cell surfaces.

C3 is the pivotal component of both the classical and alternative pathways, which generate different C3 convertases. C3b binds to specific receptors on phagocytes enhancing their ability to engulf a cell to which C3b is attached. C3b also acts as part of a positive feedback loop, by also activating the alternative pathway. In addition, several of the small fragments (e.g., C3a, C4a, C5a) generated are biologically active and are the cause of the local inflammatory response associated with the activation of complement.

Fredrikson GN, Truedsson L, Sjöholm AG. New procedure for the detection of complement deficiency by ELISA. Analysis of activation pathways and circumvention of rheumatoid factor influence. J Immunol Methods 1993;166:263–270.

Fritzler M. Immunofluorescent antinuclear antibody test. In: Rose, NR, et al., eds. Manual of Clinical Laboratory Immunology, ed 4. Washington, DC: American Society for Microbiology, 1992;724–729.

Gaillard O, Mellet D, Diemert MC, et al. Time-resolved immunofluorimetric assay of complement C3: application to cerebrospinal fluid. Clin Chem 1993;39:309–312.

Harley JB, Alexander EL, Bias WB. Anti-Ro(SS-A) and anti-La(SSB) in patients with Sjögren's syndrome. Arthritis Rheum 1986;29:196–206.

Hebert LA, Cosio FG, Neff JC. Diagnostic significance of hypocomplementemia. Kidney Int 1991;39:811–821.

Isenberg DA, Dudeney C, Williams W. Measurement of anti-DNA antibodies: a reappraisal using five different methods. Ann Rheum Dis 1987;46:448 –456.

Jennette JC, Falk RJ. ANCA—diagnostic markers or pathogenic agents. Bull Rheum Dis 1992;41(8): 3–6.

Lane AT, Watson RM. Neonatal lupus erythematosus. Am J Dis Child 1984;138:663 –666.

Lockshin MD, Gharavi A. Antiphospholipid antibody. In: Rose NR, et al., eds. Manual of Clinical Laboratory Immunology, ed 4. Washington, DC: American Society for Microbiology, 1992;875–788.

Loizou S, McCrea JD, Rudge AC, Reynold R, Boyle CC, Harris EN. Measurement of anticardiolipin antibodies by an enzyme-linked immunosorbent assay (ELISA): standardization and quantitation of results. Clin Exp Immunol 1985;62:738–745.

Love LA, Leff RL, Fraser DD, et al. A new approach to the classification of idiopathic inflammatory myopathy: myositis-specific autoantibodies define useful monogeneous patient groups. Medicine 1991;70:360–374.

Maddison PJ, Provost TT, Reichlin M. Serological findings in patients with "ANA negative" systemic lupus erythematosus. Medicine 1981;60:87–94.

McNeil HP, Simpson RJ, Chesterman CN, Krilis SA. Antiphospholipid antibodies are directed against a complex antigen that includes a lipid-binding inhibitor of coagulation: β_2-glycoprotein 1 (apolipoprotein H). Proc Nat Acad Sci USA 1990;87:4120–4124.

Miller FW. Myositis-specific autoantibodies: touchstones for understanding the inflammatory myopathies. J Am Med Assoc 1993;270:1846–1849.

Mongey AB, Hess EV. Antinuclear antibodies and disease specificity. Adv Intern Med 1991;36:151 –169.

Monier JC, Sault C, Veysseyre C, Bringuier JP. Discrepancies between two procedures for ds-DNA antibody detection: Farr test and indirect immunofluorescence on *Crithidia luciliae*. J Clin Lab Immunol 1988;25:149–152.

Paxton H, Bendele T, O'Connor L, Haynes DC. Evaluation of the RheumaStrip ANA profile test: a rapid test strip procedure for simultaneously determining antibodies to autoantigens U1-ribonucleoprotein (U1-RNP), Sm, SS-A/Ro, SS-B/La and to native DNA. Clin Chem 1990;36:792–797.

Renz M, Heim C. Braünling O, Czichos A, Wieland C, Seelig HP. Expression of the major human ribonucleoprotein (RNP) autoantigens in Escherichia coli and their use in an EIA for screening sera from patients with autoimmune disease. Clin Chem 1989;35: 1861–1863.

Roberts DE, Rubin RL. Anti-neutrophil cytoplasmic autoantibodies. In: Rose, NR, et al., eds. Manual of Clinical Laboratory Immunology, ed 4. Washington, DC: American Society for Microbiology, 1992;781–784.

Rose NR, de Macario EC, Fahey JL, Friedman H, Penn GM, eds. Manual of Clinical Laboratory Immunology, ed 4. Washington, DC: American Society for Microbiology, 1992.

Rubin RL. Enzyme-linked immunosorbent assay for anti-DNA and antihistone antibodies including anti-(H2A-H2B). In: Rose, NR, et al., eds. Manual of Clinical Laboratory Immunology, ed 4. Washington, DC: American Society for Microbiology, 1992;735–740.

Rubin RL, Waga S. Antihistone antibodies in systemic lupus erythematosus. J Rheumatol 1987;14(suppl 13): 118–126.

Steen VD, Powell DL, Medsger TA. Clinical correlations and prognosis based on serum autoantibodies in patients with systemic sclerosis. Arthritis Rheum 1988;31:196–203.

Swaak AJG, Groenwold J, Brosveld W. Predicative value of complement profiles and anti-ds DNA in systemic lupus erythematosus. Ann Rheum Dis 1986;45:359–366.

Tan EM. Antinuclear antibodies: diagnostic markers for autoimmune diseases and probes for cell biology. Adv Immunol 1989;44:93–151.

Tan EM, Christian C, Holman HR, et al. Anti-tissue antibodies in rheumatic disease: standardization and nomenclature. Arthritis Rheum 1977;20:1419–1420.

Taylor PV, Scott JS, Gerlis LM, Esscher E, Scott O. Maternal antibodies against fetal cardiac antigens in congenital heart block. New Engl J Med 1986;315:667–672.

ter Borg EJ, Horst G, Hummel EJ. Measurement of increases in anti-double stranded DNA antibody levels as a predictor of disease exacerbation in systemic lupus erythematosus: a long-term prospective study. Arthritis Rheum 1990a;33:634–643.

ter Borg EJ, Horst G, Limburg PC, van Rijswijk MH, Kallenberg CGM. C-reactive protein levels during disease exacerbation and infections in systemic lupus erythematosus: a prospective longitudinal study. J Rheumatol 1990b;17:1642–1648.

van der Woude FJ, Rasmussen N, Labatto S. Autoantibodies against neutrophils and monocytes: tools for diagnosis and marker of disease activity in Wegener's granulomatosis. Lancet 1985;1:425–429.

van Venrooy WJ, Charles P, Maini RN. The consensus workshops for the detection of autoantibodies to intracellular antigens in rheumatic diseases. J Immunol Methods 1991;140:181–189.

Ward TM, ed, Proteins and Tumour Markers, Vol 2, part 3. In: Seth J, ed. The Immunoassay Kit Discovery, Series A: clinical chemistry. Norwell, MA: Kluwer Academic Publishers, 1993.

Weiner ES, Earnshaw WC, Senecal JL, Bordwell B, Johnson P, Rothfield NF. Clinical association of anticentromere antibodies and antibodies to topoisomerase 1: A study of 355 patients. Arthritis Rheum 1988;31:378–385.

Wilson MR, Sanders RD. Immunodiffusion assays for antibodies to small nuclear ribonucleoproteins and other cellular antigens. In: Rose, NR, et al., Manual of Clinical Laboratory of Immunology, ed 4. Washington, DC: American Society for Microbiology, 1992;741–746.

CHAPTER 14

Cardiac Markers

Marian Kane

Biochemical markers have been used in the confirmation of acute myocardial infarction (AMI) since 1962 (Apple, 1992). When cardiac muscle is deprived of oxygen, cell death ensues with leakage of cellular contents. The plasma concentration time-profile of each cellular protein after a cardiac ischemic incident depends on the extent of the damage to heart tissue, its rate of leakage from the cells, and its rate of clearance from the circulation.

The enzymes aspartate transaminase, lactic dehydrogenase (LD), and creatine kinase (CK) were the earliest cardiac markers, and analysis of the isoenzyme patterns of these enzymes has become routine. Diagnosis of myocardial infarction is now confirmed, according to World Health Organization (WHO) criteria, when the presence of characteristic chest pain (and/or electrocardiographic [ECG] changes) is associated with a demonstrable increase, and subsequent fall, in the activity of the MB isoenzyme of CK.

Thrombolytic therapy is now widely given to treat AMI and, in order to be effective, it must be administered no later than 12 hours after the initial onset of symptoms and preferably within 6 hours (TIMI Study Group, 1985). However, ECG changes and/or increases in serum enzyme levels are not always apparent within this time frame. Similarly, clinical and ECG changes cannot accurately identify successful coronary reperfusion (Califf, et al., 1988). There have, therefore, been many investigations of these and many other cardiac markers to test their suitability for very early diagnosis of AMI and as markers of reperfusion. See Table 14–1 for the properties of some of the most important markers.

MARKERS AND ASSAYS

Creatine Kinase

Creatine kinase (CK) (Table 14–1) reversibly catalyzes the production of energy-rich phosphocreatine from adenosine triphosphate (ATP) and creatine (reviewed by Jones and Swaminathan, 1990), and is found predominantly in tissues that use large

235

Table 14-1 Properties of Some Cardiac Markers

Marker	Relative Molecular Mass	Location Within Myocardium	Tissue Distribution	Typical Normal Range
CK	86,000	Cytoplasm (90%), mitochondria (10%)	Ubiquitous	43–172 U/L
CK-MB	86,000	Cytoplasm	2–50% of myocardial CK; 1–8% of skeletal muscle CK	1–8 μg/L, 3–15 U/L
CK-MB isoforms	86,000			
CK-MB$_2$		Tissue isoform	Tissue isoform	Ratio: MB$_2$/
CK-MB$_1$		Formed in plasma		MB$_1$ < 1.5
CK-MM isoforms	86,000			
CK-MM$_3$		Tissue isoform	50–98% of myocardial CK; 92–99% of skeletal muscle CK	Ratio: MM$_3$/ MM$_1$ 0.3–0.8
CK-MM$_2$		Formed in plasma		
CK-MM$_1$		Formed in plasma		
LD1	135,000	Cytoplasm	57% of myocardial LD; also in kidney, red blood cells, brain	30–100 U/L
				Ratio: LD1/ LD2 > 0.76
Myoglobin	17,000	Cytoplasm	Skeletal muscle, myocardium	< 90 μg/L
Troponin I	24,000	98% in myofibrils, 2% in cytoplasm	Myocardium	< 3.1 μg/L
Troponin T	37,000	98% in myofibrils, 2% in cytoplasm	Myocardium	< 0.2 μg/L
Myosin heavy chain	200,000	Myofibrils	Myocardium	< 15 μg/L
Myosin light chain I	27,000	98% in myofibrils, 2% in cytoplasm	Myocardium	< 6.6 μg/L
Myosin light chain II	20,000	98% in myofibrils, 2% in cytoplasm	Myocardium	Not available
α-Actin	43,000	Myofibrils, cytoplasm	Myocardium	< 0.2 mg/L
S-100a$_0$	21,000	Intercalated discs	Myocardium, skeletal muscle	< 0.5 μg/L
Heart fatty acid binding protein	14,000	Cytoplasm	Myocardium	< 19 μg/L

amounts of energy. In muscle tissue, it is located mainly in the cytoplasm but is closely associated with the myofibrils.

Cytosolic CK consists of two different subunits, M and B, each having independent intrinsic enzyme activity. These subunits combine to give three different CK isoenzymes, CK-BB, CK-MB and CK-MM, the proportion of each isoenzyme varying between tissues. Cardiac muscle generally contains a higher proportion of the CK-MB isoenzyme than any other tissue, especially in diseased hearts, which can contain up to 50% CK-MB isoenzyme. The proportion of CK-MB in skeletal muscle is normally around 1% although it can be as high as 8% in marathon runners. CK-MM accounts for most of the remaining CK activity in cardiac and skeletal muscle, with only trace amounts of CK-BB.

In plasma, the CK-M subunit slowly loses its terminal lysine residue. Thus, there are three isoforms of plasma CK-MM (CK-MM$_1$, CK-MM$_2$ and CK-MM$_3$) and two of CK-MB (CK-MB$_1$ and CK-MB$_2$), depending on whether the whole or truncated form of the M subunit is present. Because of its bulk, skeletal muscle normally accounts for nearly all the plasma CK, including CK-MB. The CK isoenzyme pattern in the serum of healthy individuals is, therefore, primarily CK-MM with less than 3% CK-MB and only trace amounts of CK-BB. Following AMI, total serum CK activity and, more dramatically, CK-MB mass and activity increase, reflecting the higher CK-MB content of myocardial cells.

A variety of procedures are available for measurement of total CK activity in the serum. Total CK mass is not determined. Most of the assay procedures are carried out in the clinical laboratory by trained personnel, although dry chemistry methods using portable bench-top reflectance analyzers are now available for emergency bedside use (Downie, et al., 1993).

CK isoenzyme levels, in particular CK-MB, are traditionally measured either by ion-exchange separation and activity measurement, or by electrophoretic separation followed by activity staining and fluorescence analysis by densitometry (Marshall, et al., 1991). CK-MB levels are expressed as actual CK-MB activity or as percent of total CK activity. Electrophoresis currently remains the most popular method, and commercial systems are widely available. Analysis time has been reduced to under 1 hour and sensitivity is 1 μg/L. However, this method is not suitable for emergency room use, as sophisticated equipment is required.

CK-MB is also measured by immunoinhibition of the M subunit and measurement of the residual activity due to the B subunit. The CK-MB activity is then taken as twice the measured B activity. The presence of high CK-BB levels, variant CKs, or adenylate kinase may interfere with this assay method (Delanghe, et al., 1990a). Assay of the activity remaining after immunoprecipitation of all isoforms with the M subunit can be used to correct for this (Chan, et al., 1985), but this makes the assay more complex and less suitable for emergency room use. An alternative approach utilizes a CK-MB specific monoclonal antibody for immunocapture of CK-MB followed by measurement of enzyme activity (Landt, et al., 1988).

The recent trend in CK-MB analysis is to measure CK-MB mass rather than activity. Several sensitive immunometric assays have been described and many are now commercially available (Table 14–2). Specificity is achieved by using two different

Table 14-2 Some Commercial Immunometric Assays for CK-MB Mass Measurement

Kit	Capture antibody, solid phase	Label	Detection	Range (μg/L)	Detection limit (μg/L)	Assay time (min)
Dako Novoclone	Anti CK-MB, microtiter plate	Anti CK-MB-HRP	Colorimetric	5–150	0.8	<60
Hybritech Tandem-E CKMB II	Anti-CK-B, beads	Anti CK-M-AP	Colorimetric	0–100	0.8	90
Hybritech ICON-QSR	Anti CK-B, membrane	Anti-CK-M-AP	Colorimetric reflectance	2–50	2	10
Abbott IMx	Anti CK-MB, beads	Anti-CK-M-AP	Fluorometric	3–300	0.7	40
Baxter Stratus	Anti CK-MB, glass fiber	Anti-CK-BB-AP	Fluorometric	4–125	0.4	60
Amerlite	Anti CK-B, microtiter plate	Anti-CK-MB-HRP	Luminometric	2–300	0.3	15
Ciba Corning Magic Lite	Anti CK-BB, paramagnetic beads	Anti-CK-MB-acri-dinium ester	Luminometric	0–500	0.65	30
IIL QuiCK-MB	Anti CK-B, beads	^{125}I-anti-CK-M	Solid scintillation	2–40 EU/L	0.2 or 0.6 EU/L	120 or 30

HRP, Horseradish peroxidase; AP, alkaline phosphatase; EU, equivalent units.
Data compiled in part from Ward TM. The Immunoassay Kit Directory, Vol 1, Part 3. Proteins and Tumour Markers. Lancaster, England: Kluwer Academic Publishers, 1992.

antibodies, often monoclonal, directed against the M or B subunits, or the M-B contact region. Most such assays are comparable in overall analytic performance (Wu, et al., 1989; Wolfson, et al., 1991). However, falsely elevated CK-MB values, as a result of high molecular weight alkaline phosphatase in serum samples, have been noted with an alkaline-phosphatase-based kit (Butch, et al., 1989). Another assay failed to detect elevated CK-MB, possibly due to the characteristics of the antibodies used (Peaston and Lai, 1992). Generally, CK-MB mass results correlate well with activity measurements (Chan, et al., 1985; Van Blerk, et al., 1992), although activity decreases faster than mass with time, both in vivo (Delanghe, et al., 1990a) and in vitro (Buttery, et al., 1992). The upper limits of the linear ranges of the assays vary from 50 (Icon assay, Hybritech Corp., San Diego, CA) to 500 μg/L (Magic Lite Assay Ciba, Corning Diagnostics Corp., Medfield, MA). The analytic range of an assay influences cost and turnaround time per sample, as a narrow range requires more frequent sample dilution and duplicate or repeat assays. Overall, assays like the Icon method are suited for emergency room use, as they require minimal equipment apart from an inexpensive reader.

Whereas CK-MM is not a specific cardiac marker, measurement of the relative concentrations of its isoforms can be useful in the early diagnosis of AMI or identification of thrombolytic success. Both CK-MB and CK-MM isoforms are measured mainly by modifications of the electrophoretic technique used for isoenzyme analysis (Wu, 1989). Monoclonal antibodies capable of reacting specifically with one or other of the isoforms have been described (e.g., Suzuki, et al., 1990) and these may form the basis of sensitive immunoassays to measure levels of the isoforms of CK-MM and CK-MB. Purified isoforms are now also available for standardization (Wu, 1989).

Lactic Dehydrogenase

LD, which reversibly catalyses the interconversion of lactate and pyruvate, is a tetramer with two subunit types, M and H, giving rise to five different isomers (LD1 to LD5). LD1 (4 × H) is found in highest concentration in heart, kidney and red blood cells, and serum LD1 levels are raised after AMI (Maekawa, 1988).

LD is assayed by measurement of its enzymatic activity, and its isoenzymes are chiefly measured after electrophoresis on commercial systems. Elevated LD1 is recognized by the characteristic "LD flip," where the LD1/LD2 ratio is increased. LD1 can also be measured by immunochemical assays, which use antibodies to the M subunit to remove all but the LD1 activity from serum. In addition, chemical inhibition methods are available.

Myoglobin

Myoglobin is a cytosolic hemeprotein, which is particularly enriched in striated muscle cells and the myocardium. It functions in the intracellular transport and storage of oxygen. Serum myoglobin concentration is measured by immunoassay. RIAs have ^{125}I-myoglobin as tracer, but more recently two-site IEMA (Nishida, et al., 1985; Juronen, et al., 1988) and IFMA (Silva, et al., 1991) have been described. Commercial a says are available but are not widely used routinely because they are time-consuming.

Myoglobin can also be measured with rapid latex agglutination assays (e.g., Chapelle and Heusghem, 1985). These require no sophisticated equipment and allow qualitative or semi-quantitative analysis. However, they may occasionally give false negative results at concentrations >5000 μg/L (Toft, et al., 1988), although such high levels are only found after skeletal muscle trauma or in muscle disorders. Furthermore, while latex agglutination tests are considered to be very user-friendly, poor performance has been recorded when they are used as bedside tests (Hangaard, et al., 1987). Therefore, latex agglutination methods must be used with caution.

Immunonephelometric and immunoturbidometric assays for myoglobin have also been developed (Delanghe, et al., 1990b; Mair, et al., 1992a). They are based on shell/core polymer particles coated with antimyoglobin antibodies. When used with specialized analyzers, they can give results in 10 to 15 minutes. A turbidimetric assay has also been modified for use with a routine chemistry analyzer (Bakker, et al., 1993).

Troponin

Troponin, which participates in the regulation of the contraction process, is a complex of three nonidentical subunits located mainly on the thin filaments of the contractile apparatus with a small percentage unbound in the cytosol. Each subunit is a single polypeptide chain which exists in different isoforms with different tissue distribution. Two of the subunits, troponin I (inhibits ATPase activity) and troponin T (binds tropomyosin), have cardiac-specific isoforms and therefore have potential as truly cardiac-specific markers (Mair, et al., 1992b).

A one-step sandwich assay for cardiac troponin T is now available commercially. It uses horseradish peroxidase in the monoclonal label, and the streptavidin-biotin reaction to anchor the capture monoclonal to the solid phase. It has a detection limit of 0.1 μg/L and 1% cross-reactivity with skeletal troponin T (Katus, et al., 1992), but as its turnaround time is 90 minutes, this will need to be shortened to make the assay suitable for real-time monitoring of patients in the emergency room. At least two immunoenzymometric assays (IEMA) have been developed for cardiac troponin I, each with two matched monoclonal antibodies and with alkaline phosphatase (Bodor, et al., 1992) or horseradish peroxidase (Larue, et al., 1993) labeled antibodies. In both assays cross-reactivity with the skeletal isoform was 0.1% or lower. While the detection of the former assay was only 2 μg/L, the measurement range of the latter was 0.2 to 20 μg/L. This more sensitive assay had a short turnaround time (30 minutes) and shows much promise as a method for detecting AMI (Larue, et al., 1993).

Myosin

Myosin is the major structural protein of the thick filament of the contractile apparatus. Each myosin molecule consists of two heavy chains and two pairs each of light chain I and light chain II. All the myosin subunits exist as different isoforms but the differences are small and whether truly cardiac-specific isoforms exist is not definite. Immunoassays have been developed for the cardiac isoforms of myosin heavy chain (e.g., Larue, et al., 1991), myosin light chain I (e.g., Michel, et al., 1992), and myosin light chain II (e.g., Nagai, et al., 1979), but all show cross-reaction with the corresponding subunit from skeletal muscle. Perhaps more specific antibodies would reduce this.

CLINICAL APPLICATIONS

Early Diagnosis of Acute Myocardial Infarction

As the benefits of thrombolytic therapy are realized, early and accurate identification of AMI in patients presenting with ambiguous symptoms and signs becomes an increasingly important clinical challenge. Ideally, what is needed is a specific marker that is present in serum at concentrations above the normal range as early as possible but definitely within the first 6 hours after onset of symptoms. High cardiac specificity would enable AMI to be confidently recognized in the presence of damage to skeletal muscle, as after multiple trauma, surgery, or even intramuscular injection. When comparing the performance of cardiac markers in early diagnosis, only measurements from blood samples taken prior to the start of thrombolytic therapy should be considered, as thrombolytic therapy alters the release kinetics of several markers.

Compared with other markers for which commercial assays are available, increases of serum myoglobin levels are first to be detected after AMI, perhaps because its low molecular weight facilitates myoglobin's early leakage from the myocardium. Increases in myoglobin have been shown to aid early diagnosis (Ohman, et al., 1990), but because myoglobin is not cardiac specific, they cannot be used for confirmation of AMI. It has been suggested that simultaneous measurement of the enzyme carbonic anhydrase III, which is present in skeletal muscle but not in the myocardium, would allow the source of the increased myoglobin to be determined (Väänänen, et al., 1990). A low serum myoglobin concentration within the period of 4 to 12 hours after onset of pain allows AMI to be ruled out with a high probability (Mair, et al., 1992a).

Blood levels of CK and CK-MB begin to rise within 4 to 8 hours of an AMI. Therefore, single CK or CK-MB measurements do not compare favorably with myoglobin in detecting AMI within the first 6 hours and are not recommended for this purpose. On the other hand, serial measurements can clearly show a gradual increase in concentration with time and are more sensitive for diagnosis. Frequent serial measurements of CK and CK-MB mass have been used in the selection of additional patients for thrombolytic therapy (Downie, et al., 1993; Marin and Teichman, 1992). It must be remembered that CK-MB is not cardiac specific either.

Measurement of CK-MM and CK-MB isoforms has also been investigated for early detection of AMI (Wu, 1989). Like myoglobin, the tissue isoforms of CK-MM and CK-MB are elevated 3 to 9 hours after onset of symptoms. Although not cardiac specific, early detection of changes in the concentrations of CK-MM isoforms is often easier because of the greater quantities released. The ratio of tissue to serum isoforms is the best indicator, although realization of the full potential of these markers in early diagnosis awaits improvements in assay methodology.

The detection of elevated levels of cardiac troponin T is 100% diagnostic of cardiac damage, which would be particularly useful in patients with associated skeletal muscle injury. Concentrations begin to rise 1 to 10 hours after AMI (Mair, et al., 1992b), which gives it a diagnostic sensitivity similar to CK-MB within the first 6 to 8 hours. However, current assay time for troponin T is 90 minutes, which mitigates against its use in early diagnosis.

Although there are grounds for optimism with troponin T or troponin I, an ideal biochemical marker for early diagnosis of AMI is still not generally available. Alternatively, one of the newly described markers, α-actin (Aránega, et al., 1993), heart fatty acid binding protein (Kleine, et al., 1992), and S-100a$_0$ (Usui, et al., 1990), may prove to be what is needed.

Diagnosis of Acute Myocardial Infarction on Late Presentation

Serial measurements of CK-MB, the "gold standard," have a high sensitivity from 12 to 24 hours after onset of symptoms. However, they are not reliable for patients presenting later than 24 hours afterward. CK-MB levels may already have returned to normal at this stage. Instead, the LD isoenzyme pattern, which becomes abnormal within 12 to 24 hours and remains so for several days, is examined to aid diagnosis (Maekawa, 1988). All the proteins of the contractile apparatus are released over an extended period from the damaged myocardium and could also be used in late diagnosis. Troponin I or T, in particular, could act as more specific markers during this period.

Detection of Successful Reperfusion

Thrombolytic therapy is unsuccessful in at least 20% of AMI patients (Chesebro, et al., 1987). Identification of those in whom recanalization has not occurred, in order to allow emergency "rescue" angioplasty to be performed as soon as possible, is difficult. Measurement of some cardiac markers has potential for the noninvasive detection of reperfusion and cardiac specificity is not as important here, as AMI will already have been diagnosed before the administration of therapy.

Figure 14–1 shows the serum concentration profiles of the four markers for which commercial assays are generally available, CK, CK-MB, myoglobin, and troponin T, in a group of AMI patients given thrombolytic therapy. Successful reperfusion was associated with accelerated release of all four markers, but especially myoglobin, CK-MB, and troponin T, into the serum, and was associated with earlier peaks of myoglobin and troponin T concentrations. Clearly, myoglobin and CK-MB levels begin to rise earlier than the other two markers when reperfusion occurs and therefore have greatest potential for the rapid noninvasive detection of reperfusion.

In limited studies, both the rate of increase and the relative increase in concentration of CK-MB and myoglobin over the 1 to 2 hours following thrombolytic therapy were found useful in the prediction of reperfusion (Garabedian, et al., 1988; Ellis, et al., 1988; Laperche, et al., 1992). However, it is important to establish specific cut-

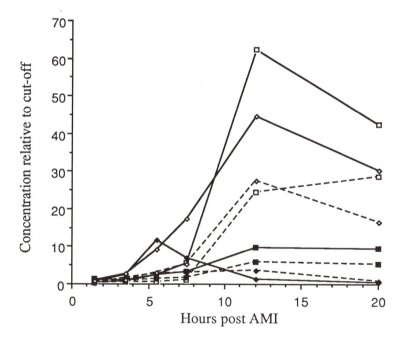

Figure 14–1. Serum concentration profiles of CK (■), CK-MB mass (◇), myoglobin (◆), and troponin T (□) in AMI patients who were given thrombolytic therapy. On the basis of clinical criteria and subsequent angiography, patients were divided into two groups: those who reperfused (17 patients, solid lines) and those who did not (9 patients, broken lines). The concentrations (median values) are plotted against the time from the initial onset of symptoms. The patients who reperfused and those who did not were admitted a mean of 2.6 hours (range 0 to 4 hours) and 4.9 hours (range 1 to 10 hours), respectively, after onset of symptoms. Thrombolytic therapy was administered as soon as possible after and definitely within 1 hour of admission. (Adapted from Lavin F, Kane M, Shah P, et al. Noninvasive assessment of infarct reperfusion by analysis of three cardiac enzyme markers—CPK, myoglobin and troponin T. Br Heart J 1993;69 (suppl):31.)

off limits for each assay method (Christenson, et al., 1990). Measurement of the iso-forms of CK-MM and CK-MB may also be useful for assessment of reperfusion (Laperche, et al., 1992; Puleo, 1992), but present methodology is not suited to bed-side use.

Prognosis of Unstable Angina

Patients with unstable angina are a heterogeneous group (Braunwald, 1989). Cardiac marker analysis has permitted identification of two sets of unstable angina patients, those showing no change in marker concentration on serial measurement and those showing serial changes similar to, but much lower than, those found in AMI. The concentration of myoglobin (Isakov, et al., 1988), CK-MB mass (Bøtker, et al., 1991), and troponin T (Hamm, et al., 1992) have each been useful in this regard, but no comparative study of these three markers in unstable angina has been reported. In each of these studies, the groups in which the concentrations of markers were elevated showed higher occurrences of subsequent coronary events. Thus the use of cardiac markers for the early classification of unstable angina patients is of clear po-tential benefit.

REFERENCES

Apple FS. Acute myocardial infarction and coronary reperfusion: serum cardiac markers for the 1990s. Clin Chem 1992;97:217–226.

Aránega AE, Reina A, Muros MA, Alvarez L, Prados, J, Aránega A. Circulating α-actin pro-tein in acute myocardial infarction. Int J Cardiol 1993;38:49–55.

Bakker AJ, Boymans DAG, Dijkstra D, Gorgels JPMC, Lerk R. Rapid determination of serum myoglobin with a routine chemistry analyzer. Clin Chem 1993;39:653–658.

Budor GS, Porter S, Landt Y, Ladenson JH. Development of monoclonal antibodies for an as-say of cardiac troponin-I and preliminary results in suspected cases of myocardial in-farction. Clin Chem 1992;38:2203–2214.

Bøtker HE, Ravkilde J, Søgaard P, Jørgensen PJ, Hørder M, Thygesen K. Gradation of unstable angina based on a sensitive immunoassay for serum creatine kinase MB. Br Heart J 1991;65:72–76.

Braunwald E. Unstable angina: a classification. Circulation 1989;80:410–414.

Butch AW, Goodnow TT, Brown WS, McClellan A, Kessler G, Scott MG. Stratus automated creatine kinase-MB assay evaluated: identification and elimination of falsely increased results associated with a high-molecular-mass form of alkaline phosphatase. Clin Chem 1989;35:2048–2053.

Buttery JE, Stuart S, Pannal PR. Stability of the CK-MB isoenzyme on routine storage. Clin Biochem 1992;25:11–13.

Califf RM, O'Neill W, Stack RS, group at TS. Failure of simple clinical measurements to predict perfusion status after intravenous thrombolysis. Ann Intern Med 1988; 108:658–662.

Chan DW, Taylor E, Frye R, Blitzer R-L. Immunoenzymatic assay for creatine kinase MB with subunit-specific monoclonal antibodies compared with an immunochemical method and electrophoresis. Clin Chem 1985;31:465–469.

Chapelle J-P, Heusghem C. Semi-quantitative estimation of serum myoglobin by a rapid latex agglutination method: an emergency screening test for acute myocardial infarction. Clin Chim Acta 1985;145:143–150.

Chesebro J, Knatterud G, Roberts R, et al. Thrombolysis in myocardial infarction (TIMI) trial, phase I: a comparison between intravenous tissue plasminogen activator and intravenous streptokinase. Circulation 1987;76:142–154.

Christenson RH, Clemmensen P, Ohman EM, et al. Relative increase in creatine kinase MB isoenzyme during reperfusion after myocardial infarction is method dependent. Clin Chem 1990;36:1444–1449.

Delanghe JR, De Mol AM, De Buyzere ML, De Scheerder IK, Wieme RJ. Mass concentration and activity concentration of creatine kinase isoenzyme MB compared in serum after acute myocardial infarction. Clin Chem 1990a;36:149–153.

Delanghe JR, Chapelle J-P, Vanderschueren SC. Quantitative nephelometric assay for determining myoglobin evaluated. Clin Chem 1990b;36:1675–1678.

Downie AC, Frost PG, Fielden P, Joshi D, Dancy CM. Bedside measurement of creatine kinase to guide thrombolysis on the coronary care unit. Lancet 1993;341:452–454.

Elli AK, Little T, Masud ARZ, Liberman HA, Morris DC, Klocke FJ. Early noninvasive detection of successful reperfusion in patients with acute myocardial infarction. Circulation 1988;78:1352–1357.

Garabedian HD, Gold HK, Yasuda T, et al. Detection of coronary artery reperfusion with creatine kinase-MB determinations during thrombolytic therapy: correlation with acute angiography. J Am Coll Cardiol 1988;11:729–734.

Hamm CW, Ravekilde J, Gerhardt W, et al. The prognostic value of serum troponin T in unstable angina. New Engl J Med 1992;327:146–150.

Hangaard J, Rasmussen O, Norregaard-Hansen K, Jorgensen N, Simonsen E, Norgaard-Pedersen B. Early diagnosis of acute myocardial infarction with a rapid latex agglutination test for semi-quantitative estimation of serum myoglobin. Acta Med Scand 1987;221:343–348.

Isakov A, Shapira I, Burke M, Almong C. Serum myoglobin levels in patients with ischaemic myocardial insult. Arch Intern Med 1988;148:1762–1765.

Jones MG, Swaminathan R. The clinical biochemistry of creatine kinase. J Int Fed Clin Chem 1990;2:108–114.

Juronen EI, Viikmaa MH, Mikelsaar A-VN. Rapid simple and sensitive antigen capture ELISA for the quantitation of myoglobin using monoclonal antibodies. J Immunol Methods 1988;111:109–115.

Katus HA, Looser S, Hallermeyer K, et al. Development and in vitro characterization of a new immunoassay of cardiac troponin T. Clin Chem 1992;38:386–393.

Kleine AH, Glatz JFC, Vannieuwenhoven FA. Release of heart fatty acid-binding protein into plasma after acute myocardial-infarction in man. Mol Cell Biochem 1992;116:155–162.

Landt Y, Vaidya HC, Porter SE, et al. Semi-automated direct colorimetric measurement of creatine kinase isoenzyme MB activity after extraction from serum by use of a CK-MB-specific monoclonal antibody. Clin Chem 1988;34:575–581.

Laperche T, Steig PG, Benessiano J, et al. Patterns of myoglobin and MM creatine kinase isoforms release early after intravenous thrombolysis or direct percutaneous transluminal coronary angioplasty for acute myocardial infarction, and implications for the early noninvasive diagnosis of reperfusion. Am J Cardiol 1992;70:1129–1134.

Larue C, Calzolari C, Bertinchant J-P, Leclercq F, Grolleau R, Pau B. Cardio-specific immunoenzymometric assay of troponin I in the early phase of acute myocardial infarction. Clin Chem 1993;39:972–979.

Larue C, Calzolari C, Léger J, Léger J, Pau B. Immunoradiometric assay of myosin heavy chain fragments in plasma for investigation of myocardial infarction. Clin Chem 1991;37: 78–82.

Lavin F, Kane M, Shah P, Forde A, Gannon F, Daly K. Noninvasive assessment of infarct reperfusion by analysis of 3 cardiac enzyme markers—CPK, myoglobin and troponin T. Br Heart J 1993;69 (suppl):31.

Maekawa M. Lactate dehydrogenase isoenzymes. J Chromatogr 1988;429:373–398.

Mair J, Artner-Dworzak E, Lechleitner P, et al. Early diagnosis of acute myocardial infarction by a newly developed rapid immunoturbidimetric assay. Br Heart J 1992a;68:462–468.

Mair J, Dienstl F, Puschendorf B. Cardiac troponin T in the diagnosis of myocardial injury. Crit Rev Clin Lab Sci 1992b;29:31–57.

Marin MM, Teichman SL. Use of rapid serial sampling of creatine kinase MB for very early detection of myocardial infarction in patients with acute chest pain. Am Heart J 1992;123:354–361.

Marshall T, Williams J, Williams KM. Electrophoresis of serum isoenzymes and proteins following acute myocardial infarction. J Chromatogr 1991;569:323–345.

Michel G, Seifert B, Ritter A. Automated microparticle capture immunoassay for the measurement of human cardiac myosin light chain 1. Clin Chem 1992;38:1104.

Nagai R, Ueda S, Yazaki Y. Radioimmunoassay of cardiac myosin light chain II in the serum following experimental myocardial infarction. Biochem Biophys Res Commun 1979;86:683–688.

Nishida Y, Kawai H, Nishino H. A sensitive sandwich enzyme immunoassay for human myoglobin using Fab-horseradish peroxidase conjugate: methods and results in normal subjects and patients with various diseases. Clin Chim Acta 1985;153:93–104.

Ohman E, Casey C, Bengtson J, Pryor D, Tormey W, Horgan J. Early detection of acute myocardial infarction: additional diagnostic information from serum concentrations of myoglobin in patients without ST elevation. Br Heart J 1990;63:335–338.

Peaston RT, Lai LC. Failure of an immunometric assay to detect elevated creatine kinase MB isoenzyme. Ann Clin Biochem 1992;29:463–464.

Puleo P. Detection of coronary artery patency after thrombolytic therapy of acute myocardial infarction using creatine kinase-MB subforms. Coronary Artery Disease 1992;3: 468–474.

Silva DP Jr., Landt Y, Porter SE, Ladenson JH. Development and application of monoclonal antibodies to human cardiac myoglobin in a rapid fluorescence immunoassay. Clin Chem 1991;37:1356–1364.

Suzuki T, Shiraishi T, Tomita K, Totani M, Murachi T. Monoclonal antibody inhibiting creatine kinase MM_3 but not isoform MM_1. Clin Chem 1990;36:153–156.

TIMI Study Group. The thrombolysis in myocardial infarction (TIMI) trial. New Engl J Med 1985;312:932–936.

Toft E, Stentoft J, Andersen PT. False-negative latex-agglutination test for myoglobin. Clin Chem 1988;34:177.

Usui A, Kato K, Sasa H, et al. S-100a$_0$ protein in serum during acute myocardial infarction. Clin Chem 1990;36:639–641.

Väänänen HK, Syrjälä H, Rahkila P, et al. Serum carbonic anhydrase III and myoglobin concentrations in acute myocardial infarction. Clin Chem 1990;36:635–638.

Van Blerk M, Maes V, Huyghens L, Derde M-P, Meert R, Gorus FK. Analytical and clinical evaluation of creatine kinase MB mass assay by IMx: comparison with MB isoenzyme assay and serum myoglobin for early diagnosis of myocardial infarction. Clin Chem 1992;38:2380–2386.

Ward TM, ed, Proteins and Tumour Markers, Vol 2 , part 3. In Seth J, ed. The Immunoassay Kit Directory, Series A: Clinical Chemistry. Norwell, MA: Kluwer Academic Publishers, 1993.

Wolfson D, Lindberg E, Su L, Farber SJ, Dubin SB. Three rapid immunoassays for the determination of creatine kinase MB: an analytical, clinical, and interpretive evaluation. Am Heart J 1991;122:958–964.

Wu AHB. Creatine kinase isoforms in ischemic heart disease. Clin Chem 1989;35:7–13.

Wu AHB, Gornet TG, Harker CC, Chen H-L. Roles of rapid immunoassays for urgent ("stat") determinations of creatine kinase isoenzyme MB. Clin Chem 1989;35:1752–1756.

CHAPTER 15

Allergy

Stella Quan

Allergies are the most common immunologic disorders and more than 1 person in 10 has been, is, or will become allergic to some substance or other. The immune response in allergic disease involves the same processes of foreign antigen recognition and the same humoral and cellular effector mechanisms as in the immunologic defense processes activated by microbial pathogens. In the person with an allergy, however, the foreign antigen, namely the allergen, causes tissue inflammation and damage and organ malfunctions. The allergen may be a pollen or dust particle which is inhaled, a food constituent, a component of insect venom, a drug, or one of the many natural or artificial chemicals in the environment.

TYPES OF ALLERGIES

There are two major types of allergic reactions, the immediate hypersensitivity reaction and delayed hypersensitivity. For immediate hypersensitivity (Fig. 15–1) the first exposure to an allergen results in the development of specific IgE antibodies that bind to the membranes of basophilic granulocytes and mast cells. Subsequent exposure to the allergen leads to stimulation of these cells to secrete histamine and other chemical mediators. These interact with surrounding tissues and elicit the allergic responses. Immediate hypersensitivity reactions occur within 24 hours after antigen challenge. Depending on the condition, localized antigen exposure leads to localized anaphylaxis such as allergic rhinitis, allergic asthma, chronic sinusitis, contact dermatitis and eczema, and allergic gastroenteritis. However, if the appropriate antigen is systemically absorbed via ingestion, injection or insect sting, an acute, life-threatening allergic reaction may occur.

The most common type of delayed hypersensitivity is contact dermatitis, in which the allergen (e.g., cathecols released by poison ivy) causes dermal inflammation on direct contact with the skin. After initial sensitization, when T memory cells encounter the specific allergen they are rapidly converted to activated CD4 T cells, which release lymphokines. These lymphokines affect macrophage function and replication, increase blood flow, increase permeability of small blood vessels, and initiate the coagulation cascades. One or more days after antigen challenge the tissues become swollen due to increased fluid and protein accumulation, leading to necrosis in severe cases. The laboratory tests generally used to evaluate delayed hypersensitivity (also called cell-mediated hypersensitivity) include appropriate skin tests, lymphocyte activation tests, methods for counting T lymphocytes (e.g., E-rosette test), and the macrophage migration inhibition test.

REGULATION OF IgE SYNTHESIS

The synthesis of IgE is tightly controlled by many interactions of immune cells and cytokines and occurs at a very low rate in the healthy individual. In culture, human peripheral lymphocytes do not spontaneously secrete IgE even when IgG secretion is easily monitored. For IgE secretion there is an apparently absolute requirement for interaction of the B cells with CD4-positive T cells and, in addition, interleukin-4 (IL-4) acts to induce IgE synthesis. Other cytokines such as interleukins-5 and -6 (IL-5 and IL-6) and α- and γ-interferon also play important roles. In contrast, peripheral lymphocytes from atopic patients (from the Greek, *atop-*, "out of place") spontaneously secrete IgE at a significant rate, and this is further increased by the addition of IL-4. Therefore, allergic sensitization must be often related to disruption of the strict control of IgE synthesis, but how this occurs is unknown. Immunoassays for specific lymphokines (e.g., Teppo, et al., 1991; Ishizuka, et al., 1992), which are implicated in both immediate and delayed sensitivity reactions, may become important in the future assessment of allergies.

DIAGNOSIS AND MONITORING

Diagnosis

In vitro methodologies that are of significance for the detection and diagnosis of most allergic disorders involve the measurement of total serum IgE, IgE specifically directed toward individual antigens, IgG blocking antibodies, and histamine release from basophils. In vivo skin testing is sensitive, simple to perform, and is the gold standard method for the identification of specific allergens. Measurement of IgG blocking antibodies is useful for the monitoring of therapy and is discussed later under Specific IgG. The use of properly standardized preparations of allergens is essential to efficient allergy testing (Yunginger and Adolphson, 1992).

Total IgE

Allergy-related physiologic changes are often associated with abnormally high amounts of IgE class antibodies. IgE binds strongly via its Fc to receptors on mast cells and basophils, thereby mediating allergic hypersensitivity.

IgE has a molecular weight of 188,000 and, compared with IgG, IgA or IgM, is normally present in only trace quantities in plasma. VanArsdel and Larson (1989)

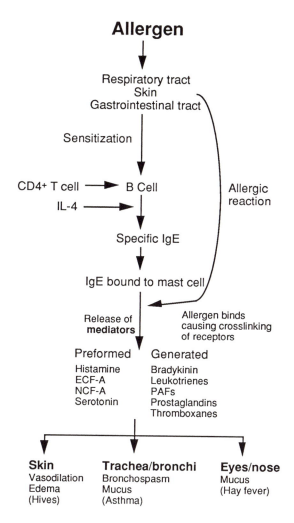

Figure 15–1.   Mechanism of immediate (type 1) hypersensitivity (anaphylaxis). First exposure to allergen results in the development of specific IgE antibodies that bind to high affinity receptors for IgE on the membranes of basophilic granulocytes and mast cells. Subsequent exposure to the allergen leads to stimulation of these cells resulting in the secretion of chemical mediators which interact with surrounding tissues and elicit the allergic responses.

The mediators listed are histamine, which increases vascular permeability and induces smooth muscle contraction; eosinophil chemotactic factor of anaphylaxis (ECF-A), which attracts and deactivates eosinophilic leukocytes; neutrophil chemotactic factor of anaphylaxis (NCF-A), which attracts and deactivates neutrophilic leukocytes; serotonin, which increases vascular permeability; bradykinin, which causes contraction of bronchioles and induces vasodilation and hypotension; leukotrienes (also called slow-reacting substance of anaphylaxis), which increase capillary permeability, stimulate contraction of bronchioles, and inhibit the mitogenic response of lymphocytes and smooth muscle contraction; platelet activating factors (PAFs), which stimulate aggregation and lysis of platelets; prostaglandins, which act as vasodilators, bronchoconstrictors, and regulators of hemostasis; and thromboxanes, which act as bronchoconstrictors.

reported a normal range of total serum IgE in a healthy population of 48 to 240 μg/L (20 to 100 IU/mL, where 1 IU equals 2.4 ng IgE protein). However, basal levels are highly variable with high levels in some individuals being inherited as a simple, recessive mendelian trait. In addition, total IgE levels are elevated in patients with parasitic infections and some immunodeficient states. IgE is low in young children, peaks about 14 years of age, and may gradually decline through adulthood and old age. In adults, IgE concentrations greater than 800 μg/L (333 IU/mL) are generally considered to be abnormally elevated (Hamilton and Adkinson, 1992). While total IgE is, in general, higher in atopic patients than in nonatopic individuals, normal and pathologic concentration ranges overlap greatly, and hence the measurement of total serum IgE alone is not a sensitive procedure for diagnosing the allergic state.

A wide range of immunometric assays, most with radioisotopic or enzymic labels, are used to determine total IgE. In these, anti-IgE is coated onto a solid phase (sp) such as a tube, a well, magnetizable particles, a glass fiber matrix, or a paper disk (sp-Ab). IgE in the serum sample binds to the solid phase anti-IgE (sp-Ab–IgE), and the amount bound is determined with labeled anti-IgE (e.g., sp-Ab–**IgE**–Ab-^{125}I). Monoclonal antibodies are used in the great majority of assays, either as matched pairs, matched pairs of "cocktails" of two or more antibodies or, as is often the case, in combination with a polyclonal antibody (Ward, et al., 1993). In these assays the monoclonal antibody is most often immobilized and the polyclonal antibody is labeled. The amount of total IgE present is obtained from a calibration curve with known IgE standards, usually prepared from WHO IRP 75/502. Immunometric assays with chemiluminescent (acridinium ester) (Roche, et al., 1991) or fluorescent (Eu^{2+}) labels promise ranges of measurement as wide as 0.8 to 48000 μg/L (0.3 to 2000 IU/mL) (Ryttman and Holmlund, 1991).

Specific IgE

Identification of the allergen causing an allergic reaction is important for the diagnosis and therapy of an allergic disease, and IgE antibodies that bind specific allergens can be detected in serum by immunometric assays with a variety of labeling substances. Since tests are available with any one of more than 350 allergens, a preliminary decision must be made as to which allergens to test, and this is usually based on clinical observations, the results of skin testing, or specific IgE multiallergen screening.

The RAST (radioallergosorbent test) and automatable CAP systems marketed by Kabi Pharmacia Diagnostics AB (Uppsala, Sweden) are widely used. In these and similar assays, allergens (Al) or allergen-protein conjugates are covalently or noncovalently bound to solid phase (e.g., cellulose disks or threads, microtiter wells, cellulose carrier encased in a capsule, soluble polymer matrix, etc.) (sp-Al). Specific antibodies present in patient serum bind to the allergen (sp-Al–**IgE,** sp-Al–IgG, sp-Al–IgA), and the bound IgE is quantitated with labeled anti-IgE (e.g., sp-Al–**IgE**–Ab-^{125}I).

Reactions between specific IgE and the allergen are usually arranged to occur on the surface of the solid phase, and having an excess of available immobilized allergen can be very important. When the amount of antigen available is relatively small, the binding of specific IgE may be susceptible to competition from major class antibodies which also bind to allergen. For example, with serum from an individual with a high concentration of IgG antibodies to the specific allergen, the IgG could compete with IgE antibodies for binding, perhaps resulting in a false negative reading. Maximizing the concentration of immobilized allergen may be achieved by the use of high-surface-area solid-phase components, such as microparticles or a porous membrane or three-dimensional capsule, and by ensuring that the coupling procedure used is suitable for the allergen in question.

Alternatively, an antibody capture approach can be used as described by Olivieri, et al. (1993). They incubated solid phase anti-IgE (sp-Ab) with sample to absorb both nonspecific and specific IgE in the sample (sp-Ab–IgE, sp-Ab–**IgE**). Biotinylated allergan (Al-biotin), which was also present, bound to the allergen-specific immobilized IgE (sp-Ab–**IgE**–Al-biotin) and the amount of analyte was quantified after addition of streptavidin-horseradish peroxidase (HRP) conjugate (sp-Ab–**IgE**–Al-biotin–avidin–HRP).

In the AlaSTAT and automated Milenia AlaSTAT systems of Diagnostics Products Corporation (Los Angeles, CA), the primary reaction between specific IgE (**IgE**) and biotinylated soluble allergen (biotin-Al) is carried out in the liquid phase (biotin-Al–**IgE**). This reaction occurs in a tube coated with biotin (sp-biotin) and the antibody-allergen complex is immobilized by addition of streptavidin (sp-biotin–avidin–biotin-Al–**IgE**). Finally, anti-IgE coupled to horseradish peroxidase (Ab-HRP) is added to allow specific quantitation of complexes containing IgE (sp-biotin–avidin–biotin-Al–**IgE**–Ab-HRP).

Most assays for specific IgE measure one type of allergen-specific IgE at a time. However, some tests can measure up to 35 specific IgEs simultaneously with multiple allergens immobilized on discrete areas of strips or disks. The luminescent, enzyme-linked MAST® system, which has each allergen coated on a separate cellulose thread (Brown, et al., 1984), and the Matrix Aero system of Abbott Laboratories (Chicago IL) (Lindberg, et al., 1991) are established examples of such an approach.

When it is desirable to compare concentrations of specific IgEs, whether in the same or different patients, it is presently essential to always use the same assay system. This is because the various assays for allergen-specific IgE are very poorly standardized, due to differences in the intrinsic compositions of the allergen preparations used, differences in the presentation of the epitopes (due to different immobilization techniques and varied solid supports), and differences in threshold and calibration criteria.

Skin Testing

During skin prick testing, a patient is challenged with small amounts of each of a panel of common allergens in order to identify that (or those) which may be producing the suspected allergic reaction of clinical interest. Each allergen is introduced into the skin and a positive allergic reaction may produce a fully developed wheal and erythema reaction within as little as 15 minutes. Quantitative results may be obtained by measurement of the mean diameter of the wheal and by repeating the test at ever greater dilutions of allergen until only a trace, or a negative, reaction is observed (Norman, 1992).

Even though there is good correlation between the results of in vitro measurements of serum-specific IgE concentrations and the results of skin tests, properly performed skin testing remains the gold standard and has been shown to be more clinically sensitive, more cost-effective, and to be completed in a shorter time (Smith, 1992). However, the greater analytic sensitivity of assays for specific IgE can be clinically significant in the special cases of anaphylactic sensitivities to drugs and hymenoptera venoms. Not every positive skin test result means that the allergen in question normally induces allergic disease in that individual. Conversely, skin tests may be negative when the patient is indeed sensitive. This last is most probable in drug or low-molecular-weight-substance allergy, as the actual allergic reaction is often caused by metabolic products of the compound, sometimes only after they have reacted with tissue components to form complete antigen.

In vitro testing for specific IgE antibodies, as opposed to skin testing, is clearly indicated when:

- Patients (particularly young children) are more apprehensive of skin testing than of venipucture
- Dermatographism or extensive dermatitis prevents proper interpretation of skin tests
- Patients are taking medications that may modify the result of skin testing (e.g., antihistamines or steroids)
- Patients have a history of apparent allergy accompanied by negative skin tests. In such cases, in vitro tests can provide independent confirmation of the absence of reaginic IgE antibodies.

Histamine

The interaction of specific allergen with IgE antibody bound to the high affinity IgE receptors on the surface of basophils results in the secretion of histamine and other mediators of immediate hypersensitivity into the extracellular fluid. As histamine is rapidly degraded by histaminases in tissue fluids and eosinophils, the accurate measurement of plasma histamine presents many technical problems related to sample taking, preparation, and storage. However, the determination of the urinary metabolite N-methylhistamine by radioimmunoassay (Kabi Pharmacia Diagnostics AB Uppsala, Sweden) is a practical alternative for the general assessment of allergic disorders.

The concentration of histamine released in vitro from washed peripheral blood leukocytes in the presence of added soluble allergens has been found to correlate well with the results of skin tests and the concentration of specific IgE, and can indicate the degree of severity of an allergic disease (Siraganian and Hook, 1992). Previously, high performance liquid chromatography (HPLC), as well as chemical and enzyme isotopic assays were used to to quantitate histamine. Quantitation of histamine release has to be performed shortly after collection of the blood, and such methods are too complicated for routine use. However, commercial histamine immunoassays are available, which simplify the procedure. Recently, a novel histamine radioimmunoassay (RIA) was developed based on the use of a monoclonal antibody specific for acyl-histamine and not for other biologic amines (Mata, 1992). This assay is based on competition between acylated histamine and labeled acylated histamine for binding to the monoclonal antibody coated on tubes. The acylation step is essential for immunorecognition of histamine and increases the sensitivity and specificity of the assay.

A close correlation is usually found in patients with hay fever between the results of skin tests with ragweed or grass pollen and in vitro histamine release. However, when skin tests are performed by the endpoint method they are 10 times more sensitive. The sensitivity of the histamine release RIA assay can also be significantly lower than in vitro specific IgE assays.

Monitoring Therapy

Immunotherapy is the controlled immunization of allergic individuals with the allergen to which they are sensitive, and the favorable effects of such immunization may be due to the generation of antibodies that neutralize the allergen and decrease the formation of sensitizing, specific IgE antibody, as well as to other poorly understood mechanisms (Creticos et al., 1987; Lucas, 1990). Effective immunotherapy may be associated with a rise in serum levels of allergen-specific IgG antibodies.

Specific IgG

IgG blocking antibody is IgG antibody present in body fluids that interferes with other manifestations of immunity, especially those that prevent association of antigen with cell-bound IgE. Although high IgG titers do not necessarily predict a favorable response to allergen immunotherapy, the failure to induce an IgG response is related to poor clinical outcome. Immunometric assays similar to those of specific IgE antibodies can be used to measure allergen specific IgG antibodies in serum.

Although IgG4 binds to mast cells and has been linked to some cases of food allergy, the measurement of IgG4 for the detection of non-IgE, mast-cell-mediated food allergies has not been adopted, as there is actually little evidence that IgG4 is responsible for the allergic reactions (Condemmi, 1991).

REFERENCES

Brown CR, Higgins KW, Frazer K, et al. Simultaneous determination of total Ig and allergen-specific IgE in serum by the MAST chemiluminescent assay system. Clin Chem 1984;31:1500–1505.

Condemmi JJ. Unproved diagnostic and therapeutic techniques. In: Metcalfe DD, Sampson HA, Simon RA, eds. Food Allergy: Adverse Reactions to Foods and Food Additives. Boston: Blackwell Scientific Publications, 1991;392–404.

Creticos PS, Norman PS. Immunotherapy with allergens. JAMA 1987;258:2874–2880.

Hamilton RG, Adkinson NF Jr. Measurement of total serum immunoglobulin E and allergen-specific immunoglobulin E antibody. In: Rose NR, deMacario EC, Fahey JL, Friedman H, Penn GM, eds. Manual of Clinical Laboratory Immunology, ed 4. Washington, DC: American Society for Microbiology, 1992;689–701.

Ishizuka T, Kawagoe M, Suzuki K, et al. An ultrasensitive system to detect IL-4-enzyme-linked immunosorbent assay (ELISA) combined with an avidin-biotin and enzyme amplification system. J Immunol Methods 1992;153:213–222.

Lindberg RE, Anawis MA, Bailey M, et al. Development of the Abbot Matrix™ Aero assay for the measurement of specific IgE. J Immunoassay 1991;12:465–485.

Lucas AH. IgG subclass-restricted immune responses to allergens. Springer Semin Immunopathol 1990;12:385–400.

Mata E, Gueent JL, Moneret-Vautrin DA, et al. Clinical evaluation of in vitro leukocyte histamine release in allergy to muscle relaxant drugs. Allergy 1992;47:471–476.

Norman PS. Skin testing. In: Rose NR, deMacario EC, Fahey JL, Friedman H, Penn GM, eds. Manual of Clinical Laboratory Immunology, ed 4. Washington, DC: American Society for Microbiology, 1992;685–688.

Olivieri V, Beccarini G, Gallucci G, Romano T, Santoro F. Capture assay for specific IgE: an improved quantitative method. J Immunol Methods 1993;157:65–72.

Roche D, Susini de Luca H, Tugendhaft N. Chemiluminescent and radioimmunology compared for 10 allergens. Clin Chem 1991; 37:474–475.

Ryttman A, Holmlund E. A wide range IgE assay. Clin Chem 1991; 37:1064.

Siraganian RP, Hook WA. Histamine release and assay methods for the study of human allergy. In: Rose NR, deMacario EC, Fahey JL, Friedman H, Penn GM, eds. Manual of Clinical Laboratory Immunology, ed 4. Washington, DC: American Society for Microbiology, 1992;709–716.

Smith TF. Allergy testing in clinical practice. Ann Allergy 1992;68:293–301.

Teppo A-M, Metsärinne, Fyhrquist F. Radioimmunoassay of interleukin-6 in plasma. Clin Chem 1991;37:1691–1695.

VanArsdel PP Jr, Larson EB. Diagnostic tests for patients with suspected allergic disease. Ann Intern Med 1989;110:304–312.

Ward TM, ed. Proteins and Tumour Markers, Vol 2, part 3. In: Seth J, ed. The Immunoassay Kit Directory, Series A: Clinical Chemistry. Norwell, MA: Kluwer Academic Publishers, 1993.

Yunginger JW, Adolphson CR. Standardization of allergens. In: Rose NR, deMacario EC, Fahey JL, Friedman H, Penn GM, eds. Manual of Clinical Laboratory Immunology, ed 4. Washington, DC: American Society for Microbiology, 1992;678–684.

CHAPTER 16

Serum Tumor Markers

Robert Stebbins

The first identification of a serum substance useful in detecting cancer was in 1938, when a phosphatase with a low optimum pH (prostatic acid phosphatase, PAP) was found in several patients with metastatic prostatic cancer. Since that time, a variety of protein and carbohydrate antigens, enzymes, hormones, etc., have been identified as being present in increased amounts in fluids and tissues of patients with a wide range of cancers.

APPLICATIONS AND ASSAYS

Applications

The most useful tumor marker would be both specific for a particular tumor type and easily detectable even when there are few marker secreting cells. In addition, that marker would continue to be produced despite the genetic alterations in tumor cells that may happen when the disease recurs after treatment. Certain hormonal tumor markers are specific for particular cancers, for example, serotonin and its by-product 5-hydroxyindole acetic acid are excreted by carcinoid tumors. The β subunit of human chorionic gonadotropin (hCGβ) is detectable when there are as few as 10,000 hCG secreting tumor cells in patients with gestational trophoblastic disease. Yet assays for 5-hydroxyindole acetic acid do not detect small numbers of carcinoid tumor cells and hCG is not specific to trophoblastic disease. Further, benign disease states may also be associated with elevated levels of tumor markers.

In practice, the major use for serum tumor marker measurements is the monitoring of response to therapy and the detection of tumor recurrence.

Immunoassays

Table 16–1 lists most of the substances measured in patient samples for the monitoring of tumor viability and growth. They constitute a very wide variety of proteins, complex carbohydrates, and low molecular weight compounds, sometimes poorly defined as chemical entities, and collectively they represent a small but significant fraction of the enormous research effort into malignant disease.

The assays used to measure tumor markers include most types of immunoassay (Table 16–1). Reagent-excess immunometric assays are much more often used than limited-reagent assays, and nonisotopic labeling substances are now more common than ^{125}I. Most of the nonisotopic assays employ enzyme labels, but there are commercial immunofluorometric assays (IFMA) and immunochemiluminometric assay (ICMA) for all the most important markers. Judging by the numbers of commercial kits available, the six most frequently assayed substances used as tumor markers are ferritin, alpha-fetoprotein (AFP), carcinoembryonic antigen (CEA), hCG, β_2-microglobulin, and prostate specific antigen (PSA), although kits for ferritin and hCG owe much of their prominence to their other applications (Ward, 1992).

Total immunoglobulin class and subclass antibodies are also measured as markers in cases of tumors derived from B cells, and these are usually determined with turbidimetric, nephelometric, and radioimmunodiffusion assay kits (Ward, 1992).

The standardization of immunoassays for individual tumor markers is often poor, particularly when the marker represents a heterogeneous, poorly defined substance. Even when the same monoclonal antibodies and standard (for calibrant preparation) are used, agreement between assays may be less than desirable, and may not markedly improve as new kits are developed to benefit from growing demand for a popular marker (e.g., CA 19-9, Zuchelli, et al., 1993).

Monoclonal antibodies used in immunoassays for cancer markers are sometimes also administered to cancer patients for immunoscintigraphic investigations of tumor location (after labeling with ^{131}I), or for therapy. OC125 is a monoclonal antibody which binds specifically to cancer antigen (CA) 125. A recent study suggested that administration of OC125 $F(ab')_2$ fragments to patients led to the development of anti-OC125 antibodies and consequently to the overestimation of CA 125 in serum samples from those patients when immunoassays with OC125 were used (Reinsberg, et al., 1993).

In the rest of this chapter the clinical applications of the main tumor markers are discussed under headings representing the most important malignant diseases.

COLORECTAL CARCINOMA

Carcinoembryonic Antigen

Since its first identification in the mucosa of colon tumors, the measurement of carcinoembryonic antigen (CEA) has been extensively evaluated in the diagnosis and treatment of colorectal carcinoma. Although not specific for this disease (significantly elevated levels of CEA are commonly found in patients with breast, lung, and other carcinomas), the highest serum levels of CEA are generally observed in patients with metastatic colon cancer. In general, serum CEA levels rise with increasing tumor cell burden. As with other tumor markers, high tumor tissue concentrations of CEA do not always produce elevated serum levels of CEA (Begent, 1987). A new immunoenzymometric assay (IEMA) for a cancer-associated mucin, CA M43, may

Table 16-1 Tumor Markers and Immunoassays for Measuring Them

Tumor Marker	Acronym	Description	Tumor Types	Method of Assay, Number of Commercial Kits							
				EIA	FIA	RIA	ICMA	IEMA	IFMA	IRMA	Total
α-Fetoprotein	AFP	63,000 mol wt glycoprotein of fetal liver and yolk sac from 10th week of gestation	Hepatocellular carcinoma hepatoblastoma, germ cell tumors, also fetal monitoring	0	0	7	3	20	1	10	41
β$_2$-Microglobulin		11,500 mol wt peptide component of class I MHC	Malignant lymphoma, allograft rejection	5	1	9	0	9	0	2	26
Bombesin		14 residue neuropeptide	Pancreatic adenomata	0	0	2	0	0	0	0	2
Breast cancer mucin		Polymorphous epithelial mucin	Breast cancer	0	0	0	0	1	0	0	1
Calcitonin		32 residue polypeptide	Medullary thyroid carcinoma	0	0	7	0	1	0	2	10
Carbohydrate antigen 50	CA 50	CA 50 and CA 19-9 are epitopes on the same high mol wt mucin	Gastrointestinal carcinoma pancreatic carcinoma, (chronic pancreatitis)	0	0	0	1	0	1	1	3
Carbohydrate antigen 125	CA 125	200,000 mol wt sialocarbohydrate of coelomic epithelium	Ovarian carcinoma, carcinomatosis peritonei, (endometriosis)	0	0	0	1	3	0	5	9
Carbohydrate antigen 15-3	CA 15-3	290,000 mol wt cell surface antigen from human breast carcinoma	Breast carcinoma	0	0	0	1	2	0	4	7
Carbohydrate antigen 19-9	CA 19-9	See CA 50	Gastrointestinal tumors, pancreatic carcinoma, mucinous adenocarcinomata	0	0	0	1	3	0	4	8
Carbohydrate antigen 195	CA 195	High mol wt mucin	Gastrointestinal carcinoma, pancreatic carcinoma	0	0	0	0	0	0	1	1

Table 16-1 (*continued*)

Tumor Marker	Acronym	Description	Tumor Types	Method of Assay, Number of Commercial Kits							
				EIA	FIA	RIA	ICMA	IEMA	IFMA	IRMA	Total
Carbohydrate antigen 72-4	CA 72-4	GIT tumor-associated antigen	Gastric carcinoma, colo-rectal carcinoma, lung carcinoma	0	0	0	1	1	0	1	3
Carbohydrate antigen 549	CA 549	Acidic glycoprotein of polymorphous epithelial mucins found in breast cancer tumors	Metastatic breast carcinoma, pancreatic carcinoma, biliary tract carcinoma, gastrointestinal tract carcinoma	0	0	0	0	1	0	1	2
CAR-3		Polymorphous epithelial mucin	Carcinoma of pancreas, biliary or GIT	0	0	0	0	0	0	1	1
Carcinoembryonic antigen	CEA	200,000 mol wt acidic glycoproteins of surface glycocalyx of gastrointestinal and related epithelia	Gastrointestinal and related malignancies	0	0	2	2	19	1	9	33
Cathepsin-D		52,000 mol wt lysosomal protease present in most cells	Marker of tumor invasiveness, e.g., for breast cancer	0	0	0	0	0	0	1	1
CD 8 (soluble)		Detached accessory cell surface proteins of lymphocytes	Some lymphomas	0	0	0	0	1	0	0	1
CD 23 (soluble)		See CD 8	Lymphomas and leukemias	0	0	0	0	1	0	1	2
Human chorionic gonadotropin, intact	hCG	39,000 mol wt glycoprotein hormone with 30% carbohydrate, consisting of 2 subunits α and β, of which β is specific for hCG	Choriocarcinoma, gonadal teratomas	0	0	0	2	5	1	5	13

Analyte	Abbreviation	Description	Clinical association								
Human chorionic gonadotropin, intact + free β subunit	hCG + hCGβ	hCGβ has an X amino acid residue, glycoslyated extension at the C-terminal not found in the other glycoprotein hormones	Choriocarcinoma, gonadal teratomas	0	0	0	1	9	0	8	18
Epithelial mucin core antigen	EMCA	400,000 glycoprotein core antigen of epithelial mucin	Breast cancer	0	0	0	0	1	0	0	1
Estrogen receptor		Intracellular receptor mediating estrogen action	Tumor tissue marker of hormone responsiveness	0	0	0	0	1	0	0	1
Ferritin		450,000 mol wt iron storage protein	Acute leukemia, Hodgkin's disease	0	0	4	2	20	2	17	45
α-Glycoprotein hormone subunit, free		Common glycoprotein subunit of FSH, hCG LH, and TSH	Pituitary adenomata, germ cell tumors, hydatiform mole, choriocarcinoma	0	0	1	0	0	0	2	3
Neurone specific enolase		γγ and αγ forms of dimeric glycolytic enzyme. ββ form is found in skeletal muscle	Neuroblastoma, small-cell carcinoma of lung, melanoma, pancreatic islet cell carcinoma	0	0	1	1	3	0	1	6
Parathyroid hormone related peptide	PTH-r	141 residue PTH-like polypeptide hormone	Malignancies with hypercalcemia	0	0	2	0	0	0	0	2
Placental alkaline phosphatase	PLAP	Placental and placental-like isoenzymes of enzyme	Testicular seminoma, ovarian dysgerminoma, epithelial ovarian carcinoma, (pineal germinoma, PLAP in CSF)	0	0	0	0	2	0	0	2

Table 16–1 Tumor Markers and Immunoassays for Measuring Them (*continued*)

Tumor Marker	Acronym	Description	Tumor Types	Method of Assay, Number of Commercial Kits							
				EIA	FIA	RIA	ICMA	IEMA	IFMA	IRMA	Total
Progesterone receptor		Intracellular receptor mediating progestagen action	Tumor tissue marker of hormone responsiveness	0	0	0	0	1	0	0	1
Prostate specific antigen	PSA	34,000 mol wt monomeric glycoprotein of the serine protease family	Prostatic carcinoma, (prostatic hypertrophy), (prostatitis), (forensic semen marker)	0	0	0	1	8	1	6	16
Prostate specific protein		94 residue protein produced by prostate epithelial cells	Prostatic carcinoma	0	0	0	0	1	0	0	1
Prostatic acid phosphatase	PAP	Isoenzymes 2 and 4 (deglycosylated) of prostatic tissue	Prostatic carcinoma	1	0	6	0	5	0	2	14
Protein S-100		21,000 mol wt acidic calcium-binding protein found throughout nervous system	Cerebral tumors, melanoma, (nervous system damage)	0	0	0	0	0	0	1	1
Serotonin		5-Hydroxytryptamine, produced in chromaffin cells of GIT	Carcinoid tumors	1	0	0	0	0	0	0	1
Squamous cell carcinoma associated antigen	SCC	48,000 mol wt glycoprotein, subfraction of TA-4 antigen	Squamous carcinoma of cervix uteri, lung, and esophagus	0	0	0	0	0	0	1	1

Marker	Abbrev.	Description	Associated malignancy								
Tumor-associated glycoprotein-72	TAG-72	1,000,000 mol wt mucin-like glycoprotein	Adenocarcinomata of colon, breast, endometrium, lung, stomach, and pancreas	0	0	0	0	3	0	0	3
Tumor-associated glycoprotein-551	TAG-551	Mucin-like glycoprotein		0	0	0	0	1	0	0	1
Thyroglobulin		660,000 mol wt iodo-protein of thyroid	Thyroid follicular carcinoma	0	0	6	2	1	1	4	14
Tissue polypeptide antigen		Produced normally during S and G2 phase of cell cycle	Nonspecific malignancy	0	0	0	1	1	0	3	5
Tumor-associated trypsin inhibitor	TATI	6000 mol wt inhibitor of trypsin and acrosin	Ovarian carcinoma, etc.	0	0	1	0	0	0	0	1
Urinary gonadotropin peptide	UGP	10,400 mol wt protein with identical sequence to hCG-β	Nonspecific malignancy	0	0	0	0	1	0	0	1

Abbreviations: MHC, major histocompatability complex; GIT, gastrointestinal tract; PTH, parathyroid hormone; CSF, cerebrospinal fluid; FSH, follicle-stimulating hormone; LH, luteinizing hormone; TSH, thyroid-stimulating hormone; HCG-βcf, core fragment of HCG-β (see Chap. 9).

Data from Ward TM, ed. Proteins and Tumour Markers, Vol 1, part 3. In: Seth J, ed. The Immunoassay Kit Directory, Series A: Clinical Chemistry. Norwell, MA: Kluwer Academic Publishers, 1992.

be complementary to CEA measurement and when combined they were found to yield 87% positivity in metastatic disease (van Kamp, et al., 1993).

Although serum CEA levels are elevated in only 5% to 28% of patients with localized stage A or B colorectal carcinoma, preoperative CEA levels provide useful prognostic information. Within each pathologic stage, those patients with elevated CEA levels generally experience earlier recurrence and shorter survival as compared with other patients in the same cohort.

The serum half-life of CEA in normal individuals is 1 to 2 days, but may be prolonged in patients with hepatic or renal dysfunction. In patients with localized primary colorectal carcinoma and elevated serum CEA concentrations, those levels quickly fall within the normal range following successful surgical resection. In patients with persistent elevation of serum CEA after primary surgery, however, standard chemotherapy does not significantly improve survival. A rising serum CEA level in a postresection patient signals tumor recurrence. In 50% of patients, this change is the first sign of recurrence and may precede detection of clinical disease by 6 to 8 months. In patients with rising CEA levels only, second-look surgical procedures to detect potentially resectable disease have been advocated. About 10% to 15% of patients with second resection may experience long-term survival or cure, and the 5-year survival rate may approach 33% (Martin, et al., 1985).

Immunoscintigraphy with radiolabeled antibody to CEA can localize tumor in patients with new or recurrent colorectal carcinoma, and this may help identify candidates for surgical resection of primary or metastatic tumor (Begent, et al., 1986).

Serum CEA concentrations may also be elevated in patients who do not have malignant disease. Five percent of patients who smoke have serum CEA levels above the normal range upper limit. Liver disease, pancreatitis, inflammatory bowel disease, and renal failure may all be associated with elevated CEA levels.

PANCREATIC CANCER

Almost all persons who contract ductal pancreatic carcinoma in the United States die from it, and it is the fourth ranked cause of cancer mortality. In contrast, Japanese investigators have reported a 5-year survival rate of up to 30% and, with early detection, even probable cure (Tsuchiya, et al., 1986).

CA 19-9

CA 19-9 is a serum tumor marker that was originally detected in a colorectal carcinoma cell line. It has shown sensitivity and specificity exceeding 80% in detecting pancreatic carcinoma (Pleskow, et al., 1989; Steinberg, 1990). However, although there is a significant correlation of elevated serum levels of CA 19-9 with tumor grade and site, fewer than 50% of potentially resectable tumors less than 20 mm in diameter can be detected by CA 19-9 measurement alone. Twenty percent to 50% of patients with colorectal, gastric, and hepatocellular carcinoma may also have elevated serum CA 19-9 levels, and elevated levels may be observed in patients with pancreatitis and liver disease.

Combining ultrasound examination and CA 19-9 measurements improves detection of pancreatic carcinoma, with a sensitivity of 97% and specificity approaching 90%. In a surgically documented study, 85% of carcinomas less than 3 cm were identified by a combination of the two techniques (Iishi, et al., 1986).

CA 50 antigen appears to have similar sensitivity and specificity to CA 19-9 for pancreatic carcinoma, which is not surprising because they may represent different epitopes on the same high molecular weight mucin. Serum CEA levels are frequently elevated in pancreatic carcinoma, but the low specificity of CEA for this tumor renders its measurement of limited value.

With successful resection serum CA 19-9 levels fall to the normal range and a subsequent rise may be the first sign of recurrent disease. The interval between the first detection of an elevated CA 19-9 level and the appearance of clinical disease may be several months (Safi et al., 1990), but such early detection does not generally prolong life, as no useful treatment for recurrent disease exists. However, patients with non-resectable stage II-III disease, whose preoperative CA19-9 levels were less than 370 U/ml, had significantly prolonged survival compared to those with higher levels (Lundin, et al., 1994). A recent study compared the behavior of CA 19-9, CA 195, CAM 43, CA 242, and tissue polypeptide epitope (TPS) in the diagnosis and surveillance of pancreatic cancer (Banfi, et al., 1993). They found that CA 19-9 gave good clinical sensitivity (70%) and high specificity (60% to 100%) and that CA 195 was similar. CAM 43 had high specificity, while TPS gave high sensitivity in cases of recurrence, so that these may prove useful when used in combination with CA 19-9 or CA 195.

HEPATOCELLULAR CARCINOMA

Hepatocellular carcinoma (HCC) is one of the most common cancers, with 1.3 million deaths per year worldwide. In the United States, no fewer than 10,000 new cases are observed annually. The most important risk factor for developing HCC is chronic hepatitis B infection, and new evidence suggests that infection or co-infection with hepatitis C virus may be an additional major contributor (Tanaka, et al., 1991). Environmental risk factors include malnutrition, excessive alcohol intake, parasitic infections, and aflatoxin ingestion. Emigrants from high risk areas of Asia retain that risk after moving to a low risk area, while black immigrants from Africa do not. The reason for this difference is unknown.

Alpha-Fetoprotein

Measurements of serum AFP concentrations have been used to screen high risk populations for HCC, to follow response to therapy, and to detect tumor recurrence. However, AFP is not specific for HCC and about 40% of patients with HCC have normal levels (Yeh, et al., 1987). Elevated AFP levels are also observed in cirrhosis and chronic active hepatitis, as well as in trophoblastic disease and nonseminomatous testicular carcinoma.

Patients with chronic liver disease are particularly at risk, and for them the predictive value of an elevated AFP value may approach 9%, that is, 1 in 11 patients with elevated AFP will actually have HCC. Finding an elevated AFP value in this population encourages regular monitoring of such patients. Tumors as small as 10 mm may be detected by ultrasound and these can be successfully removed. Combining ultrasound and AFP screening further improves the detection of early HCC (Cottone, et al., 1988), and for high risk patients AFP should be measured and scanning done every 3 to 6 months. An assay validated for the measurement of AFP in saliva samples has recently been developed to facilitate screening (Yio, et al., 1992).

Although some anaplastic hepatocellular carcinomas produce little or no AFP, an elevated AFP level generally confers a poorer prognosis. More exactly, poor prognosis tumors demonstrate shorter AFP concentration doubling times. Occasionally, HCC patients display a spontaneous decrease in serum AFP levels despite tumor persistence or growth. In some studies, up to 40% of HCC patients are found to have normal AFP levels, but they generally do not have cirrhosis, which improves prognosis.

AFP serum levels fall rapidly following successful tumor resection, and a subsequent rise indicates tumor recurrence. If early and limited recurrent disease is localized by a scanning procedure, second hepatic resection is sometimes successful. However, even when AFP was secreted by the primary tumor, it may not be secreted by the recurrent tumors. A change in the biology of the recurrent tumor or the development of a nonsecreting second primary HCC may explain this observation.

Other Markers

Serum ferritin levels are elevated in nearly all patients with hepatocellular carcinoma, but they are also high in 85% of patients with cirrhosis. CA 50 is detectable in patients with hepatobiliary carcinomas, but for the diagnosis or monitoring of treatment in HCC it offers no advantage over AFP. An abnormal prothrombin, termed "protein induced by vitamin K absence-II" (PIVKA-II), is elevated in serum in two thirds of patients with HCC. Serum PIVKA levels correlate with tumor bulk and may be useful in monitoring response to treatment of HCC patients with low or normal AFP levels (Fujiyama, et al., 1986).

Differentiating the sugar-chain structures of circulating forms of AFP may allow improved discrimination of hepatocellular carcinoma from hepatic cirrhosis. Serial measurements may also be useful for predicting the subsequent development of HCC in patients with cirrhosis (Sato, et al, 1993). Elevated concentrations of serum tumor necrosis factor-α (TNF-α) may be detected earlier than abnormal AFP in recurrent HCC patients following resection (Nakazaki, 1992; Kasahara, et al., 1993).

LUNG CANCER

Lung cancer is the leading cause of death due to cancer in men older than 35 years and is the second fatal cancer in adult women. Lung cancer is increasing in women, probably because of increased tobacco use, and may become the major cause of cancer mortality in women in the next 10 years. At diagnosis, lung cancer has spread to regional nodes or distant sites in 70% of cases, and 5-year survival rates are approximately 10%. Efforts to improve early detection of lung cancer, whether by chest radiography, sputum cytology, or tumor markers, have proved futile (Järvisalos, et al., 1993).

In patients with non–small cell lung cancer, there is no reliable tumor marker for diagnosis or following response to treatment. Serum CEA and CA 19-9 may be elevated in 50% of patients with non–small cell cancer but clinical and radiographic measurements provide the best guide to response to treatment.

Both tumor promotor and tumor suppressor gene activity appear to be implicated in the initiation and progression of certain types of lung cancer. Serum levels of *ras* oncogene product were found to be elevated in 7 of 11 subjects previously exposed to asbestos or silica more than one year preceding the clinical diagnosis of cancer or mesothelioma (Brandt-Rauf, et al., 1992). Elevated serum levels of c-erbB-2 oncogene-encoded p185 protein have also been detected on pnuemoconiosis patients who developed lung cancer. Positive serum samples were detected an average 35 months prior to cancer diagnosis (Brandt-Rauf, et al., 1994).

Small Cell Lung Cancer

Small cell lung cancer (SCLC), a tumor of neuroendocrine origin, is marked by rapid cell proliferation and is prone to recurrence. SCLC tumors secrete many substances that would qualify as tumor markers but most are nonspecific hormonal peptides and are not helpful in diagnosis.

Neuron Specific Enolase

Neuron specific enolase (NSE) has been reported elevated in 69% of newly diagnosed SCLC patients, including 39% of patients with local disease and 87% with extensive disease. NSE levels reflect tumor burden and are higher in extensive than limited disease (Carney, et al., 1982). NSE concentrations also correlate with response to combination chemotherapy. Sequential serum NSE measurements can be used to monitor response to therapy. Elevated levels of NSE are seen in 95% of SCLC patients with carcinomatous meningitis and in greater than 50% with parenchymal brain disease.

Other Markers

Other proposed serum tumor markers for SCLC include creatine kinase BB and circulating chromogranin A levels, as well as CEA, LDH, α_1-acid glycoprotein and neural cell adhesion molecule (Ganz, 1987; Jacques, et al., 1993). Although the serum concentrations of such markers tend to correlate with tumor mass and response to treatment, in general they have no greater clinical sensitivity or specificity than NSE.

Numerous hormones are produced in excess in patients with small cell lung cancer. Twenty-seven percent of patients with SCLC produce excessive adrenocorticotropic hormone (ACTH), and 65% of patients produce elevated serum levels of antidiuretic hormone. Clinically, these patients may exhibit Cushing's disease or the syndrome of inappropriate secretion of antidiuretic hormone, respectively. Calcitonin levels are increased in the majority of SCLC patients, but do not respond to pentagastrin stimulation as in patients with medullary carcinoma of the thyroid. In the patient with high levels of a particular hormone, serial measurements can provide useful information.

BREAST CANCER

One in 10 American women will develop breast cancer, and 40,000 die of the disease each year. Earlier detection of smaller, and frequently noninvasive, breast cancer tumors has followed increasing use of better mammographic techniques. Whether earlier discovery and more aggressive use of adjuvant therapy will translate into improved survival remains to be established. There is no reliable serum tumor marker for early breast cancer.

Carcinoembryonic Antigen

Serum CEA levels are elevated in only 20% of patients with localized breast cancer, but the presence of an elevated CEA level at diagnosis confers a poorer prognosis. Sixty percent of patients with metastatic breast cancer have elevated serum levels of CEA, and continued increases in CEA levels correlate well with progressive metastatic disease. If initially elevated, the serum CEA level can be useful in following response to treatment.

CA 15-3

Serum CA 15-3 assay, with a monoclonal antibody against a cell surface antigen from breast cancer cells, may prove more useful in the management of breast cancer patients. However, like CEA, CA 15-3 has both low sensitivity and specificity for the initial detection of breast cancer. Only 20% of stage I breast cancer patients have elevated CA 15-3 levels, and it is elevated in 20% of patients with benign breast disease (Hayes, et al., 1986).

With the development of metastatic disease, 50% to 80% of patients exhibit elevated serum levels of CA 15-3, and tumor volume appears to correlate with the level of the circulating antigen. When compared with CEA, serum CA 15-3 levels are more frequently elevated in patients with metastasis to lymph nodes, liver, and bone (Hayes, et al., 1986). Seventy percent of women with metastatic breast cancer combined with normal CEA levels have elevated CA 15-3 levels.

Serum CA 15-3 levels do not always follow the clinical response to treatments for metastatic breast cancer. In general, significant differences in CA 15-3 levels are detectable among patients with complete response, stable disease, and progressive disease following treatment. Serum levels increase in 75% of patients who are not responding to treatment, but CA 15-3 may fall in only 40% of patients responding well to treatment.

Other Markers

Several other serum tumor markers have been studied in breast cancer patients. Epithelial mucin core antigen (EMCA) measurements may help distinguish breast cancer from other cancers, especially if combined with measurement of CA 15-3 levels, but they are insensitive to early breast cancer. However, EMCA alone may prove as useful as CA 15-3 in monitoring response to therapy in patients with metastatic breast cancer (Dixon, et al., 1993). Elevated levels of mammary-specific antigen (MSA), another breast cancer–derived antigen, may be seen in 70% of stage I patients (Tjandra, et al., 1988). Serum levels of c-erbB-2 and myc oncoproteins are elevated in some preoperative patients with breast cancer, and these levels return to normal after the operation. However, serum oncoprotein levels do not always correlate with tissue overexpression. It is not yet clear whether tissue overexpression or detectable serum levels of c-erbB-2 or myc oncoprotein predict for more aggressive disease or earlier tumor recurrence (Pupa, et al., 1993; Breuer, et al., 1994). Many other serum markers have been proposed as tumor markers for breast cancer, but their utility is unproved.

OVARIAN CARCINOMA

Ovarian carcinoma is the fourth most common cause of cancer death in women living in industrialized countries, except in Japan where death rates are very low. The reason for this difference is unknown. It is the most common cause of death from gynecologic cancer, being more than twice as important as cervical and endometrial cancers combined. Nearly 90% of ovarian carcinomas are epithelial in origin; the remainder derive from stromal or germ cell lines.

Ovarian carcinoma usually eludes early detection. Seventy-five percent of patients have tumor spread beyond the ovary at diagnosis; in over 60% tumor has spread beyond the pelvis. Ultrasound and tumor marker measurement offer little improvement over history and physical examination in enabling an early diagnosis. Evidence of familial ovarian cancer in relatives and a history of breast cancer increase the risk, while oral contraceptive use and childbearing can protect women from developing ovarian carcinoma.

CA-125

The large glycoprotein CA-125 is found on fetal coelomic epithelium and in adult pleura, pericardium and mesothelium. It is also present in the epithelium of the endometrium, endocervix and fallopian tube. CA-125 is not found in normal ovary but may be present in benign ovarian cysts. OC-125 monoclonal antibody reacts with multiple antigenic determinants on the CA-125 antigen, and using OC-125 for immunoassay elevated serum CA-125 concentrations are detected in over 80% of patients with epithelial ovarian carcinoma (Bast, et al., 1983). Serum CA-125 levels may also be raised in patients with cancers of breast, lung, colon and of endometrium, fallopian tube and cervix, as well as in patients with endometriosis and pelvic inflammatory disease, and in 1% of normal individuals. Non-ovarian carcinoma metastatic to liver may produce very high serum levels of CA-125.

Measurement of serum CA-125 is a poor screening test for ovarian carcinoma because of its lack of sensitivity and specificity. Screening 5550 women Einhorn and coworkers found elevated CA-125 in 175. Following further thorough evaluation, 12 patients of the 5550 underwent laparotomy, and ovarian cancers were detected in nine. Six of these nine had normal CA-125 levels at the time of diagnosis and three had normal levels. Four of the six with raised CA-125 had early, stage I or II disease (Einhorn, et al., 1990).

Elevated CA-125 levels after surgery or chemotherapy accurately predicts finding residual disease at second-look surgery. Even with normal CA-125 levels, however, residual disease may be found in 60% of cases at surgery. Changes in CA-125 levels correlate with disease regression or progression in 90% of patients (Bast, et al., 1987). Elevation of a previously normal CA-125 level in a treated patient may precede clinical detection of recurrent disease by several months, and serum CA-125 is generally measured every two-to-three months following primary treatment.

Other Markers

CEA levels are elevated in approximately 60% of patients with stage III disease. CEA is not effective as a screening test and its measurement adds little to CA-125 when monitoring disease progression or recurrence. Serum inhibin may also become a useful tumor marker for mucinous and granulosa cell ovarian carcinoma (Healy, et al., 1993). Other markers, including macrophage colony-stimulating factor (M-CSF), ovx1, CA15-3, and TAG72-3 have been proposed as complements to the use of CA-125 and transvaginal Doppler ultrasound to improve the early diagnosis and treatment of ovarian carcinoma. None has yet proven superior (Woolas, et al., 1993).

GESTATIONAL TROPHOBLASTIC DISEASE

Gestational trophoblastic disease (GTD) encompasses benign hydatidiform mole, invasive mole, and choriocarcinoma, all of which secrete hCG. Most trophoblastic tumors develop after a molar pregnancy, but they can occur after a normal pregnancy or following an abortion or ectopic pregnancy. Treatment of GTD, which is usually effective, is based on disease type, and serum hCG concentrations can be used to guide decisions regarding type, duration, and changes of therapy (Goldstein, 1991).

Human Chorionic Gonadotropin

HCG, which is usually produced by syncytiotrophoblasts of the placenta, is dimeric with an α- and a β-subunit. The assays used for cancer monitoring can be specific for intact hCG, intact hCG *and* free hCG-β, free α-subunit, hCG-β core fragment (hCG-βcf, also called urinary gonadotropin peptide), and free hCG-β. Commercial immunoassays are available for the determination of all of these (Table 16–1); free hCG-β assays are now available from Medgenix Diagnostics (Brussels, Belgium) and CIS Bio International (Gif-sur-Yvette, France). Note that immunoassays that measure both free hCG-β and intact hCG are sometimes misleadingly referred to as β-hCG or β-subunit determinations. Because different hCG immunoassays measure different species individually or in combination, care should be taken to use appropriate and reliable reference ranges when arriving at diagnostic decisions (Stenman, et al., 1993). For further information on glycoprotein hormone structure and immunoassays for hCG see Chapter 9.

As few as 10,000 cancer cells may produce a detectable rise in serum hCG levels, and there is a good correlation between tumor burden and hCG concentration (Goldstein, et al., 1978). Patients may be stratified into good risk and high risk on the basis of their serum hCG concentration together with a general assessment of the extent of the disease (Bagshawe, 1976). If hCG levels do not show progressive decline after evacuation of a hydatidiform mole, chemotherapy is necessary. For other gestational neoplasms, single agent chemotherapy is usually curative for low risk patients; high risk patients require combination chemotherapy. The half-life of hCG is about 36 hours, and serum hCG should fall by 25% with each chemotherapy treatment. If hCG levels plateau or rise, this is a signal of failure of the current treatment. Following remission, hCG levels should be measured monthly for 3 months, and then less frequently for 1 or 2 years to assure persistent remission (Goldstein, 1991).

TESTICULAR CARCINOMA

Testicular carcinoma is the most common malignancy in men from ages 15 to 35 years and is the leading cause of death in ages 29–35. Overall survival rates are 90% and approach 100% in patients with low-stage disease. This success in treatment has been aided by highly sensitive tumor markers, AFP and hCGβ, that permit accurate diagnosis, staging and monitoring of treatment.

Alpha-fetoprotein

Over 90% of testicular cancers are of germ cell origin, and these are classified as seminomas or non-seminomatous tumors. AFP is produced by the fetal yolk sac, gastrointestinal tract and liver. It is thought not to be produced by pure siminomas and this may allow reclassification of a tumor identified pathologically as a seminoma that is associated with elevated AFP. AFP concentration is correlated with tumor volume and raised levels predict for poorer prognosis (Stoter, et al., 1987). AFP is also discussed above under Hepatocellular Carcinoma.

Human Chorionic Gonadotropin β-subunit

HCGβ is produced by trophoblastic tissue and elevated levels are found at diagnosis in 40% to 60% of patients with non-seminomatous tumors and in 10% of men with pure seminoma. Other cancers, including breast, lung, liver, pancreas and kidney may also secrete hCGβ. Because of the short serum half-life of hCG and hCGβ, their serum levels can be used to monitor the course of treatment in advanced disease. Several methods for calculating appropriate response to therapy have been proposed. These may define an adequate response to therapy as at least one log (90%) decline in tumor marker concentration with each treatment cycle (Picozzi, et al., 1984). Following orchiectomy persistent elevation of marker indicates residual disease. Surgical resection of selected patients with persistently elevated markers may offer these patients their only possible chance for cure (Eastham, et al., 1994). However, up to 40% of patients with negative normal levels may have residual disease in the retroperitoneum. HCGβ and hCG are also discussed below under Gestational Trophoblastic Disease.

PROSTATE CANCER

Prostatic carcinoma is the most common malignant tumor and the second cause of cancer mortality in men. According to Armbruster (1993), in 1992 in the United States 132,000 new cases of prostate cancer were projected, with 34,000 mortalities, afflicting more than 50% of males above 70 years. The cheapest and most important prostate screening method is digital rectal examination. If suggestive of cancer, transrectal ultrasonagraphy and appropriate biopsies should be performed; regardless of prostate specific antigen (PSA) level. Prospective trials are underway to determine the value of digital examination, ultrasonography and serum PSA concentration in screening for early cancer. However, although a specific and sensitive tumor marker screening assay or other test may diagnose early prostate cancer, there is as yet no evidence that early diagnosis increases survival.

Prostatic Acid Phosphatase (PAP)

While 85% to 90% of patients with metastatic prostate cancer have high levels of serum PAP, less than 30% exhibit elevated levels in stage A and B disease. Use of PAP as a marker is also limited by the restricted detection limit and susceptibility to interference of the traditional enzyme assay test; but even when measured by immunoassay it has no advantages over PSA measurements for the detection of disease in situ. Serum levels are also increased in patients with benign prostatic hypertrophy. However, the less expensive PAP enzyme assay test continues to be used throughout the world for the monitoring of metastatic cancer. For this reason, and to help improve the standardization of assays of PAP activity, a new PAP reference preparation has recently been prepared (Francis, et al., 1992).

Prostate specific antigen

PSA is generally recognized as the premier tumor marker for prostatic cancer, and its biochemistry, methods of measurement, and clinical applications have recently been reviewed (Armbruster, 1993). PSA is synthesized in the rough endoplasmic reticulum, stored in vesicles and vacuoles, and released in the glandular lumina by exocytosis. Its cellular location is the same in normal, benign prostatic hypertrophy, and in malignant tissues. PSA is not found in women, and may be elevated in both benign prostatic hypertrophy and malignant disease. In patients with localized cancer, it falls quickly to undetectable levels following radical prostatectomy.

Serum PSA levels correlate closely with cell mass in men with benign prostate disease and with tumor volume in patients with prostatic adenocarcinoma. Nonetheless, it is not possible by use of PSA measurement to distinguish stage A and B prostate cancer from benign prostatic hypertrophy (Stamey, et al., 1987). However, by combining the PSA measurement and Gleason score of prostate biopsy, Roach, et al. (1994) discriminate between low risk and high risk groups for lymph node metastasis. Based on these data, they omit whole pelvic irradiation in patients identified as low risk.

Serial PSA measurements are used to monitor patients with prostate carcinoma. PSA levels indicate stable or progressive diseases with a sensitivity of 93% and a specificity of 97%. A rapid decline in PSA with hormonal treatment may predict longer disease-free survival. PSA is more sensitive than PAP for predicting recurrence, and the combination of the two assays adds no additional clinical benefit compared with measuring PSA alone (Ercole, et al., 1987; Dupont, et al., 1991).

Persistent elevation of serum PSA following prostatectomy implies residual disease. Elevated PSA levels after pelvic radiotherapy are sometimes observed and do not always appear to signify persistent disease. This may represent either distant or radioresistant disease or persistent benign PSA-secreting tissue (Schellhammer, et al., 1991). In a patient previously treated for prostate carcinoma, a rising PSA level is indicative of tumor recurrence, but 1 to 5 years may elapse before clinically detectable disease is apparent. Generalized prostate cancer is not curable by present methods, and therefore treatment may be delayed until there are signs of rapid growth, pain, or organ compromise.

Combining serum PSA determinations with other measurements may become useful in the future for screening older men. For example, the PSA concentration may be divided by the measured prostate volume (determined by transrectal ultrasonography) to obtain a "PSA density," or annual PSA measurements may be used to compute a "rate of change," with a high PSA density or high positive rate of change indicating a higher probability of cancer (Armbruster, 1993).

Prostate Specific Protein

Prostate specific protein (PSP) is, with PAP and PSA, one of the three most abundant secretory proteins of the prostate gland. It also is claimed to be useful as a marker for prostate cancer and has been well characterized immunologically (Huang, et al., 1992).

MULTIPLE MYELOMA

Multiple myeloma is a monoclonal plasma cell neoplasm derived from B lymphocytes. Approximately 80% of myeloma neoplasms secrete immunoglobulin (M-protein) that may be detected in serum as a narrow band or spike on electrophoresis. About 20% of patients have light chain (Bence Jones protein) secretion only, and 1% of tumors release no immunoglobulins or light chain.

β_2-Microglobulin

β_2-Microglobulin, an accessory protein of the HLA antigen (the class I major histocompatibility complex, MHC), is synthesized by nucleated cells, including myeloma cells. β_2-Microglobulin is found in serum and is excreted in the urine. Elevated urine levels are observed in renal failure.

β_2-Microglobulin levels, when corrected for renal function, are an accurate indicator of tumor mass and prognosis. Individuals with low-elevated initial serum levels survive, on average, for more than 50 months, while patients with high levels survive for about 12 months. However, its concentration does not accurately reflect response to treatment, and does not reliably distinguish between multiple myeloma and monoclonal gammopathy of uncertain significance (MGUS), a normally benign condition with an isolated, constant serum M-protein concentration. Treatment of multiple myeloma with alpha interferon may produce a persistent and significant increase in β_2-microglobin levels that can interfere with assessment of tumor response to therapy (Tienhaara, 1991). (See also Chap. 12.)

M-Protein

For multiple myeloma, serum M-protein levels also correlate well with tumor cell burden. The doubling time of M-protein concentrations is typically 4 to 6 months at the time of diagnosis, but in the late stages of disease the cell mass doubling time (and consequently the M-protein concentration doubling time) progressively shortens. At diagnosis, serum M-component levels alone offer little prognostic information. During treatment, the serial assessment of M-protein levels generally provides an accurate measure of response to therapy or disease progression. Because IgG half-life is longer with lower numbers of tumor cells (28 to 30 days as compared with 8 to 10 days with high tumor mass), assessing response by measuring M-protein levels requires longer intervals in low tumor mass myeloma. Survival improvement strongly correlates with reduction in M-component synthetic rate.

Significantly elevated serum lactate dehydrogenase (LD) levels predict drug resistance and shortened survival (9 months) in patients with multiple myeloma. Affected patients frequently have plasma cell leukemia or lymphoma-like extaosseus disease (Dimopoulos, et al., 1991).

As myeloma becomes increasingly refractory to treatment, tumor cells may become more primitive and lose their ability to secrete immunoglobulin. Measuring serum M-protein levels in these patients is not helpful but is, in fact, misleading.

Immunoglobulin light chains (Bence Jones protein) are catabolized by the kidney and excreted in the urine. Differences in renal function and light chain excretion rate, which depends on serum light chain concentration, make urinary Bence Jones protein measurements an unsatisfactory marker of myeloma cell burden and response to treatment. (See also Chap.12.)

MULTIPLE ENDOCRINE NEOPLASIA SYNDROMES

Multiple endocrine neoplasia (MEN) is characterized by the occurrence of tumors involving two or more endocrine glands. It may be inherited in association with autosomally dominant alleles or may occur sporadically. MEN-1 (located at chromosome 11q13) is characterized by the occurrence of tumors of the parathyroid glands (secreting parathyroid hormone with resulting hypercalcemia), the pancreatic islets (secreting gastrin more often than insulin), and the anterior pituitary. MEN-2 (located at chromosome 10cen-10q11.2) is associated with medullary carcinoma of the thyroid C-cells (secreting calcitonin) and occurs in a number of variants. Hyperparathyroidism may also be associated with MEN-2.

Since both hypercalcemia and gastrin stimulate calcitonin secretion by neoplastic C-cells, intravenous infusion of pentagastrin (0.5 mg/kg), alone or in combination with calcium, accompanied by blood sampling (at 2.5, 10, and 30 minutes) and calcitonin measurement (see Chap. 10), may be used as a screening procedure for family members suspected to be at risk from MEN-2 (McLean, et al., 1984). Calcitonin concentrations (normal stimulated calcitonin is ≤300 pg/mL for males and ≤150 for females) greater than 1000 pg/mL are diagnostic of medullary carcinoma of the thyroid (Pommier, 1992). With children at risk, screening should be regular and begin in infancy. Specific DNA probes for relevant genetic loci will become available for screening of both MEN-1 and MEN-2 (Thakker, 1993). (See also Chap. 11.)

Conclusion

Serum tumor markers have five potential uses: population screening, diagnosis, prognosis, monitoring treatment response, and detecting recurrence.

As a population screening tool, the clinical sensitivity of a serum tumor marker is increased by preselection of the population to be screened, for example, AFP concentrations to screen for hepatoma in patients with hepatitis B infection. However, such a selection process also increases the percent of false positive results. Diagnostic precision is increased when the range of diseases associated with a particular serum tumor marker is small, and combinations of tumor marker measurements can increase the statistical probability of correctly diagnosing a particular disease. Moreover, most tumor markers do not permit very early detection of small volume tumors (hCG in gestational trophoblastic disease is an exception), and this constitutes another important limitation in benefit-effective population screening.

For a tumor marker to convey accurate prognostic information, serum levels must generally correlate with tumor cell burden, as prognosis for most patients with cancer depends on extent and location of disease. Some patients with highly responsive cancers such as gestational trophoblastic disease may have extensive disease and markedly elevated serum tumor marker levels and yet be curable. In this situation, the elevated serum tumor marker level is less important in establishing prognosis than in guiding the choice of therapy.

Serial tumor marker measurements are frequently used to monitor response to disease treatment in patients who had elevated marker levels at diagnosis. Failure of tumor marker level to fall with treatment is usually a reliable indicator of treatment failure. However, levels may remain elevated for months to years after primary treatment without evidence of clinical disease recurrence, as may be seen with persistently elevated PSA levels following pelvic irradiation for prostate carcinoma.

Serum tumor markers are also used to detect recurrence of disease but, unfortunately, most recurrent cancers are rarely curable with current therapeutic protocols. Nevertheless, more intense therapy, such as bone marrow transplantation, may help cure some previously incurable diseases. Ultimately, the analysis and manipulation of genes and gene products may allow both better diagnosis and treatment of neoplastic disease.

REFERENCES

Armbruster DA. Prostate-specific antigen: biochemistry, analytical methods, and clinical application. Clin Chem 1993;39:181–195.

Bagshawe KD. Risk and prognostic factors in trophoblastic neoplasms. Cancer 1976;38:1373–1385.

Banfi G, Zerbi A, Pastori S, Parolini D, Di Carlo V, Bonini P. Behaviour of tumor markers CA19.9, CA195, CAM43, CA242 and TPS in the diagnosis and follow-up of pancreatic cancer. Clin Chem 1993;39:420–423.

Bast RC Jr, Klug TL, St John E, et al. A radioimmunoassay using a monoclonal antibody to monitor the course of epithelial ovarian cancer. N Engl J Med 1983;309:883–887.

Bast RC, Hunter V, Knapp RC. Pros and cons of gynecologic tumor markers. Cancer 1987;60:1984–1989.

Begent RHJ. The value of carcinoembryonic antigen in clinical practice. Br J Hosp Med 1987;April:335–338.

Begent RHJ, Keep PA, Searle F, et al. Radioimmunolocalization and selection for surgery in recurrent colorectal cancer. Br J Surg 1986;73:64–67.

Brandt-Rauf PW, Luo JC, Carney WP, et al. Detection of increased amounts of the extra-cellular domain of c-erbB-2 oncoprotein in the serum during pulmonary carcinogenesis in humans. Int J Cancer 1994;56:383-386.

Brandt-Rauf PW, Smith A, Hemminski K et al. Serum oncoproteins and growth factors in as-bestos and silicosis patients. Int J Cancer 1992;50:881–885.

Breuer B, DeVivo I, Luo JC, et al. Erb-2 and myc oncoproteins in sera and tumors of breast cancer patients. Cancer Epidem Biomarkers and Prevention 1994;3:63–66.

Carney DN, Linde DC, Cohen MH. Serum neuron-specific enolase: a marker for disease ex-tent and response to therapy of small cell lung cancer. Cancer 1982;137:583–585.

Cottone M, Turri M, Caltagione M, Maringhini M, Seiarrino E, Virdone R. Early detection of hepatocellular carcinoma associated with cirrhosis by ultrasound and alpha fetoprotein: a prospective study. Hepatogastroenterology 1988;35:101–103.

Dimopoulos MA, Benlogie B, Smith TC, Alexandrian R. High serum lactate dehydrogenase level as a marker for drug resistance in multiple myeloma. Ann Int Med 1991;115:931–935.

Dixon AR, Price MR, Hand CW, et al. Epithelial mucin core antigen (EMCA) in assessing therapeutic response in advanced breast cancer—a comparison with CA15-3. Br J Can-cer 1993;68:947–949.

Dupont A, Cusan C, Gomez JC, Thibeault M-M, Tremblay M, Labrie F. Prostate specific anti-gen and prostatic acid phosphatase for monitoring therapy of carcinoma of the prostate. J Urol 1991;146:1064–1068.

Eastham JA, Wilson TG, Russell C, et al. Surgical resection in patients with nonseminomatous germ cell tumor who fail to normalize serum tumor markers after chemotherapy. J Urol 1994;43:74–80.

Einhorn N, Sjovall K, Schienfeld DA, et al. Prospective evaluation of the specificity of serum CA-125 levels for detection of ovarian carcinoma in a normal population. Ann Soc Clin Oncol 1990;9:157–163.

Ercole CJ, Lange PH, Mathisen M, Chiou RK, Vessella RL. Prostate specific antigen and prostatic acid phosphatase in the monitoring and staying of patients with prostatic cancer. J Urol 1987;138:1181–1184.

Francis JM, Moss DW, Colinet E, Calam DH, Bullock DG. A reference preparation of human prostatic acid phosphatase: purification, characterization and field trials. Ann Clin Biochem 1992;29:176–183.

Fujiyama S, Morishita T, Sagawa K. Clinical evaluation of plasma abnormal prothrombin (PIVKA-II) in patients with hepatocellular carcinoma. Hepatogastroenterology 1986;33:201–205.

Goldstein DP. Endocrine assay in chorionic tumors. Clin Obstet Gynecol 1978;18:41–60.

Goldstein DP. Gestational trophoblastic neoplasia in the 1990s. Yale J Biol Med 1991;64:639–651.

Ganz PA, Ma PY, Wang HJ, Elashoff RM. Evaluation of three biochemical markers for seri-ally monitoring the therapy of small-cell lung cancer. J Clin Oncol 1987;5:472–479.

Hayes D, Zurawski VR, Kufe DW. Comparison of circulating CA 15-3 and carcinoembryonic antigen levels in patients with breast cancer. J Clin Oncol 1986;4:1542–1550.

Healy DL, Burger HG, Mamers P, et al. Elevated serum inhibin concentrations in post-menopausal women with ovarian tumors. N Engl J Med 1993;329:1539–1542.

Huang C-L, Liang HM, Brassil D, et al. Two-site monoclonal antibody-based immuno-radiometric assays for measuring prostate secretory protein in serum. Clin Chem 1992;38:817–823.

Iishi H, Yamamura H, Tatsuta M, Okuda S, Kitamura T. Value of ultrasonographic examination combined with measurement of serum tumor markers in the diagnosis of pancreatic cancer less than 3 cm in diameter. Cancer 1986;57:1947–1951.

Jacques G, Auerbach B, Pritsch M, et al. Evaluation of serum neural cell adhesion molecule as a new tumor marker in small cell lung cancer. Cancer 1993;72:418–425.

Järvisalos J, Hakama M, Knekt P, et al. Serum tumor markers CEA, CA 50, TATI and NSE in lung cancer screening. Cancer 1993;71:1992–1998.

Kasahara A, Hayashi N, Susamoto H, et al. Clinical evaluation of plasma des-gamma-carboxy prothrombin as a marker protein of hepatocellular carcinoma in patients with tumors of various sizes. J Digestive Dis and Sci 1993;38:2170–2176.

Lundin J, Roberts PJ, Kuusela P, Haglund C. The prognostic value of preoperative serum levels of CA19-9 and CEA in patients with pancreatic cancer. Br J Cancer 1994;69:515–519.

McLean GW, Rabin D, Moore L, Deftos L, Lorber D, McKenna TJ. Evaluation of provocative tests in suspected medullary carcinoma of the thyroid: heterogeneity of calcitonin responses to calcium and pentagastrin. Metabolism 1984;33:790–796.

Martin EW Jr, Minton JP, Carey CC. CEA-directed second-look surgery in the asymptomatic patient after primary resection of colorectal carcinoma. Ann Surg 1985;202:310–317.

Nakasaki H. Preoperative and postoperative cytokines in patients with cancer. Cancer 1992;70:790–796.

Picozzi VS, Freiha FS, Heinnigan JF, et al. Prognostic significance of a decline in serum chorionic gonadotropin levels after initial chemotherapy for advanced germ cell carcinoma. Ann Int Med 1984;100:183–186.

Pleskow DK, Berger HS, Gyves J, Allen E, McLean A, Podolsky DK. Evaluation of a serologic marker, CA 19-9, in the diagnosis of pancreatic cancer. Ann Intern Med 1989;110:704–709.

Pommier RF. Medullary thyroid cancer. The Endocrinologist 1992;2:393–405.

Pupa SM, Menard S, Morelli D, et al. The extracellular domain of c-erbB-2 oncoprotein released from tumor cells by proteolytic cleavage. Oncogene 1993;8:2917-2923.

Reinsberg J, Schultes B, Wagner U, Krebs D. Monitoring cancer antigen 125 in serum of ovarian cancer patients after administration of ^{131}I-labeled F(ab')$_2$ fragments of OC125 antibody. Clin Chem 1993;39:891–896.

Roach M 3rd, Marquez C, Yua HS, et al. Predicting the risk of lymph node involvement using the pre-treatment prostate specific antigen and Gleason score in men with clinically localized prostate cancer. Int J Rad Onc Biophys 1994;28:33–37

Safi F, Roscher R, Beger HG. The clinical relevance of the tumor marker CA 19-9 in the diagnosing and monitoring of pancreatic carcinoma. Bull Cancer (Paris) 1990;77:83–91.

Sato Y, Nakata K, Kato Y, et al. Early recognition of hepatocellular carcinoma based on altered profiles of alpha-fetoprotein. N Engl J Med 1993;328:1802–1806.

Schellhammer PF, Schlossberg SM, El-Mahdi AM, et al. Prostate specific antigen levels after definitive irradiation for carcinoma of the prostate. J Urol 1991;145:1008–1011.

Stamey TA, Yang N, Hay AR, McNeal JE, Freina FS, Reduive E. Prostate-specific antigen as a serum marker for adenocarcinoma of the prostate. N Engl J Med 1987;317:909–916.

Steinberg W. The clinical utility of the CA 19-9 tumor-associated antigen. Am J Gastroenterol 1990;85:350–355.

Stenman U-H, Bidart J-M, Birkin S, Mann K, Nisula B, O'Connor J. Standardization of protein immunoprocedures: Choriogonadotropin (CG). Scand J Clin Lab Invest 1993;53 (suppl 216):42–78.

Stoter G, Sylvester R, Sleijfer DT et al. Multivariate analysis of prognostic factors in patients with disseminated nonseminomatous testicular cancer: results from a European Organization for Research on Treatment of Cancer multiinstitutional phase III study. Cancer Res 1987;47:2714–2718.

Tanaka K, Hirohata T, Koga S, et al. Hepatitis-C and hepatitis-B in the etiology of hepatocellular cancer in the Japanese population. Cancer Res 1991;51:2842–2847.

Thakker RV. The molecular genetics of the multiple endocrine neoplasia syndromes. Clin Endocrinol 1993;38:1–12.

Tienhaara A, Remes K, Pellinieri T-T. Alpha interferon raises serum beta-2-microglobulin in patients with multiple myeloma. Br J Hematol 1991;77:335–338.

Tjandra SS, McLaughlin PJ, Russell IS, Collins JP, McKenzie IF. Comparison of mammary serum antigen with B2M and carcinoembryonic antigen (CEA) assays in patients with breast cancer. Eur J Cancer Clin Oncol 1988;24:1633–1640.

Tsuchiya R, Noda T, Harada N, et al. Collective review of small carcinomas of the pancreas. Ann Surg 1986;203:77–81.

van Kamp HJ, von Mesdorff-Pouilly S, Kenemans P, et al. Evaluation of colorectal cancer-associated mucin CA M43 assay in serum. Clin Chem 1993;39:1029–1032.

Ward TM, ed, Proteins and Tumor Markers, Vol 1, part 3. In: Seth J, ed. The immunoassay Kit Directory, Series A: Clinical Chemistry. Norwell, MA: Kluwer Academic Publishers, 1992.

Woolas RP, Xu FJ, Jacobs IJ, et al. Elevation of multiple serum markers in patients with stage I ovarian cancer. J Natl Cancer Inst 1993;85(21):1748–1751.

Yeh YC, Tsai JF, Chuang LY, et al. Elevation of transforming growth factor alpha and its relationship to the epidermal growth factor and alpha-fetoprotein levels in patients with hepatocellular carcinoma. Cancer Res 1987;47:896–901.

Yio XY, Jiang J, Yin FZ, Ruan K-H. Highly sensitive sandwich enzyme immunoassay for alpha-fetoprotein in human saliva. Ann Clin Biochem 1992;29:519–522.

Zuchelli GC, Pilo A, Chiesa MS, et al. Growing use of nonisotopic CA 19-9 immunoassays increases between laboratory variability. Clin Chem 1993;39:909–911.

CHAPTER 17

Infectious Disease

Stella Quan

Vast numbers of bacteria coexist peacefully with their vertebrate hosts and most viruses that can be detected in humans cause no detectable illness under normal circumstances. However, when the delicate balance between the host and microorganisms is upset, infection of the host may occur. The term *infectious disease* is applied when the physiology of the host is altered and damage occurs. It is the consequence of the interaction of a mildly virulent microorganism and a host with impaired defense function, or of a highly virulent microorganism and a normal host, or a situation somewhere between these extremes.

INFECTION AND THE IMMUNE RESPONSE

The interaction between host and microorganism is initiated by the microbe's attachment to particular molecular structures ("receptors") on host cells, and the spread of infection may occur in tissues, via the lymphatic system, or through the bloodstream. Microbial pathogens have offense/defense mechanisms, including toxins, enzymes, and phagocyte resistant capsules, which help them resist immobilization and destruction long enough to attain large enough numbers to establish infection. The host's defenses involve nonspecific mechanisms, such as mucocutaneous barriers, phagocytosis, and the alternative pathway of the complement system, as well as specific mechanisms dependent on exact recognition of antigenic determinants on the invader.

The inflammatory reaction involves cells such as neutrophils, macrophages, lymphocytes, and plasma cells that, individually or cooperatively, attempt to contain the infection by phagocytosis (see Chap. 12 for further information on phagocytes and immunocytes). The humoral immune response mechanism generates specific binding molecules (the immunoglobulins) that mark the pathogen for destruction by phagocytosis or by means of the complement system. By augmenting the cellular reaction against microbial invasion, the classical pathway of the complement system plays important roles in both the humoral immune response and the inflammatory reaction.

281

Humoral Immune Response

B lymphocytes, or B cells, are specialized leukocytes carrying an enormous diversity of membrane-bound, cell-specific immunoglobulin M (IgM) molecules which act as receptors. Many millions of specific B cells roam the circulation and strong binding of a pathogen by the membrane-bound IgM on a B cell stimulates the cell to divide and differentiate. This gives rise to a clone of cells (plasma cells), each secreting a soluble form of the original specific IgM, which is capable of specifically binding the antigen that mediated the original interaction with the pathogen. IgM also has special binding sites on its constant region which interact with phagocytes and complement, so that the coating of pathogen by IgM aids in its destruction.

Two additional aspects of humoral immunity make it a very powerful defense mechanism. The genes coding for the selected, specific IgM are prone to rearrangement and selective mutation, and the original B cell clone gives rise to subclones secreting antibodies with different constant regions (class switching) suited to a comprehensive defense reaction, and antibodies with improved affinity for the pathogenic antigen (affinity maturation). Second, some participating B cells (memory cells) continue in the circulation, so that subsequent invasions are quickly met by the appearance of large amounts of high affinity antibodies of classes (usually including IgG1) suited to a rapid quenching of the infection (Fig. 17–1).

Antibodies are glycoproteins with at least two specific antigen binding sites (see Chap. 1 for further detail of immunoglobulin structure in general and IgG structure in particular, and for discussion of the Ig binding site). There are nine immunoglobulin classes and subclasses: IgA1, IgA2, IgD, IgG1, IgG2, IgG3, IgG4, IgE, and IgM, each class being determined by the constant region of its heavy chain; their general properties and functions are summarized in Table 17–1.

Cellular Immune Response

Cell mediated immunity, which involves the interaction of T lymphocytes with phagocytes and B lymphocytes, is essential for the prevention and control of cancer and of infection by intracellular pathogens. T cells display on their surfaces an enormous variety of specific receptors (T cell receptor, TCR), only one binding specificity being present per cell. Like immunoglobulins, these are generated by the joining of gene segments selected at random from libraries with multiple copies of each segment. Mature T cells also carry either CD4 or CD8 molecules on their plasma membranes, and these determine the kinds of antigen bearing cells with which they can interact. CD8+ cells only recognize antigen in conjunction with cells with HLA class I surface proteins, found on all nucleated cells, while CD4+ cells only recognize antigen presented by cells with HLA class II, present only on B cells, activated T cells, macrophages, monocytes, and a limited number of other cell types.

Killer T cells are CD8+ and cytotoxic; they directly kill virus-infected HLA class I+ cells, thereby preventing virus replication. On the other hand, the roles of CD4+ cells are largely regulatory. CD4+ helper T cells activate macrophages and killer T cells, and stimulate the differentiation of antibody secreting cells by releas-

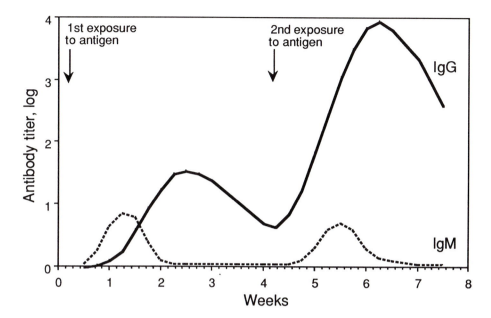

Figure 17–1 Primary and secondary humoral immune responses. In the primary response there is an early burst of antigen-specific IgM secretion which dies off rapidly. Specific IgG antibody synthesis takes longer to reach a maximum rate. On secondary exposure to antigen, the time profile of serum IgM concentration is unchanged, but the concentration of antigen-specific IgG antibodies rapidly increases to reach a much higher titer than after first exposure, and there is a much slower falling off in concentration. In addition, the binding affinities of the IgG antibodies synthesized later in the primary response and in the secondary response are significantly higher. The pattern of IgA synthesis resembles that for IgG and these two antibody classes combined constitute the immediate humoral defense against future penetrations by pathogens carrying the now familiar antigen. Clinically, finding an elevated titer of specific IgM antibodies or only low affinity IgG antibodies indicates that exposure was relatively recent.

ing lymphokines, thereby amplifying the host's response to infection. CD4+ suppressor T cells, which develop from helper cells, suppress the activities of helper cells, acting as a brake and preventing an excessive reaction.

Epidemiology and Etiology

In investigating the epidemiology of an infectious disease, the clinical condition under study must be clearly defined and the etiologic agent precisely identified. Beyond classic cultural techniques and biochemical characterization methods, the range of immunoassay methods described below can be used to identify and demonstrate the presence of pathogenic microorganisms associated with infectious diseases in clinical or pathologic specimens.

Table 17–1 Immunoglobulin classes, their physiochemical properties, and physiologic functions

Property	IgG	IgA	IgM	IgD	IgE
Mol wt	150,000	395,000	900,000	185,000	200,000
Component chains	2γ, 2κ or λ	4α, 4κ or λ, J-chain, secretory component*	10μ, 10κ or λ, J-chain	2δ, 2κ or λ	2ε, 2×κ or λ
% Carbohydrate	3	8	12	13	12
Binds to macrophages	++	±	–	–	±
Binds to mast cells	–	–	–	–	++
Fixes complement (classical)	++	–	+++	–	–
Crosses placenta	++	–	–	–	–
% Total Ig	80	13	6	0–1	0.002
Serum concentration g/L	8–16	1.4–4	0.5–2	0–0.4	17–450 ng/mL
Subclasses	IgG1, IgG2, IgG3, IgG4,	IgA1, IgA2,	None	None	None
Functions	Major Ig of the general circulation where it combats microorganisms and their toxins. IgG1 is the dominant subclass (65%). IgG4 exhibits reduced binding to monocytes and complement, but binds to mast cells.	As the main Ig in seromucous secretions IgA guards external body orifices and surfaces.	First antibody of the immune response and firstline defense against bacteremia. It is a very effective agglutinator.	Function has not been defined. Most is bound to the outer surface of the lymphocyte.	Raised in parasitic infections. Helps in the protection of external surfaces by promoting a strong inflammatory response. Mediates allergic reactions and is raised in atopic disease.

*IgA also exists as a monomer with 2α and 2κ or2λ.

IMMUNOASSAYS

Classically, the identity of a pathogen causing a disease was established by complex procedures often involving preliminary purification, culture, differential staining, and microscopic evaluation; equivalent procedures today are still the only methods accepted as definitive for most pathogens. However, immunoassays have become very important in the routine diagnosis and monitoring of the majority of infectious diseases. Such assays are designed to detect and measure pathogen, the specific immune response, the inflammatory response (e.g., C-reactive protein [see Chap. 16] and amyloid protein A [Nakayama, et al., 1993]) and tissue damage (e.g., β_2-microglobulin [see Chap. 16]).

Measurement of Antibodies

Antibody tests include the full range of immunoassay procedures used for the detection and quantitation of specific antibodies, including complement fixation, hemagglutination assays, latex agglutination assays, gel diffusion assays, immunofluorescent staining, immunoblot, and Western blot assays (Fig. 17–2), reagent excess sandwich immunoassays, and competitive immunoassays (Rose, et al., 1992; Kemeny, 1992). Complement fixation and hemagglutination assays are decreasing in popularity because the complex biologic reagents used are very difficult to control and the specificity is sometimes compromised. Reagent excess sandwich assays (particularly microtiter plate immunoenzymometric assay [IEMA], also called enzyme-linked immunosorbent assay [ELISA]) are used to specifically determine antibodies of a certain class or subclass combined with a certain antigenic specificity (e.g., Dolan, et al., 1991). These are of two main types: "antibody capture" and "antigen capture." Antigen capture assays are often more suitable for minor class antibodies (see Chap. 1 for further details).

As described above, the affinity of the immunoglobulin synthesized in response to an infection increases as the infection develops and is then conquered or controlled. Therefore, both IgM and early IgG antibodies have, in general, lower affinity for pathogen antigens than IgG antibodies, that represent past immunity. This situation is exploited by the use of "protein denaturing immunoassay" or "avidity ELISA," both of which are designed to detect only high affinity antibodies (e.g., Thomas and Morgan-Capner, 1991; Ward, et al., 1993; Lappalainen, et al., 1993). To explain briefly, diluted patient sera are placed in contact with solid phase coated with pathogen antigen and, instead of the usual washing step, a protein denaturant solution such as 6 M urea is used to elute both nonspecifically adsorbed proteins *and* lower-affinity specific antibodies, before thorough washing and the determination of the remaining bound antibody with labeled anti-Ig or anti-IgG antibody (sp-Ag–**Ab**–Ab-Enz, where **Ab** represents only high affinity antibody) (Lappalainen, et al., 1993). Such procedures have the further potential advantage that interference from cross-reacting antibodies against related or other antigens may be excluded (Ward, et al., 1993). Two recent studies emphasize possible problems (Underwood, 1993) and the importance of thorough validation (Goldblatt, et al., 1993) with such assays.

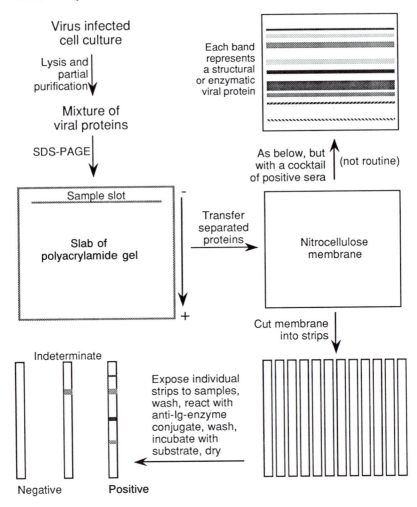

Figure 17–2 Western blot technique for the detection of specific antibodies against a range of antigens from a virus or bacterium.

The diagram is largely self-explanatory but some extra information may be useful. Transfer of the separated proteins from the slab of polyacrylamide gel to the nitrocellulose membrane may be aided by creating an electric gradient between the two (electrophoretic elution), or by simple diffusion, by which the membrane is "blotted" with the separated proteins by being laid on top of the gel. The membrane is then usually treated with neutral protein to reduce subsequent nonspecific adsorption of detection agents. Commercially prepared Western blot kits contain a number of strips prepared by cutting up the carefully dried membrane sheet. The final immune complexes detected on the strips take the form sp-Ag–**Ab**–Ab-Enz, where the solid phase (sp) is the membrane and the antibody-enzyme (Ab-Enz) is anti-human IgG (or anti-IgM or anti-Ig) conjugated to alkaline phosphatase or horseradish peroxidase. Ab-^{125}I with autoradiographic detection is also used.

A crucial part of Western blot analysis is the visual scoring of the results. Few if any seropositive samples give bands corresponding to all the potential antigens and a certain min-

Competitive assays for specific antibodies, with a labeled monoclonal anti-body specific for a selected epitope on the antigen of interest, can determine patient antibodies specific for that epitope (Kemeny, 1992). An alternative format for competitive determination of specific antibodies has been described (Berry, et al., 1993). In an assay for antibodies against HIV-2, a recombinant fusion protein (β-galactosidase/immunodominant region of the transmembrane glycoprotein of HIV-2 [ANT 53], BGAL/ANT53) and immobilized antibody against β-galactosi-dase (sp-AntiBGAL) are used. Patient antibodies specific for ANT 53 (**Ab**) compete with the sp-AntiBGAL for the soluble BGAL/ANT 53 to give either sp-AntiBGAL and BGAL/ANT 53–**Ab** or sp-AntiBGAL–BGAL/ANT 53, so that the amount of enzyme activity bound is inversely proportional to the amount of specific antibody present.

Immunoassays for specific antibodies are also discussed in Chapters 1, 13, and 15.

Measurement of Antigens

Immunoassays for the detection and measurement of pathogens, and proteins, etc., derived from pathogens, include the same assay designs and formats used for the de-termination of hormones, tumor markers, etc. (Rose, et al., 1992 [various chapters]; Guinet, et al., 1991; Gupta, et al., 1992; Pujol, et al., 1993; Yamashiki, et al., 1993). Unlike in the endocrine laboratory, few of the early immunoassays routinely used in bacteriology had radiolabels. This tradition has continued, with microtiter plate im-munoenzymometric assays (e.g., ELISA) being very popular.

However, while immunoassays for antigens will long continue to be used, DNA probe assays with a polymerase chain reaction (PCR) amplification step are much more sensitive and may become the method of choice for the routine identification of many specific pathogens (e.g., Al, et al., 1993; Pedneault and Katz, 1993).

INFECTIOUS AGENTS AND DISEASES

Because of limitations of space the selection of infectious agents and associated dis-eases included below is limited. Inevitably, important areas of interest to many read-ers are ignored, but it is hoped that the most important aspects of the application of immunoassays to the diagnosis and monitoring of infectious diseases are discussed in the context of at least one disease.

---

imum number of specific bands is defined as a positive result. Samples giving some bands, but insufficient for a positive diagnosis, are defined as indeterminate, and samples giving no bands are defined as negative. For example, for the serodiagnosis of Lyme disease Dressler, et al. (1993) recommend that a positive result should require at least 2 of the 8 most common IgM bands in early disease and at least 5 of the 10 most frequent IgG bands after the first weeks of infection.

Adenovirus

Adenoviruses are nonenveloped, double-stranded DNA viruses 70 to 90 nm in diameter, with 10 structural proteins. The capsid proteins are arranged in an icosahedron shape. Each virion has 240 hexons and 12 pentons with an individual base and a fiber. The hexon contains the immunodominant epitopes.

Human adenoviruses presently consist of 47 serotypes grouped into six subgroups, and are important clinically because they cause acute infections of the respiratory system and conjunctiva, and are associated with a fatality rate of 60% in patients with pneumonia and 50% in those with hepatitis. They can also infect the eye, gastrointestinal tract, and the bladder. About 10% of all respiratory illnesses in children are caused by adenovirus, and some types of gastrointestinal illness, characterized by severe diarrhea, are etiologically associated with enteric adenovirus types 40 and 41. Infections in immunosuppressed patients constitute a new and severe problem, with the defective host immune response leading to persistent infections (Hierholzer, 1992).

Adenoviruses are endemic in all populations throughout the year. Transmission of the gastrointestinal disease occurs via the oral/fecal route. The incubation period is 1 to 2 days. Most of the symptoms are self-limiting, and the illness usually resolves within a week. There are no specific drugs or therapeutic measures, and vaccines are not available for general administration.

A definitive diagnosis of adenovirus infection is made with visualization of the virus by electron microscopy, isolation of the virus in tissue culture, or demonstration of the presence of antibodies by indirect immunofluorescence. Test antigen used to detect antibodies against all 47 serotypes is stable and is commercially available. Isolated adenovirus can be grouped by hemagglutination inhibition testing followed by specific serotyping. Serologic diagnosis of adenovirus infection involves the demonstration of a fourfold rise in antibody titer by complement fixation, neutralization, hemagglutination inhibition, and by ELISA (Hierholzer, 1991). However, complement fixation assay is not very sensitive, especially in children, and enzyme linked assays are gaining popularity.

A two-site assay for the free viral hexons has been developed and applied to the measurement of virus production rates in culture (Everitt and Varga, 1993).

Chlamydia

Chlamydiae are small (200 to 1500 nm in diameter), nonmotile, obligate intracellular microbes resembling gram-negative bacteria, and the infectious particle is a 0.3μm structure termed the elementary body (EB). Three species are recognized as clinically important. *Chlamydia psittaci* causes psittacosis in humans and many animal diseases. *Chlamydia pneumonaie,* TWAR strain (Hyman, et al., 1991), the most recently identified species, causes respiratory tract infections. *Chlamydia trachomatis* is one of the most common human pathogens causing blinding trachoma in hundreds of millions of people. It is also the most prevalent sexually transmitted pathogen currently recognized. It causes urethritis, epididymitis, cervicitis, pelvic in-flammatory disease, urethral syndrome, lymphogranuloma venereum, salpingitis, pneumonitis, and inclusion conjunctivitis. See Bowie, et al. (1990) for a comprehen-sive survey of current knowledge of chlamydial infections.

Chlamydiae usually induce chronic infections in which a balance between host and parasite is established. Although antibodies to chlamydiae are produced, they do not protect against reinfection, but prevent penetration of susceptible host cells, thus limiting the spread of infection. Chlamydial infections are often asympto-matic or nonspecific in their clinical course, and many progress to produce sequelae. Several antimicrobial drugs, particularly tetracycline and erythromycin, can suppress chlamydial growth, provided that a reliable diagnosis is made.

The diagnosis of chlamydial infection is based mainly on culture techniques and, given fresh samples and adequate time and money, they are still the methods of choice. Immunoassay procedures are also used to detect chlamydial antigens in clin-ical specimens (Chernesky, et al., 1986), and these have the advantage that the sam-ples to be analyzed are not as susceptible to deterioration during storage and transport. The immunofluorescence test is a sensitive and specific detector of antichlamydial antibodies, but requires an experienced microscopist who can distinguish between fluorescing chlamydial particles and nonspecific fluorescence. When a range of chlamydia species and serovars are available, antibodies specific for individual species or serovars may be detected (Schachter, 1992).

Colorimetric and chemiluminescent immunoassays with either monoclonal or polyclonal antibodies to the cell wall lipopolysaccharide (LPS) characteristic of chlamydiae are commercially available and should detect all types of chlamydiae. They are best documented for diagnosis of infections with *C. trachomatis*. Abbott's enzyme immunoassay (Chlamydiazyme; Abbot Laboratories, North Chicago, IL) is comparable to Syva's direct fluorescence assay (Microtrak DFA; Syva Company, San Jose, CA) in performance with respect to sensitivity and specificity. They are ap-proximately 75% to 85% sensitive and approximately 97% to 98% specific in de-tecting current chlamydial infection.

Immunoassays in general are less sensitive than culture methods and have a specificity of about 97%. Thus, they are not suitable for screening low prevalence populations because of the presence of false positives and, in high risk populations, single positive results for *C. trachomatis* are seldom diagnostic, on their own, for cur-rent genital infection. However, immunoassays do have the advantages of rapid turn-around and do not require viable bacteria.

Herpesviruses

Cytomegalovirus

Human cytomegalovirus (CMV) is a member of the family Herpesviridae, with an approximate size of 200 nm. Complete CMV particles consist of a core contain-ing double-stranded DNA and an icosahedral capsid, surrounded by a lipid contain-ing envelope.

The incidence of individuals seropositive to CMV in the general U.S. population is estimated to be 50% to 70%. Most cytomegalovirus-affected healthy individuals are asymptomatic, with the virus remaining latent. Infections are due to reactivation of latent virus during any period of immunosuppression, or due to primary infection because of organ transplant or blood transfusion. Infection may also be congenital. Symptoms include fever, malaise, myalgias, leukopenia, thrombocytopenia, colitis, pneumonitis, hepatitis, retinitis, and encephalitis. CMV is a major cause of severe disease in patients with impaired immune defenses such as during therapy for neoplastic disease, and is one of the most important causes of morbidity and mortality in acquired immune deficiency syndrome (AIDS) (Griffiths, 1990).

Hyperimmune anti-CMV globulin from seropositive donors has been given to bone marrow and renal transplant recipients for the prevention of the CMV related disease in numerous studies, but the results obtained are controversial. However, the individual globulin preparations used may have contained greater or lesser proportions of neutralizing and non-neutralizing antibodies. The use of an immunoenzymometric assay (IEMA) specific for neutralizing antibodies to ensure the potency of the globulin preparations used (Kropff, et al., 1993) may lead to more consistent results, alone or in combination with antiviral drugs.

Diagnosis of CMV disease is difficult (Drew, 1988), since virologic or serologic detection of CMV indicates active infection but does not establish that such infection is responsible for symptomatic illness. In combination with pathologic documentation of the disease, virus isolation by conventional cell culture or the shell viral assay (Cleaves, et al., 1984), including staining with a fluorescent monoclonal antibody specific for immediate early antigen, is most useful. Monoclonal antibodies directed against CMV proteins, CMV immediate-early, or early antigens can be used in the immunofluorescent detection of CMV-infected human leukocytes (Ehrnst, et al., 1993), and such tests may be useful in identifying post-transplant patients who would benefit from antiviral treatment.

Assays for CMV-specific IgG and total immunoglobulin have been developed and include indirect hemagglutination, indirect immunofluorescence, anticomplement immunofluorescence, latex agglutination, radioimmunoassay (RIA), and ELISA. However, both acute and convalescent serum samples are required, which delays diagnosis. CMV-specific IgM assays offer rapid serologic diagnosis of primary CMV infections, but significant discordant results are seen amongst different commercial kits. Negative IgG and IgM results should be interpreted with caution in patients who are immunosuppressed or who might be experiencing recurrent infections. Serologic tests are useful primarily in seroepidemiologic studies.

The presence of CMV antibody as evidence of past or present infection is the most valuable indicator of a potentially infective blood or organ donor. The serologic screening of potential donors by IgG-specific or total antibody assays is therefore an essential step in the prevention of acquired CMV disease (Hopson, et al., 1992; Kraat, et al., 1992).

Epstein-Barr Virus

Epstein-Barr virus (EBV) is classified as a herpesvirus, based on its size, structure, and the composition of its genome. It is composed of a lipoprotein envelope and a nucleocapsid with double-stranded DNA and is 150 to 170 nm in diameter. Eighty percent to 90% of all adults have been exposed to the virus, which is transmitted principally by way of saliva. EBV infects human B lymphocytes and, as with other herpesviruses, causes a persistent, latent infection with intermittent reactivations.

EBV is the etiologic agent of infectious mononucleosis (Henle, et al., 1968), which is a self-limiting, lymphoproliferative disease characterized by fever, pharyngitis and cervical lymphadenopathy, lasting for 1 to 4 weeks. It can, however, be complicated by splenomegaly, hepatitis, pneumonitis, pericarditis, myocarditis, aseptic meningitis, and encephalitis. There is no specific treatment, but short-term administration of corticosteroids can be helpful. EBV is implicated in the etiology of nasopharyngeal carcinoma and Burkitt's lymphoma, and has been associated with B cell lymphomas in immunosuppressed patients (e.g., Pedneault and Katz, 1993).

In patients with symptoms of mononucleosis, the initial diagnosis is usually made by a nonspecific serologic test for heterophilic antibody, which is an IgM antibody unrelated to those antibodies directed to specific EBV antigens. The heterophilic antibody of infectious mononucleosis agglutinates sheep and horse erythrocytes and is absorbed by bovine red cells and by guinea pig kidney cells. Heterophilic antibody test kits which use horse erythrocytes and incorporate an absorption step with guinea pig kidney or beef red cells are to be recommended (Sumaya and Jenson, 1992). Determination of EBV-specific antibodies can rule out false positive heterophilic results and decipher EBV infection from other similar illnesses, in cases where the test for heterophilic antibody is negative but clinical symptoms clearly indicate EBV infection.

Specific antibodies against four viral antigens, or antigen complexes, can be detected by indirect immunofluorescence assay, anticomplement immunofluorescence, or ELISA. These include viral capsid antigen (VCA), early antigen-diffuse component (EA/D), early antigen-restricted component (EA/R), and nuclear antigen (EBNA, composed of six distinctive polypeptides), and both purified viral antigens and antigens produced with recombinant DNA methods have been used in the assays (Pearson, 1988; Hille, et al., 1993). Separate detection of EBNA-1 and EBNA-2 antibodies may be of value for the diagnosis of acute and chronic infectious mononucleosis. The use of recombinant antigens to serologically differentiate between infections by two EBV subtypes (type A and type B) that have two different EBNA 2 proteins (EBNA-2A and EBNA-2B) and may have different oncogenic potential, may also be clinically useful (Hille, et al., 1993).

Interpretation of results is based on the observed reactivities to the different antigens. The immune responses in acute mononucleosis are characterized by raised IgG and IgM antibody titers to VCA and detectable titers of IgM antibodies to EBNA. VCA-IgM usually disappears 1 to 2 months after onset, while VCA-IgG persists for life. Anti-EBNA IgG usually gradually increases during convalescence and also persists for life. Antibodies to EA/D usually rise during the acute phase and disappear 3 to 6 months after onset. Moderate to high levels of anti-EBV antigens called restricted components (anti-EBV[R]) of the IgG class can appear by themselves during the later stage of convalescence and are seen in cases of Burkitt's lymphoma. Nasopharyngeal carcinoma patients in general have a unique additional high titer to IgA-VCA and IgA-EA/D.

Herpes Simplex Viruses

The herpes simplex virus (HSV) is 180 to 200 nm in diameter and consists of a DNA-containing core within an icosadeltahedral capsid which is, in turn, enclosed by a fibrous tegument structure and an envelope. Herpes simplex virus type 1 (HSV-1) is responsible for herpes gingivostomatitis, an infection of the oral mucosa referred to as fever blisters or cold sores, and neonatal encephalitis. Herpes simplex virus type 2 (HSV-2) (and sometimes type 1) causes a sexually transmitted disease of the genitalia in which the lesion appears after a week and causes a burning sensation. Females are more likely to be asymptomatic and may infect their children at birth (Rawls, 1985).

HSV infection of the newborn infant is associated with significant morbidity and mortality, in addition to malformations such as microphthalmia, microcephaly, or hydranencephaly in cases of intrauterine infections. In general, when epithelial surfaces are involved, prolonged shedding of viruses may occur, leading to infection of persons in close contact.

A number of tests have been developed for the detection and identification of HSV, including conventional tissue culture, latex agglutination, immunofluorescence, immunoperoxidase staining, and ELISA. Immunofluorescence staining of cultured virus with fluorescein isothiocyanate-labeled monoclonal antibodies is the most cost-effective and least time-consuming method of confirming and differentiating HSV-1 and HSV-2.

In cases where isolation and culture were not successful or not performed, a significant rise in the titer of serum IgM antibodies specific for HSV may be diagnostic. However, assays for IgM HSV antibodies cannot be used to distinguish primary from recurrent infections because the host response to reactivation can also include IgM antibody production. False positive IgM results can occur when rheumatoid factor and specific IgG antibodies are present together. In addition, many current tests cannot reliably distinguish HSV-1 and HSV-2 antibodies (Ashley, et al., 1991), but Western blot analysis can demonstrate reactivity with type-specific viral proteins (Ashley, et al., 1988).

Human Immunodeficiency Viruses

Human immunodeficiency viruses type 1 and 2 (HIV-1 and HIV-2) belong to the family of Retroviridae. They are spheric and measure 80 to 130 nm in diameter. The nucleocapsid complex at the center of the virus, containing the single-stranded positive-sense RNA, is enclosed within the capsid, which is in turn surrounded by a host cell membrane–derived envelope from which project viral protein spikes. AIDS, resulting after a prolonged latent infection with HIV-1, was first recognized as a new disease from reports of the unusual occurrence of *Pneumocystis carinii* pneumonia and Kaposi's sarcoma in urban male homosexuals. Most HIV-2 infected individuals are asymptomatic and there is a longer incubation period than with HIV-1. Currently, it is estimated that about 1 million residents of the United States are infected with HIV-1, while less than 50 are infected with HIV-2.

HIV is transmitted through intimate sexual contact, contaminated blood and blood products, and passage from mother to child during perinatal events. HIV infections can result in a variety of disease states, including acute mononucleosis–like syndrome, prolonged asymptomatic infection, AIDS-related complex, and AIDS. HIV infected individuals remain asymptomatic for an average of 10 years after exposure to the virus. Most histopathologic changes in AIDS are caused by secondary, opportunistic infections or neoplasms. No vaccine is currently available. Treatment is of necessity multifaceted prophylaxis, therapy for opportunistic infections and malignancies, erythropoietin therapy for use in patients with anemia, and antiviral drugs (e.g., zidovudine).

The diagnosis of HIV infection is based on the detection of specific antibodies to HIV, detection of viral antigens, isolation of virus, or detection of viral RNA (Roberts, 1991; Sloand, 1991). Following infection with HIV, antibodies are often detected in plasma from 1 week to 3 months later. Viral lysate, recombinant antigens, or peptides corresponding to the envelope proteins of HIV are used in IEMA for the measurement of specific antibodies. Combination assays for the simultaneous detection of antibodies to HIV-1 and HIV-2 are commonly used for screening of blood donations (see Chap. 1).

Because HIV antibody screening assays are configured to give very few false negative results, false positive results (e.g., after influenza vaccination [Hsia, 1993]) are a recurring problem. Specimens that are found to be repeatedly reactive for HIV-1 by one or more screening assays should be reassayed with a confirmatory assay in which the sample is analyzed for specific antibodies to a range of viral antigens, for example, Western blot assay, immunofluorescence assay, or radioimmunoprecipitation antibody test. HIV-specific IgM antibodies are not always detectable in closely monitored infected patients, but when detected usually appear before specific IgG (Simmonds, et al., 1991).

Serum anti-HIV IgA testing provides a specific and fairly sensitive method for the detection of HIV in infants, since maternal anti-HIV IgG is passively transferred across the placenta and may persist through 15 months of age in uninfected infants, whereas maternally derived IgA does not cross the placental barrier (Quinn, et al., 1991). HIV antibody tests validated for saliva and urine samples have been developed and, while some preliminary data show that sensitivity and specificity with urine and saliva samples are inferior to serum or plasma samples, newer assays with special saliva collection devices under field trial may be more than accurate enough to complement serum assays.

Effective assays for HIV antigen could be very useful for the detection of peri-natally acquired HIV infection, and for the general detection of infection prior to the presence of antibody. Immunoassays for the *gag*-derived product, p24, and other HIV antigens are available for research purposes. Recently it has been reported that acid treatment of serum samples to promote dissociation of immune and other complexes improves the diagnostic utility of p24 detection in infected babies (Quinn, et al., 1993). It is extremely rare for an adult sample to test negative in the antibody assay and yet positive in an antigen assay and the Food and Drug Administration does not recommend antigen testing for routine blood donor screening. Viral load was shown to be closely associated with CD4+ cell count by flow cytometry and has been proved to be a better predictor of the progression to AIDS than virus isolation and culture techniques (O'Shea, et al., 1991).

Human T-Cell Lymphotrophic Viruses

Human T- cell Lymphotrophic viruses types I and II (HTLV-I and HTLV-II) are retroviruses antigenenically and genetically closely related to each other but only distantly related to HIV. HTLV-I is associated with adult T cell leukemia (Poiez, et al., 1980) and also with "HTLV-I associated myelopathy/tropical spastic paraparesis," which is characterized by progressive weakness in the lower extremities and sensory disturbances. HTLV-II was first isolated from two patients with T-cell hairy leukemia (Kalyanaraman, et al., 1982), but there is little evidence of pathologic consequence from HTLV-II infection.

HTLV-I is endemic but rare in Japan, the Caribbean, the southeastern United States and west Africa, and its incidence in high risk populations may be underesti-mated by the use of serologic as opposed to PCR assays (Al, et al., 1992). Viruses from both groups preferentially infect CD4+ T lymphocytes. HTLV-I is a persistent infection, with the latency between infection and disease estimated to be between 10 to 40 years. The modes of transmission of HTLV and HIV are similar, and dual infection of HIV-1 with HTLV-I or HTLV-II may be associated with a more rapid prognosis than for HIV-1 alone.

Detection of anti-HTLV-I and HTLV-II antibodies is most often accomplished through initial screening of serum or plasma by IEMA, with confirmation by Western blot, radioimmunoprecipitation, or immunofluorescence (Anderson, et al., 1989). Western blot analysis may not always be sensitive enough to detect antibodies to en-velope products, and in the absence of clear envelope protein reactivity in Western blot assay, the specimen should be further tested by radioimmunoprecipitation. ELISA is based on viral lysate, recombinant antigens, or peptides from conserved re-gions between HTLV-I and HTLV-II or type-specific regions from the envelope of the virus. The most reliable technique used to differentiate between HTLV-I and HTLV-II is PCR. Since infection with HTLV-I, in contrast to HTLV-II, is often as-sociated with the development of serious illness, it is important to identify which virus is present for appropriate patient counseling. New IEMA tests have been developed which utilize a panel of synthetic peptides for the simultaneous detection of antibodies against HIV-1, HIV-2, HTLV-I, and HTLV-II.

Lyme Disease

Lyme disease is a tick-transmitted infection caused by the spirochete *Borrelia burgdorferi* (Burgdorfer, et al., 1982), a helical-shaped bacterium (10 to 25 μm by 0.2 to 0.4 μm, cross-sectional diameter) that shows a characteristic undulating motility. Lyme borreliosis has been reported with increasing frequency during the last few years, and is now the most common tickborne infection in the United States and in Europe.

Early localized infection occurs 3 to 30 days after the tick bite and is characterized by an expanding circular red rash with a partial clearing at the site of the bite (erythema chronicum migrans) in 60% to 83% of cases. Other symptoms during the early phase include headache, fever, stiff neck, arthralgia, myalgias, malaise, and fatigue or swelling of the lymph nodes, but the presence of erythema migrans is the best clinical marker. However, it is not always observed and making a reliable diagnosis from clinical observations only is sometimes difficult. The initial phase of the disease is benign and can be treated with antibiotics. The later, chronic phase of the disease is difficult to treat and may result in progressive encephalomyelitis, chronic arthritis, acrodermatitis chronica atrophicans, and cardiac abnormalities. Therefore, early diagnosis is essential to allow effective treatment.

Laboratory confirmation of infection is established when diagnostic levels of IgM and IgG to the spirochete are detected in serum or cerebrospinal fluid sample, or when an important change in antibody titer in paired acute and convalescent sera samples is detected (Rahn, et al. 1991). A specific immune response against *B. burgdorferi* is usually detected by immunofluorescence assays or IEMA within weeks of the onset of the disease. However, due to the absence of any standardization procedure and the variability of the antigen preparations used, tests supplied by different suppliers or performed in different laboratories may differ in sensitivity and specificity, making the interpretation of results difficult. Western blotting (Ma, et al., 1992; Dressler, et al., 1993) aids in the identification of false positive ELISA results and criteria for immunoblot analysis have been proposed (Dressler, et al., 1993).

However, infected patients may be seronegative during any phase of Lyme disease. Serum antibodies to *B. burgdorferi,* as determined by IEMA, are frequently not present when erythema migrans first appears but usually develop in association with the later cutaneous manifestations of Lyme disease. The rate of false positive and false negative results in antibody assays with crude antigen preparations has meant that misdiagnoses occur. However, clinical accuracy of IEMA may be significantly improved by the use of flagellin-enriched antigens together with absorbants to remove cross-reactants (Lin, et al., 1991), or by the use of recombinant protein preparations (Fawalt, et al., 1993; Rasiah, et al., 1994).

Parvovirus B19

Parvovirus B19 is a recently discovered 20 nm, single-stranded DNA virus (Clewley, 1984) associated with erythema infectiosum, aplastic crises in chronic hemolytic anemia, arthritis, and intrauterine infections with hydrops fetalis. Erythema infectiosum has an incubation period of 4 to 14 days, is common in children, and occurs in focal and community-wide outbreaks. The initial manifestation of the illness is a distinctive fiery red appearance of the cheeks, with circumoral pallor. It usually resolves in 4 weeks, but may last for months. Diagnosis is usually based on clinical observations, but may be confirmed by an elevated titer of anti-parvovirus IgM antibodies.

Serologic diagnosis of acute or past parvovirus B19 infection is based on the detection of specific IgG and IgM anti-B19 antibodies against one of a range of antigen preparations, e.g. viral particles obtained from plasma of viremic patients in the acute phase of infection, recombinant B19 capsid proteins, or immunodominant peptides corresponding to parts of virus protein 1 (VP1) and virus protein 2 (VP2) (Anderson, et al. 1986; Cotmore, et al., 1986; Fridell, et al., 1991; Soderlund, et al., 1992). Specific IgA antibodies are too persistent to be a useful indicator for recent parvovirus B19 infection (Erdman, 1991). Specific IgM antibodies are the most sensitive indicator of acute parvovirus B19 infection in immunologically healthy persons but can persist up to 6 months. At the onset of erythema infectiosum, anti-B19 IgM is detected. Anti-B19 IgG is detected in clinical specimens 1 week after onset of erythema infectiosum and persists throughout the convalescent period. Sera containing high concentrations of anti-IgM rubella virus antibody may give low false positive results (Kurtz and Anderson, 1985).

Diagnosis of the early viremic stage of parvovirus B19 infection may be possible by measuring VP1 and VP2 proteins in patient serum with a well-characterized specific monoclonal antibody (R92F6) that binds to a conserved epitope on both VP1 and VP2 (Loughrey, et al., 1993).

Rickettsial Diseases

Rickettsial diseases (rickettsioses) occur with considerable frequency all over the world. The rickettsiae are small, gram-negative, obligate intracellular bacteria that are natural parasites of arthropods and some of these arthropods transmit disease to animals, including humans. Four groups of rickettsiae are pathogenic for humans: the spotted fever group (*Rickettsia rickettsii*), the epidemic typhus group (*Rickettsia prowazekii*), the scrub typhus group (*Rickettsia tsutsugamushi*) and the Q fever group (*Coxiella burnetii*). The clinical picture is variable, but usually includes a prodromal stage followed by fever, headache, prostration, and often a rash. Treatment usually consists of giving tetracycline, chloramphenicol or quinolones, and removal of vectors from patients (Wisseman, et al., 1986, Yeaman, et al., 1987). The immunoserology of the rickettsial diseases is reviewed by Hechemy (1992).

Rickettsioses have nonspecific clinical manifestations, making them difficult to diagnose in a clinical setting. The isolation of rieckettsiae from the blood or tissues of a patient is hazardous and usually does not yield results in time to influence patient management. Serologic testing remains the most frequently used approach to diagnosis. The Preteus OX19 and OX2 (Weil-Felix) febrile agglutination test is not very sensitive nor specific, and the antibodies detected are largely of IgM class and are produced for only a very short time after infection (Kaplan, et al., 1986). ELISA assays, particularly IgM capture assays, are sensitive, but the general unavailability of specific diagnostic antigens reduces the specificity of the test. Complement fixation and the microimmunofluorescence tests are the standard methods (Kaplan, et al., 1986). However, since antibodies often persist after the organisms disappear, discrimination between current and past infection requires the demonstration of a significant rise in specific antibody titer in successive specimens. It is advisable to obtain serum specimens during acute illness and another 2 to 4 weeks afterward.

The complement fixation test is specific but very insensitive in the first 3 weeks after onset of infection, is labor intensive, and strongly IgG dependent. The microimmunofluorescence assay (microIFA) can be used as an Ig class-specific test and can simultaneously detect antibodies to a number of different antigens, from 7 to 9 days after onset of the disease. MicroIFA is currently the method of choice for the serodiagnosis of rickettsial diseases (Hechemy, 1992).

Rubella

Rubella virus is a member of the family Togaviridae. The diameter of the virus particle is 50 to 70 nm, with two heavily glycosylated envelope proteins, a nonglycosylated capsid protein, and single-stranded RNA. Live attenuated rubella virus is routinely used as vaccine.

Rubella is a mild, self-limited disease of 3 to 4 days duration which imparts lifetime immunity, but it is clinically very important because it can induce congenital malformation and persistent infection in the human fetus. About 20% of infants born to mothers infected during the first trimester have signs of congenital rubella. The rash of rubella results from viral replication, and occurs with symptoms of fever, malaise, myalgia, and headache. The incubation period is 14 to 21 days. Maternal immunity protects against intrauterine infection.

Demonstration of the presence of specific IgG in serum is evidence of immunity to rubella. Primary rubella infection is confirmed by the presence of IgM-specific antirubella antibody. A correct differential diagnosis between primary rubella and immunity to rubella is crucial for the management of pregnant patients in contact with rubella. However, false positive rubella-specific IgM reactivity is found in some cases of parvovirus B19 infection, infectious mononucleosis, and toxoplasma infection. Increasing emphasis has recently been placed on the measurement of the relative avidity of rubella-specific IgG by assays carried out with and without a step with denaturing reagents for the disruption of low affinity antigen-antibody complexes. Low avidity specific IgG is found in sera of cases of recent primary rubella infection or recent rubella immunization (Thomas and Morgan-Capner, 1991). Virus isolation is reserved for confirmation of congenital rubella from amniotic fluid.

Toxoplasmosis

Toxoplasma gondii, a coccidian protozoan parasite of worldwide distribution, is the causative agent for toxoplasmosis infection in humans, mammals, and birds. It exists in three forms: tachyzoite, cystizoites, and oocyst; both tachyzoites and cystizoites are found in apparently normal individuals, but oocysts only develop in (and are excreted by) members of the cat family, which are the only definitive hosts.

The majority of toxoplasmal infections are asymptomatic and persist for life. Human infection is frequently by ingestion of tissue cysts in raw or uncooked meat. Toxoplasmosis can occur in the immunosuppressed host as a result of the reactivation of preexisting infection, and the resulting illness can be fatal. Characteristic manifestations of the disease in AIDS include encephalitis, pneumonitis, and myocarditis. Acute infections are usually treated with a combination of pyrimethamine and trisulfapyrimidines.

Congenital infections also occur, almost always due to primary infection of the mother during pregnancy. Infection of the fetus increases in probability with gestational age, but with severe neonatal disease being associated with transmission early in pregnancy. Most infected children are initially asymptomatic but, without treatment, by early adulthood the majority show symptoms such as chorioretinitis or neurologic defects.

Diagnostic tests for toxoplasma infection include isolation of toxoplasma, demonstration of tachyzoites in tissue sections or smears of body fluid, antigen assay (Lindenschmidt, 1985), Sabin-Feldman dye test (Sabin and Feldman, 1948), indirect fluorescence antibody test, agglutination test (Suzuki, et al., 1988), complement fixation test, IgG- and IgM-specific ELISA and double sandwich IgM assay. The usefulness of a given diagnostic method may differ with the category of infection in specific clinical situations.

With the immunocompetent patient, most infections are acute and mild, with lymphadenopathy the most common symptom, and most patients recover over 1 to 2 months. A negative dye or immunofluorescence assay (IFA) test titer virtually excludes a positive diagnosis, but infection is confirmed by seroconversion from negative to positive, or by a serial rise from a low to high titer in two serum samples drawn 3 weeks apart. Complement fixation and indirect hemagglutination tests give positive results later in the course of the illness. If both IgM and IgG titers are high, acute infection is probable. However, a negative IgM-IFA test titer does not rule out acute infection. Diagnosis of ocular toxoplasmosis with retinochoroiditis is based on the characteristic retinal lesions and positive serologic titer. In the immunodeficient host serodiagnosis is difficult due to the depressed immune response or the existence of IgG from past infection. The presence of IgM antibody is rare. The presence of tachyzoites or antigen in the tissue, as determined by immunohistologic staining, is usually needed to confirm active infection, but antibiotic treatment is generally started when presumptive evidence is obtained by computed tomography (CT) scan or magnetic resonance imaging (MRI).

Postnatal diagnosis of *Toxoplasma* infection is complicated by the diversity or absence of symptoms in the mother and/or baby, by the variability of specific IgM expression during infancy, and by the presence of maternal IgG. During pregnancy, IgM-specific antibodies should indicate acute infection, but they have a tendency to persist for a long time, even at high titers. Lappalainen, et al. (1993) evaluated assays for specific IgM, IgA and IgE, a differential agglutination test for acute-stage specific antigens, and a specific IgG avidity assay as part of a prenatal screening program that involved 16,733 mother and 44,181 serum samples. They concluded that the measurement of the avidity of specific IgG antibodies was a highly specific and sensitive method for the verification of acute primary toxoplasma infection during pregnancy.

Treponema pallidum Infection

Treponemes are delicate, slender, corkscrew-shaped spirochetes, 6 to 14 μm by 0.09 to 0.18 μm wide, which exhibit characteristic motility. *Treponema pallidum,* the causative agent of syphilis, can penetrate mucous membrane or abraded skin, and enter the lymphatics and bloodstream. Syphilis is acquired by sexual contact or kissing with infected persons, transfusion of contaminated blood, or by passage through the placenta. The incubation period is from 3 to 90 days.

Primary infection causes skin or mucous membrane lesions called chancres accompanied by regional lymphadenopathy. The secondary stage occurs with fever, a generalized hyperpigmented papular rash on the trunk and proximal extremities, and generalized lymphadenopathy. Syphilis causes death in more than 20% of infected fetuses. Untreated infection can result in severe sequelae of tertiary syphilis, affecting all organs including the central nervous system. Definitive diagnosis of the stage of infection is based on visualization of *T. pallidum* on direct darkfield microscopic examination or direct fluorescent antibody test. The best specimens are from moist lesions or a mucous patch. *T. pallidum* cannot be cultivated in vitro. Antibiotic treatment is very effective if given at the primary stage of infection, but monitoring of treatment is important to ensure proper dosage, especially when there is immune suppression as in AIDS patients (Hook, 1989).

Serologic testing is a critical aspect in the diagnosis of syphilis and is performed on diagnostic samples, samples from antenatal programs and on all blood donations (De Schryver and Meheus, 1990). The primary serologic tests for syphilis are the Venereal Disease Research laboratory (VDRL) test, the rapid plasma reagin card test (RPR), or the automated reagin test (ART). "Syphilis reaginic" antibodies are IgG and IgM immunoglobulins directed against a mixture of cardiolipin, cholesterol and lecithin, which are associated with syphilis but are not specific. Titers are high during clinical infection and then decrease during latency or after antibiotic therapy. Positive results must be confirmed by the fluorescence treponemal antibody test employing *T. pallidum* harvested from rabbit testes to distinguish between true-positive nontreponemal results from false positive results.

A valuable application of serologic tests for treponemal infection is the accurate identification of truly uninfected newborn babies born to infected mothers. Stoll, et al. (1993) examined the clinical efficacy of the fluorescent treponemal antibody-absorption (FTA-ABS) 19S IgM test, and a treponemal-specific IgM capture IEMA.

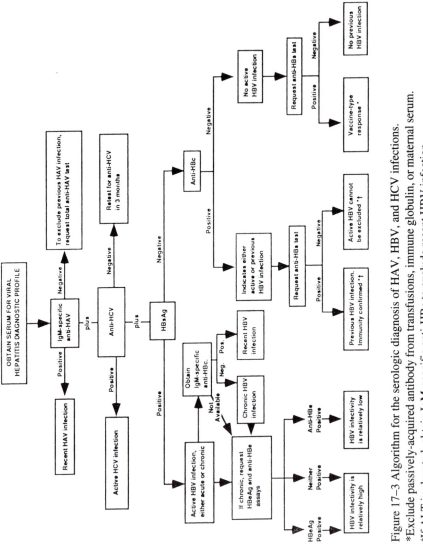

Figure 17–3 Algorithm for the serologic diagnosis of HAV, HBV, and HCV infections.

*Exclude passively-acquired antibody from transfusions, immune globulin, or maternal serum.

†If ALT is elevated, obtain IgM-specific anti-HBc to exclude recent HBV infection.

(Hollinger FB, Dreesman GR. Hepatitis viruses. In: Rose NR, deMacario EC, Fahey JL, et al.. eds. Manual of Clinical Laboratory Immunology, ed 4. Washington, DC: American Society for Microbiology, 1992;634–650. Reproduced with permission.)

They concluded that while such assays are highly specific, accuracy (88% IgM IEMA; 73% FTA-ABS) needs to be improved to allow the confident identification of uninfected babies and prevent unnecessary hospitalization.

Viral Hepatitis

Since the agents of viral hepatitis produce characteristic but generally indistinguishable clinical symptoms and cannot be exactly diagnosed on the basis of normal clinical observations alone, an algorithm describing the differential diagnosis of the major forms found in general clinical practice (hepatitis A, B, and C) is given in Figure 17–3.

Hepatitis A Virus

Hepatitis A virus (HAV) is a 27 to 32 nm picornavirus with single-stranded RNA and four major structural polypeptide antigens. There is one serotype and one principal antigenic component, designated HAV antigen. It is among the most rugged of human viruses and is transmitted mainly through the fecal-oral route. Infection is often asymptomatic.

Hepatitis A is an acute infection of the liver that occurs sporadically and in epidemics and is clinically indistinguishable from other forms of hepatitis. The incubation period is from 2 to 4 weeks, but may be shorter after ingestion of large quantities of contaminated food. It is characterized by the abrupt onset of fever, malaise, anorexia, abdominal discomfort, and jaundice. As in other types of hepatitis, elevated serum levels of liver alanine transaminase (ALT) activity occurs within a few days of the development of symptoms. Liver-type arginase, an alternative specific marker for liver damage, can be determined by IEMA (Ikemoto, et al., 1993). There is currently no antiviral agent against HAV, with most patients not requiring hospitalization unless complications occur, which is rare.

Diagnosis of hepatitis A is mainly through the use of serologic tests detecting the presence of IgM-specific anti-HAV and total anti-HAV antibodies, which are present at the onset of acute hepatitis A. The presence of anti-HAV IgM, which persists for 3 to 12 months, indicates ongoing or recent infection by HAV, and in a jaundiced patient, confirms the diagnosis as hepatitis A. Anti-HAV (including IgG) is a reliable marker for immunity to hepatitis A and persists for life.

HAV has the ability to agglutinate some kinds of red blood cells and this property has been used to develop simple hemadherence tests which can determine HAV-specific IgG or HAV-specific IgM antibodies in serum or urine specimens (Perry and Parry, 1993).

Hepatitis B Virus

Hepatitis B virus (HBV) is a 42-nm, double-shelled DNA virus of the class hepadnaviruses (Tiollais, et al., 1985). It has an outer component called hepatitis B surface antigen (HBsAg) and an inner component containing hepatitis B core antigen

(HBcAg), double-stranded DNA, and an endogenous DNA polymerase. HBeAg is a secreted product of the nucleocapsid gene. The incubation period for HBV is 1 to 6 months and infection may result in an acute self-limiting disease. Infection with HBV is marked by production of intact infectious virus particles and incomplete noninfectious particles made up of HBsAg, which are detectable in most body fluids.

Hepatitis B is a viral infection of the liver transmitted by contaminated blood or blood products (less common since the advent of sensitive immunoassay screening tests), congenitally, and by sexual or oral contact. High risk groups include intravenous drug abusers, hemophiliacs, homosexuals, and dialysis patients. In 5% to 10% of cases (but 90% in neonates), the infection becomes chronic, resulting in an HBV carrier state or chronic hepatitis of the persistent or active type. Fulminate acute hepatitis or progressive chronic hepatitis results in about a 1% rate of mortality. A late sequela of chronic disease is hepatic cell carcinoma. In some patients, the disease is aggravated by superinfection with hepatitis delta virus (see later in text). Therapeutic agents include recombinant interferon alone or in combination with steroid or anti-viral agents. Most current vaccines use purified or recombinant HBsAg and have better than 90% efficacy, which is associated with the prolonged presence of serum anti-HBsAG IgG.

Routine serologic testing to detect hepatitis B infection commonly involves agglutination assay, RIA or IEMA for HBsAg (e.g., Pujol, et al., 1993; Yamashiki, et al., 1993), and antibodies to HBcAg (anti-HBcAg). In a typical HBV infection, the presence of HBsAg in serum is indicative of acute or chronic HBV infection. HBsAg appears 2 to 4 weeks before the elevation of ALT and 3 to 5 weeks before the patients develop jaundice. Anti-HBcAg IgM appears when serum liver enzyme levels begin to rise and its presence is a reliable indicator of an acute HBV infection (Hess and Arnold, 1980). Anti-HBc IgM can be found alone during a period between the disappearance of HBsAg and the appearance of anti-HBsAg (Hollinger and Dreesman, 1992).

Ultimately, anti-HBc IgG and anti-HBsAg become the markers of past infections. Serum HBeAg may appear a few days after the appearance of HBsAg and is indicative of viral replication. HBeAg also indicates infectivity and continues in persons with chronic infection. Anti-HBe becomes detectable when HBeAg is lost and indicates the resolution of infection. Most chronic HBV patients with anti-HBe have resolving, minimal, or no liver disease. A clear diagnosis of acute hepatitis B is generally made on the basis of the presence of the clinical features of acute hepatitis with serum HBsAg and/or anti-HBc IgM. The absence of anti-HBc IgM is suggestive of underlying chronic hepatitis B or an HBsAg carrier state.

Hepatitis C Virus

Hepatitis C virus (HCV) is an incompletely characterized, small-enveloped, single-stranded virus 30 to 60 nm in diameter with properties similar to pestivirus and flavivirus. The different HCV isolates characterized to date show significant sequence heterogeneity suggesting the existence of a number of closely related, but nevertheless distinct, HCV genotypes. This recently named virus has been identified as the major cause of blood transfusion–associated non-A, non-B hepatitis, formerly the most frequent infectious disease transmitted by blood transfusion (Choo, et al., 1989). HCV is rarely transmitted by familial, sexual, or maternal-infant exposure.

Although symptoms in the acute phase of hepatitis C are generally milder than in hepatitis A or B, it is more likely to develop into a persistent, chronic state, and can develop into hepatic cirrhosis and possibly hepatocellular carcinoma. There is currently no vaccine available for HCV. Alpha-interferon has been shown to be effective in the treatment of chronic HCV in 50% of cases.

The discovery of HCV and the development of serologic tests for HCV infection were interdependent (Choo, et al., 1989). First-generation tests for anti-HCV antibodies use an antigen designated as C-100, which contains 363 amino acid residues representing nonstructural aspects of HCV and is produced in recombinant yeast culture (Choo, et al., 1989; Hollinger and Dreesman, 1992). Subsequently, a range of recombinant proteins and synthetic polypeptides representing the capsid region, core protein, and nonstructural epitopes from NS3 and NS5 regions were prepared and are included in multispecific second-generation screening assays and confirmatory assays, which have improved sensitivity. Seroconversion with the generation of anti-HCV antibodies occurs in 60% to 90% of blood recipients who develop post-transfusion hepatitis C (Esteban, et al., 1990), and prospective studies clearly show that anti-HCV antibodies indicate infectivity rather than immunity. Some second-generation assays for anti-HCV antibodies are susceptible to interference from raised IgG, making them prone to false positives when analyzing samples from a wide range of conditions, including rheumatoid arthritis (Borque, et al., 1993).

Anti-HCV is detected late in the course of acute HCV infection, after the appearance of elevated levels of ALT and generally between 4 to 24 weeks after the onset of symptoms. Individuals with chronic HCV infection exhibit persistent antibody reactivity, whereas those that resolve the infection show diminishing antibody reactivity over the duration of a few years. Ten percent to 20% of the patients infected with HCV do not have antibody reactivity. False positive results have been detected in patients with alcoholic liver disease and autoimmune chronic active hepatitis due to hyperglobulinemia. Therefore, confirmatory immunoblot assays have been developed to identify antibodies against a range of specific HCV antigens, and a multiple pattern of reactive dots provides added confidence to the ELISA results. However, a pattern of negative or indeterminant reactions cannot always be interpreted as negative, especially earlier in the course of the disease.

Testing for IgM-specific anti-HCV has not been routine, but Hellström, et al. (1993) have developed an IEMA for IgM antibodies specific for an immunologically active region (sp75) of the core protein of HCV. They found a striking association between the presence in serum of anti-sp75 IgM and HCV RNA and suggest such antibodies as a marker of chronic infection.

HCV antigen has been detected in hepatocyes by immunofluorescence microscopy and its presence precedes the appearance of anti-HCV in serum, but the clinical sensitivity and specificity tests for HCV antigen have not been well documented.

Hepatitis Delta Virus

Hepatitis delta virus (HDV) is a spheric, 36-nm defective hepatotropic RNA virus, containing delta antigen and single-stranded RNA, and coated by HBsAg. It only replicates in hosts who are concurrently infected with HBV. Coinfection of HDV with HBV may be more severe than hepatitis B, but superinfection of an already existing HBV infection can result in chronic active hepatitis and cirrhosis (Hoofnagle, 1989). Since HDV is linked to HBV, its mode of transmission is similar to that for HBV. The Middle East, Romania, and Venezuela have high rates of HDV infection. The time course of combined hepatitis B and D often exhibits two peaks of serum ALT indicating two bouts of liver damage. This may be due to HBV coming from one source and "rescue" HDV from another or, alternatively, may be due to clearance of HDV infected cells, followed by elimination of HBV infected cells (Hollinger and Dreesman, 1992).

Diagnostic laboratory tests for HDV infection involve concurrent testing for HBsAg, anti-HBc IgM, and anti-HDV. Both acute and chronic phase sera should be tested. The presence of anti-HBc IgM is suggestive of coinfection of HBV and HDV. The lack of anti-HBc IgM in the serum of a patient with acute HBsAg-positive hepatitis would raise suspicion of HDV superinfection. Anti-HDV arises late during acute HDV infection. Detection of HBsAg and a high titer of anti-HDV along with the clinical features of chronic hepatitis are strongly suggestive of chronic HDV infection. Specific IgM anti-HDV appears approximately 2 weeks after the onset of symptoms and its presence is indicative of acute HDV infection.

The primary marker of early acute infection is delta antigen which persists for about 21 days after the onset of symptoms. HDV antigen is detected by ELISA, RIA, and Western blotting, with Western blotting offering better sensitivity. HDV antigen is detected in the nuclei of hepatocytes in almost all patients with chronic HDV infection, and a decrease of serum levels is associated with improvements in the chronic state.

Hepatitis E Virus

Hepatitis E is referred to as waterborne, epidemic, or enterically transmitted non-A, non-B hepatitis, and is the major form of viral hepatitis found in the developing countries. The agent responsible has been designated as hepatitis E virus (HEV) (Bradley, 1990; Tam, et al., 1991; Ticehurst, 1991). It is 27 to 34 nm in diameter and has biophysical properties similar to caliciviruses, but partial amino acid sequence analysis revealed little similarity. The viral genome is a positive-sense RNA. Although the fecal-oral route is predominant, close contact has also been suggested as a means of transmission.

HEV infection is in general self-limiting, but a high mortality rate of 10% to 20% has been documented in pregnant women who are infected during the third trimester of pregnancy. Hepatitis E does not lead to chronic hepatitis or a carrier state.

Antibodies to HEV can usually be detected during the course of the disease and antibody capture assays employing recombinant antigens or peptides can be used for their detection (Dawson, et al., 1992; Paul, et al., 1994). IgG class, anti-HEV antibodies are long-lived.

REFERENCES

Al B, Visser S, van den Hoek A, van Doornum G, Coutinho R, Huisman H. Incidence of HTLV-I/II infection in seronegative high-risk individuals. J Med Virol 1993;39:260–265.

Anderson DW, Epstein JS, Lee TH, et al. Serological confirmation of human T-lymphotropic virus type-I infection in healthy blood and plasma donors. Blood 1989;74: 2585–2591.

Anderson LJ, Tsou C, Parker RA, et al. Detection of antibodies and antigens of human parvovirus B19 by enzyme-linked immunosorbent assay. J Clin Microbiol 1986;24: 522–526.

Ashley R, Cent A, Maggs V, Nahmias A, Corey L. Inability of enzyme immunoassays to discriminate between infections with herpes simplex virus type 1 and 2. Ann Intern Med 1991;115:520–526.

Ashley RL, Militoni J, Lee F, Nahmias A, Corey L. Comparison of western blot (immunoblot) and glycoprotein G-specific immunodot enzyme assay for detecting antibodies to herpes simplex virus type 1 and 2 in human sera. J Clin Microbiol 1988;26:662–667.

Berry N, Pepin J, Gaye I, et al. Competitive EIA for anti-HIV-2 detection in the Gambia: use as a screening assay and to identify possible dual infections. J Med Virol 1993;39: 101–108.

Borque L, Maside C, Rus A, Elena A, del Cura J, Gastañares MJ. IgG interference in second generation enzyme immunoassays for anti-hepatitis C virus antibodies. J Immunoassay 1993;14:183–189.

Bowie ER, Caldwell HD, Jones RP, et al., eds. Chlamydial Infections, Proceedings of the Seventh International Symposium on Human Chlamydial Infections. Cambridge: Cambridge University Press 1990.

Bradley DW. Enterically-transmitted non-A, non-B hepatitis. Br Med Bull 1990;46:442–461.

Burgdorfer W, Barbour AG, Hayes SF, Benach JL, Grunwaldt E, Davies JP. Lyme disease—a tick borne spirochetosis? Science 1982;216:1317–1319.

Chernesky MA, Mahony JB, Castriciano S, et al. Detection of *Chlamydia trachomatis* antigens by enzyme immunoassay and immunofluorescence in genital specimens from symptomatic and asymptomatic men and women. J Infect Dis 1986;134:141–148.

Choo QL, Kuo G, Deiner J, Overby LR, Bradley DW, Houghton M. Isolation of a cDNA clone derived from a blood-borne non-A, non-B viral hepatitis genome. Science 1989;244:359–362.

Cleaves CA, Smith TF, Shuster EA, Pearson GR. Rapid detection of cytomegalovirus in MRC5 cells inoculated with urine specimens by use of low-speed centrifugation and monoclonal antibody to an early antigen. J Clin Microbiol 1984;19:917–919.

Clewley JP. Biochemical characterization of a human parvovirus. J Gen Virol 1984;65: 241–245.

Cotmore SF, Mackie VC, Anderson LJ, Astell CR, Tattersall P. Identification of the major structural and non-structural proteins encoded by human parvovirus B19 and mapping of their genes by procaryotic expression of isolated genomic fragments. J Virol 1986;60:548–557.

Dawson GJ, Chau KH, Cabal CM, Yarbrough PO, Reyes GR, Mushahwar IK. Solid-phase enzyme-linked immunosorbent assay for hepatitis E virus IgG and IgM antibodies utilizing recombinant antigens and synthetic peptides. J Virol Methods 1992; 38:175–186.

Deschryver A, Moheng A. Syphilis and blood-transfusion: a global perspective. Transfusion 1990;30:844–847.

Dolan KT, Staub JM, Schofield TL, Ahonkhai KL, Ellis RW, Vella PP. An enzyme-linked immunosorbent assay for quantification of *Haemophilus influenzae* Type b polysaccharide-specific IgG1 and IgG2 in human and infant rhesus monkey sera. J Immunoassay 1991;12:543–564.

Dressler F, Whalen JA, Reinhardt BN, Steere AC. Western blotting in the serodiagnosis of Lyme disease. J Infect Dis 1993;167:392–400.

Drew WL. Diagnosis of cytomegalovirus infection. Rev Infect Dis 1988;10(suppl 3): S468–S476.

Ehrnst A, Barkholt L, Brattström C, et al. Detection of CMV-matrix pp65 antigen in leukocytes by immunofluorescence as a marker of CMV disease. J Med Virol 1993; 39:118–124.

Erdman DD, Usher MJ, Tsou C, et al. Human parvovirus B19 specific IgG, IgA and IgM antibodies and DNA in serum specimens from persons with erythema infectiosum. J Med Virol 1991;35:110–115.

Esteban JI, Gonzalez A, Hernandez JM, et al. Evaluation of antibodies to hepatitis C virus in a study of transfusion-associated hepatitis. N Engl J Med 1990;323:1107–1112.

Everitt E, Varga MJ. A capture enzyme-linked immunosorbent assay for virus infectivity titrations as exemplified in an adenovirus system. J Immunoassay 1993;14:1–19.

Fawcett PT, Rose C, Gibney KM, Chase CA, Kiehl B, Doughty RA. Detection of antibodies to the recombinant p39 protein of Borrelia-Burgdorferi using enzyme-immunoassay and immunoblotting. J Rheumatol 1993;20:734–738.

Fridell E, Cohen BJ, Wahren B. Evaluation of a synthetic-peptide enzyme-linked immunosorbent assay for immunoglobulin M to human parvovirus B19. J Clin Microbiol 1991;29:1376–1381.

Goldblott D, van Etten L, van Milligen FJ, Aolberse RC, Turner MW. The role of pH in modified ELISA procedures used for the estimation of functional antibody affinity. J Immunol Methods 1993;166:281–285.

Griffiths PD. Cytomegalovirus. In: Zuckerman AJ, Banatvala JE, Pattison JR, eds. Principles and Practice of Clinical Virology, ed 2. London: Wiley, 1990;69–102.

Guinet R, Bruneau S, Marlier H. Rapid identification of Candida albicans by dot-enzyme immunoassay. J Immunoassay 1991;12:225–231.

Gupta R, Talwar GP, Gupta SK. Rapid antibody capture assay for detection of group-A streptococci using monoclonal antibody and colloidal gold-monospecific polyvalent antibody conjugate. J Immunoassay 1992;13:441–455.

Hechemy KE. The immunoserology of Rickettsiae. In: Rose NR, deMacario EC, Fahey JL, Friedman H, Penn GM, eds. Manual of Clinical Laboratory Immunology, ed 4. Washington, DC: American Society for Microbiology, 1992;667–675.

Hellström UB, Sylvan SPE, Decker RH, Sönnerborg A. Immunoglobin M reactivity towards the immunologically active region sp75 of the core protein of hepatitis C virus (HCV) in chronic HCV infection. J Med Virol 1993;39:325.

Henle G, Henle W, Diehl V. Relation of Burkitt's tumor-associated herpes-type virus to infectious mononucleosis. Proc Nat Acad Sci USA 1968;59:94–101.

Hess G, Arnold W. The clinical relevance of the antibody to hepatitis B core antigen (anti-HBc): a review, J Virol Methods 1980;2:107–117.

Hierholzer JC, Adenoviruses. In: Balows A, Hausler WJ Jr, Herrmann KL, Isenberg HD, Shadomy HJ, eds. Manual of Clinical Microbiology, ed 5. Washington, DC: American Society for Microbiology, 1991;896–903.

Hierholzer JC. Adenoviruses in the Immunocompromised host. Clin Microbiol Rev 1992;5: 262–274.

Hille A, Klein K, Bäumler S, Grässer FA, Mueller-Lantzsch N. Expression of Epstein-Barr virus nuclear antigen 1, 2A and 2B in the baculovirus expression system: serological evaluation of human antibodies to these proteins. J Med Virol 1993;39:233–241.

Hollinger FB, Dreesman GR. Hepatitis viruses. In: Rose NR, deMacario EC, Fahey JL, Friedman H, Penn GM, eds. Manual of Clinical Laboratory Immunology, ed 4. Washington, DC: American Society for Microbiology, 1992;634–650.

Hoofnagle JH, Type D (delta) hepatitis. JAMA 1989;261:1321–1325.

Hook EW. Syphilis and HIV infection. J Infect Dis 1989;160:530–534.

Hopson DK, Niles AC, Murray PR. Comparison of the Vitek immunodiagnostic assay system with three immunoassay systems for detection of cytomegalovirus-specifc immunoglobulin G. J Clin Microbiol 1992;30:2893–2895.

Hsia J. False-positive ELISA for human immunodeficiency virus after influenza vaccination. J Infect Dis 1993;167:989–990.

Hyman CL, Augenbraun MH, Roblin PM, Schachter J, Hammerschlag MR. Asymptomatic respiratory tract infection with *Chlamydia pneumoniae* TWAR. J Clin Microbiol 1991; 29:2082–2083.

Ikemoto M, Ishida A, Tsunekawa S, et al. Enzyme immunoassay of liver-type arginase and its potential clinical application. Clin Chem 1993;39:794–799.

Kalyanaraman VS, Sarngadharan MG, Robert-Guroff M, et al. A new subtype of human T-cell leukemia virus (HTLV-II) associated with a T-cell variant of hairy cell leukemia. Science 1982;218:571–573.

Kaplan JE, Schonberger LB. The sensitivity of various serologic tests in the diagnosis of Rocky Mountain spotted fever. Am J Trop Med Hyg 1986;35:840–844.

Kemeny DM. Titration of antibodies. J Immunol Methods 1992;150:57–76.

Kraat YJ, Hendrix RM, Landini MP, Bruggeman CA. Comparison of four techniques for detection of antibodies to cytomegalovirus. J Clin Microbiol 1992;30:522–524.

Kropff B, Landini M-P, Mach M. An ELISA using recombinant proteins for the detection of neutralizing antibodies against human cytomegalovirus. J Med Virol 1993;39:187–195.

Kurtz JB, Anderson MJ. Cross-reactions in rubella and parvovirus specific IgM tests. Lancet 1985;2:1356.

Lappalainen M, Koskela P, Koskiniemi M, et al. Toxoplasmosis acquired during pregnancy: improved serodiagnosis based on avidity of IgG. J Infect Dis 1993;167:691–697.

Lin T-M, Schubert CM, Shih FF, Ahmad P, Lopez M, Horst H. Use of flagellin-enriched antigens in a rapid, simple and specific quantitative enzyme immunoassay for Lyme disease antibodies in human serum samples. J Immunoassay 1991;12:325–346.

Lindenschmidt EG. Enzyme-linked immunosorbent assay for detection of soluble *Toxoplasma gondii* antigen in acute phase toxoplasmosis. Eur J Clin Microbiol 1985;4:488–492.

Loughrey AC, O'Neill HJ, Coyle PV, DeLeys R. Identification and use of neutralizing epitope of parvovirus B19 for the rapid detection of virus infection. J Med Virol 1993; 39:97–100.

Ma B, Christen B, Leung D, Vigo-Pelfrey C. Serodiagnosis of Lyme borreliosis by western immunoblot: reactivity of various significant antibodies against *Borrelia burgdorferi*. J Clin Microbiol 1992;30:370–376.

Nakayama T, Sonoda S, Urano T, Yamada T, Okada M. Monitoring both serum amyloid protein A and C-reactive protein as inflammatory markers in infectious diseases. Clin Chem 1993;39:293–297.

O'Shea S, Rostron T, Hamblin AS, Palmer SJ, Banatvala JE. Quantitation of HIV: correlation with clinical, virological and immunological status. J Med Virol 1991;35:65–69.

Paul DA, Krigge MF, Ritter A. Determination of hepatitis E virus prevalence by using recombinant fusion proteins and synthetic peptides. J Infectious Disease 1994;169: 801–806.

Pearson GR. ELISA tests and monoclonal antibodies for EBV. J Virol Methods 1988;21: 97–104.

Pedneault L, Katz BZ. Comparison of polymerase chain reaction and standard Southern blotting for the detection of Epstein-Barr virus DNA in various biopsy specimens. J Med Virol 1993;39;33–43.

Perry KR, Parry JV. Simple hemadherence test for the detection of class-specific immunoglobulins to hepatitis A virus. J Med Virol 1993;39:23–27.

Poiesz BJ, Riscetti FW, Gazdor AF, Bunn PA, Minna JD, Gallo RC. Detection and isolation of type C retrovirus particles from fresh and cultured lymphocytes for a patient with cutaneous T-cell lymphoma. Proc Nat Acad Sci USA 1980;77:7415–7419.

Pujol FH, Rodriguez I, Devesa M, Rangel-Aldao R, Liprandi F. A double sandwich monoclonal enzyme immunoassay for detection of hepatitis B surface antigen. J Immunoassay 1993;14:21–31.

Quinn TC, Kline RL, Halsey N, et al. Early diagnosis of perinatal HIV infection by detection of viral-specific IgA antibodies. JAMA 1991;266:3439–3442.

Quinn TC, Kline R, Moss MW, Livingston RA, Hutton N. Acid dissociation of immune complexes improves diagnostic utility of p24 antigen detection in perinatally acquired human immunodeficiency virus infection. J Infect Dis 1993;167:1193–1196.

Rahn D, Malawista SE. Lyme disease: recommendations for diagnosis and treatment. Ann Intern Med 1991;114:472–481.

Rasiah C, Rover S, Gassman GS, Vogt A. Use of a hybrid protein consisting of the variable region of the *Borrelia burgdorferi* flagellin and part of the 83 rDa protein as antigen for serodiagnosis of lyme disease. J Clin Microbiol 1994;32:1011–1017.

Rawls WE. Herpes simplex virus. In: Fields B, ed. Virology. New York: Raven Press 1985;527–561.

Roberts CR. Laboratory diagnosis of retroviral infections. Dermatol Clin 1991;9:453–464.

Rose NR, deMacario EC, Fahey JL, Friedman H, Penn GM, eds. Manual of Clinical Laboratory Immunology, ed 4. Washington, DC: American Society for Microbi-ology, 1992.

Sabin AB, Feldman HA. Dyes as microchemical indicators of a new immunity phenomenon affecting a protozoan parasite (toxoplasma). Science 1948;108:660–663.

Schachter J. Chlamydiae. In: Rose NR, deMacario EC, Fahey JL, Friedman H, Penn GM, eds. Manual of Clinical Laboratory Immunology, ed 4. Washington, DC: American Society for Microbiology, 1992;661–666.

Simmonds P, Beatson D, Cuthbert RJG, et al. Determination of HIV disease progression: Six year longitudinal study in the Edinburgh haemophilial/HIV cohort. Lancet 1991;338: 1159–1163.

Sloand EM, Pitt E, Chiarello RJ, Nemo GJ. HIV testing. JAMA 1991;266:2861–2866.

Soderlund M, Brown KE, Meurman O, Hedman K. Prokaryotic expression of a VP1 polypeptide antigen for diagnosis by a human parvovirus B19 antibody enzyme immunoassay. J Clin Microbiol 1992;30:305–311.

Stoll BJ, Lee FK, Larsen S, et al. Clinical and serologic evaluation of neonates for congenital syphilis: a continuing diagnostic dilemma. J Infect Dis 1993;167:1093–1099.

Sumaya CV, Jenson HB. Epstein-Barr virus. In: Rose NR, deMacario EC, Fahey JL, Friedman H, Penn GM, eds. Manual of Clinical Laboratory Immunology, ed 4. Washington, DC: American Society for Microbiology, 1992;568–575.

Suzuki Y, Isaraelski DM, Danneman BR, Stepick-Biek P, Thulliez P, Remington JS. Diagnosis of toxoplasmic encephalitis in patients with acquired immunodeficiency syndrome by using a new serologic method. J Clin Microbiol 1988;26:2541–2543.

Tam AW, Smith MM, Guerra ME, et al. Hepatitis E virus (HEV): molecular cloning and sequencing of the full-length viral genome. Virology 1991;185:120–131.

Thomas HIJ, Morgan-Capner P. The use of antibody avidity measurements for the diagnosis of rubella. Rev Med Virol 1991;1:41–50.

Ticehurst J. Identification and characterization of hepatitis E virus. In: Hollinger FB, Lemon SM, Margolis HS, eds. Viral Hepatitis and Liver Disease. Baltimore: Williams & Wilkins 1991;501–513.

Tiollais P, Pourcel C, Dejean A. The hepatitis B virus. Nature 1985;317:489–495.

Underwood PA. Problems and pitfalls with measurement of antibody affinity using solid phase binding in the ELISA. J Immunol Methods 1993;164:119–130.

Ward KN, Gray JJ, Joslin ME, Sheldon MJ, Avidity of IgG antibodies to human herpes-virus-6 distinguishes primary from recurrent infection in organ transplant recipients and excludes cross-reactivity with other herpesviruses. J Med Virol 1993;39:44–49.

Wisseman CL Jr, Ordonez SV. Actions of antibiotics on *Rickettsia rickettsii.* J Infect Dis 1986;153:626–628.

Yamashiki M, Nishimura A, Kishioka H, Takase K, Kosaka Y. Rapid determination of hepatitis B surface antigen (HBsAg) by latex agglutination using an integrating sphere turbidimetric assay. J Immunol Methods 1993;158:251–256.

Yeaman MR, Mitscher LA, Baca OG. In vitro susceptibility of *Coxiella burnetti* to antibiotics, including several quinolones. Antimic Agents Chemother 1987;31:1079–1084.

CHAPTER 18

Drug Monitoring

James H. McBride, PhD

The fields of therapeutic drug monitoring and clinical toxicology have expanded greatly over the last 10 years, due largely to the application of immunoassay techniques. First, some general principles concerned with drug measurements are reviewed briefly.

To be effective, a therapeutic drug must reach the site of intended activity, which is governed by many factors, including: (1) dosage and route of administration; (2) patient compliance; (3) bioavailability of the drug; (4) pharmacokinetics of the drug; (5) the type of disease being managed; (6) patient-specific genetic and acquired physiologic factors; and (7) interactions with other drugs. Therefore, when a drug is given, the serum or whole blood level is not always predictable from the dose, and, to ensure administration of an adequate but not excessive dose, levels of the drug in body fluids may be measured.

The related complex fields of clinical toxicology and drug abuse management are further complicated by the fact that the drug(s) to be monitored may be initially unknown, by the huge numbers of potential drugs that may be taken in overdose or for recreation, and by the urgency of many requests for analyses. The application of immunoassays to the detection of drugs of abuse has increased greatly, especially in the Unites States, where the National Institute for Drug Abuse (NIDA) in 1988 recommended the testing of five analyte groups in urine and specified cutoff concentrations.

Suspected drug abusers, military and other personnel in positions of great responsibility, employees in general, and applicants for insurance policies are sometimes screened for illegal and legal drug usage. While such measurements are often carried out by methods similar to those discussed here, discussion of these applications is beyond the scope of this book.

IMMUNOASSAYS FOR DRUGS

General Requirements

Therapeutic drugs should be measured in samples drawn when a steady-state drug concentration has been reached. When oral medications are given, samples should be obtained both during steady-state and just before the next drug dose. If the dose is changed the usual protocol is to allow five half-lives of the drug to pass after the change before assuming that a new steady-state has been achieved. For those patients receiving continuous infusion, specimens should be obtained at approximately one half-life after the beginning of infusion or when apparent toxicity is demonstrated. It is also useful to consider if there have been any late or missed doses, if dosing intervals are unchanged, if renal or liver function is impaired, and at what time the serum specimen was obtained in relation to the last dose (Ackerman and Pappas, 1991).

In cases of suspected drug overdose, interaction between the attending physician, nursing staff, and laboratory personnel is essential and specimens submitted for analysis should be accompanied by complete details concerning patient status, substance ingested, and time of ingestion. In addition, the laboratory should report any preliminary findings immediately to enable rapid patient treatment.

It is also important for laboratory personnel to understand the limitations of the procedures used in their laboratories. For immunoassays, it is important to know the specificities, and hence crossreactivities, of the various in-house methods and commercial kits used. Other properties of the methods such as lower detection limits and potential interferences must be understood. For example, hemolyzed samples, high bilirubin concentration, and various endogenous factors are capable of causing interferences in commonly used immunoassays (Blecka and Jackson, 1987). In addition, the operator, and particularly the clinician, should be aware that particular patient physiologic factors and coadministered drugs may directly affect drug concentrations, or interfere with the method in use.

Analytic Methods

Almost all common drugs have small molecular weights and immunogenically must be treated as haptens. Thus in the preparation of antibodies to drugs, it is normally essential to couple the drug (hapten) to a protein carrier molecule such as bovine serum albumin in order to confer antigenicity. This holds whether one is producing polyclonal or monoclonal antibodies (see also Chaps. 1 and 2). When monitoring the binding of drugs to antibodies, it is necessary to employ a label or tracer to indicate the presence of hapten and differentiate between unbound drug and drug which is bound to antibody. Currently, the most common labeling substances include radioactive isotopes, enzymes, and fluorophores.

Immunoassays for drugs are almost all competitive reagent-limited assays and most employ labeled-analyte. Thereafter, they may usefully be categorized as separation-free (homogeneous) or requiring a separation step (heterogeneous). For separation-free assays all the necessary reagents are added to the reaction and no separation or washing procedures are required; they are, therefore, simpler to set up and perform and are easy to automate. However, it should be stressed that assays with a separation step can have much lower detection limits and may be more specific because unbound reactants are removed as part of the assay procedure. Their incubation times are much longer compared with separation-free assays. Commercially produced immunoassays are now available for every major class of therapeutic drug and metabolite. The two most common type of immunoassay for toxicology screening of drugs of abuse in clinical laboratories are enzyme-multiplied immunoassay technique (EMIT) and fluorescence polarization immunoassay (FPIA), which have been applied to dedicated automated analyzers. Frequently monitored drugs and drug metabolites are listed in Table 18-1.

Table 18–1   Therapeutic Drugs and Ranges Measured by Immunoassay

Drug	*Therapeutic Range*	
Analgesics		
Acetaminophen	31–124 μmol/L	(5–20 μg/mL)
Salicylate	1.1–2.2 mmol/L	(15–30 mg/dL)
Antiarrhythmics		
Amiodarone	1.6–3.9 μmol/L	(1–2.5 μg/mL)
Disopyramide	5.9–11.8 μmol/L	(2–4 μg/mL)
Flecainide	0.5–1.4 μmol/L	(0.2–0.6 μg/mL)
Lidocaine	6.4–21.4 μmol/L	(1.5–5 μg/mL)
N-Acetylprocainamide	38–94 μmol/L	(10–25 μg/mL)
Procainamide	17–42.5 μmol/L	(4–10 μg/mL)
Propanolol	193–386 nmol/L	(50–100 ng/mL)
Quinidine	6.2–15.4 μmol/L	(2–5 μg/mL)
Antibiotics/Aminoglycosides		
Amikacin	0–8.6 μmol/L	(0–5 μg/mL) trough
	42.8–54.8 μmol/L	(25–32 μg/mL) peak
Chloramphenicol	0–15.5 μmol/L	(0–5 μg/mL) trough
	46.4–77.4 μmol/L	(15–25 μg/mL) peak
Gentamicin	0–4 μmol/L	(0–2 μg/mL) trough
	10–24 μmol/L	(5–12 μg/mL) peak
Kanamycin	2–8 μmol/L	(1–4 μg/mL) trough
	52–72 μmol/L	(25–35 μg/mL) peak
Tobramycin	0–4.3 μmol/L	(0–2 μg/mL) trough
	10.7–25.7 μmol/L	(5–12 μg/mL) peak
Vancomycin	5.5–13.8 μmol/L	(8–20 μg/mL) trough
	20.7–27.6 μmol/L	(30–40 μg/mL) peak
Anticonvulsants		
Carbamazepine	25–51 μmol/L	(6–12 μg/mL)
Ethosuximide	283–708 μmol/L	(40–100 μg/mL)
Phenobarbital	65–172 μmol/L	(15–40 μg/mL)
Phenytoin	70–140 μmol/L	(10–20 μg/mL)
Primidone	23–55 μmol/L	(5–12 μg/mL)
Valproic acid	690–1040 μmol/L	(100–150 μg/mL)

TABLE 18–1   (*continued*)

Drug	Therapeutic Range	
Antidepressants		
Amitriptyline	433–903 nmol/L	(120–250 ng/mL)
Desipramine	280–600 nmol/L	(75–160 ng/mL)
Doxepin	107–537 nmol/L	(30–150 ng/mL)
Imipramine	446–893 nmol/L	(125–250 ng/mL)
Antineoplastics		
Methotrexate	2 µmol/L	(0.91 µg/mL)
Bronchodilators		
Theophylline	55.5–111 µmol/L	(10–20 µg/mL)
Caffeine	15–77 µmol/L	(3–15 µg/mL)
Cardiac Glycosides		
Digoxin	1.9–2.6 nmol/L	(1.5–2 ng/mL)
Digitoxin	19–39 nmol/L	(15–30 ng/mL)
Immunosuppressants		
Cyclosporin A	124–250 nmol/L	(150–300 ng/mL)
Cyclosporin A metabolites	42–83 nmol/L	(50–100 ng/mL)
Cyclosporin G	80–250 nmol/L	(100–300 ng/mL)
FK506 (plasma)	Tentative: 0.5–2.5 ng/mL	
(whole blood)	15–30 ng/mL	

Radioimmunoassay

Despite the rapid change from the use of radioactivity to nonisotopic methods in the clinical laboratory, radioimmunoassays (RIAs) are still employed, especially in the monitoring of cardiac glycosides and aminoglycosides. RIAs for digoxin have proved to be cost-effective and can be used on instrumentation available wherever steroid, protein, and polypeptide hormone assays are determined by RIA. Unfortunately, RIA kits with ^{125}I labels have limited shelf lives, special licensure is required for the use of isotopes, and nuclear waste must be disposed of in accordance with strict regulations. This, coupled with the fact that some digoxin RIA kits have antibodies which display cross-reactivity with digoxin-like substances (Valdes, 1985), has directed laboratories toward the implementation of nonisotopic methods, at least for digoxin determinations.

Enzyme Immunoassay

Both separation and separation-free enzyme immunoassay (EIA) methods are available for drug measurements (Price, 1984). Separation assays are generally used to measure drugs found at lower concentrations, for example, theophylline and methotrexate. The most commercially successful and commonly utilized separation-free method for therapeutic drug monitoring is EMIT (Syva Corp., Palo Alto, CA).

EMIT has been adapted to both manual and automated systems and EMIT kits for over 30 drugs are available. Basically, the assay system employs two reaction components. The first is an enzyme-hapten (-drug) conjugate (drug-Enz*, where Enz* indicates active enzyme) whose activity is lost when it is bound to a specific antidrug antibody. The second is antidrug antibody, which when it binds conjugate, inhibits its enzyme activity. Labeled drug and drug from the patient sample compete for binding sites on a limited concentration of the antibody:

$$Ab + drug\text{-}Enz^* + drug \leftrightarrow Ab\text{--}drug\text{-}Enz + Ab\text{--}drug$$

The drug in a sample competes with the conjugate, reducing antibody induced inhibition of enzyme activity. Therefore, enzyme activity is directly related to drug concentration and is measured by an absorbance change resulting from the catalytic action of enzyme on substrate (Berk, et al., 1986). In other EMIT assays the enzyme activity of the drug-enzyme conjugate is enhanced by binding to antibody.

Separation-free, inhibition immunoassay methods have been developed for use on a number of analyzers (Blecka, et al., 1983), for example, a theophylline assay for use on a device called VISION (Abbott Laboratories, Chicago, ILL), in which two-dimensional centrifugation is used to separate whole blood, measure reagent and plasma volumes, and then complete the procedural steps necessary (Schultz, et al., 1985). The assay utilizes haptens labeled with an irreversible enzyme inhibitor which prevents substrate hydrolysis by enzyme. Drug concentration is determined by its interaction with inhibitor-labeled analyte and a limited amount of antibody coupled to enzyme.

Enzyme immunochromatography combines enzyme-channeling immunochromatography and capillary migration and does not require any instrumentation (Zuk, et al., 1985). Briefly, whole blood or plasma may be quantitated by measuring the height of migration on a test strip and the height related to a conversion table to obtain concentration. The test strip contains absorbed antibody while an enzyme reagent containing glucose oxidase and horseradish peroxidase-drug conjugate are also provided in the kit. Another reagent contains the substrate glucose and 4-chloro-1-naphthol which, when oxidized, produces a blue product on the test strip. This system has been applied successfully to drug monitoring, especially for theophylline and digoxin, where it can be readily used at the patient's bedside or in the physician's office.

Immunoassays with Recombinant-Enzyme Fragments

Another separation-free enzyme immunoassay system is called combined enzyme donor immunoassay (CEDIA) (Khanna, et al., 1989). Recombinant DNA technology was used to produce new strains of *Escherichia coli* that synthesize large inactive fragments of β-D-galactosidase (enzyme acceptors, that may be symbolized by "Enz") or small inactive fragments of the same enzyme (enzyme donors, D), which are capable of associating to give fully active enzyme (D-Enz*). For CEDIA, a pair of stable complementary fragments were selected such that a drug or other hapten could be readily conjugated to the donor (drug-D) without inhibiting its ability to reassociate with excess acceptor. However, the binding of antibody to the conjugate inhibits reassociation, so that as analyte concentration increases more antibody becomes available and the total enzyme activity increases.

$$Ab + drug\text{-}D + drug = \leftrightarrow Ab\text{-}drug\text{-}D + Ab\text{-}drug$$

Simultaneously,

$$drug\text{-}D + Enz \leftrightarrow drug\text{-}D\text{-}Enz^*$$

With this novel approach, the CEDIA assays (like EMIT and some other separation-free systems) can be performed with routine clinical chemistry analyzers such as Hitachi 736/717, Olympus AU-500 and, Technicon DAX.

Fluoroimmunoassay

Fluoroimmunoassays (FIA) used in therapeutic drug n... nitoring offer good sensitivity, and reagent stability is impressive when compared with both RIA and EIA. However, there remains the disadvantage that background interferences arising from endogenous serum fluorescence can be a major analytic problem (Shaykh, et al., 1985). Fluorescence polarization immunoassay (FPIA) is the most frequently used FIA for drug measurements and has been successfully applied to automated instruments, the Abbott TDx and IMx (Abbott Laboratories, Chicago, ILL).

Briefly, FPIA is a separation-free, competitive technique (Jolley, 1981) in which fluorescein-drug conjugate (tracer), when excited by linearly polarized light, emits fluorescence with a degree of polarization inversely related to the molecule's rate of rotation. The lifetime of the excited state of fluorescein is 4 ns and the tracer in the assay solution has a rotational relaxation time of 1 ns, so that light emitted from the free tracer becomes highly depolarized as the complex rotates in solution. When the tracer is bound to antibody (relaxation time 100 ns), the emitted light remains polarized because of the slower rate of rotation. In the assay, drug molecules in a sample compete with tracer for a limited number of antibody binding sites so that the amount of tracer bound, and the consequent retention of polarization, are inversely related to drug concentration.

An automated fluorescence endpoint EIA system for drug measurements with a separation step based on the principle of radial partition (Giegel, 1985) has been developed for use on a dedicated instrument, Stratus (Baxter, Miami, FL). The assay is based on competitive binding of drug antibodies immobilized on glass fiber paper to drug in the patient's sample or to alkaline phosphatase-drug conjugate. After a short incubation period, usually 5 minutes, all unbound species are radially eluted by addition of a wash and further addition of a nonfluorescent substrate 4-methylumbelliferyl phosphate. Bound alkaline phosphatase-drug complex converts the substrate to a fluorescent entity, 4-methylumbelliferone which emits light at 453 nm. With this approach, individual drug measurements can be completed within 10 minutes.

Endogenous Interference in Immunoassays for Therapeutic Drug Monitoring

Various aspects of endogenous interference in immunoassays have been recently reviewed (Gosling, 1990, Weber, et al., 1990). Particular interferences are of interest in therapeutic drug monitoring, especially in RIA for digoxin, where endogenous digitalis-like factors can be a problem (Graves, 1986). Although the main component of the interferent has been demonstrated to be lipid in nature (Sandrzadeh, et al., 1988), insufficient specificity for antibodies for digoxin must also be considered. Much of the interference can be removed by chromatography (Longerich, et al., 1988), which can increase analysis time in the monitoring of digoxin. However, such interference is most commonly encountered with neonates, renal failure, hepatic disease, pregnancy, and cases of essential hypertension.

Interference in immunoassays for drugs may also be caused by the presence of heterophilic antibodies (anti-IgG antibodies) which are capable of reacting with the antibodies used in the drug assay. It has been reported that as much as 30% to 40% of patient samples tested in the United States may have heterophilic antibodies present (Boscato and Stuart, 1988). However, it is considered that this type of interference can be eliminated by the addition of nonimmune mouse or bovine serum, while horse, rabbit, and especially porcine sera are less efficient (Weber, et al., 1990).

THERAPEUTIC DRUGS

Drugs that are routinely monitored are conveniently classified according to the kind of therapy for which they are used (e.g., control of epilepsy, management of cardiac function). Therapeutic ranges for various drugs are given in Table 18-1.

Anticonvulsants

Carbamazepine. (Tegretol). Carbamazepine is structurally related to the tricyclic antidepressants and is effective in the treatment of generalized tonic-clonic, partial, and partial-complex seizures and pain associated with trigeminal neuralgia. Monitoring of carbamazepine by immunoassay is usually best achieved by obtaining trough specimens because of the drug's long half-life. However, peak values may be more useful in cases of mild toxicity (Moyer, et al., 1987). Toxicity is associated with blurred vision, nystagmus, ataxia, drowsiness, and diplopia.

With carbamazepine and other anticonvulsant drugs there is considerable drug-drug interaction. They induce the metabolism of oral contraceptives, warfarin, and doxycycline and hence reduce the effects of these drugs. Also, propoxyphene and erythromycin interfere with carbamazepine metabolism leading to its accumulation with resultant toxicity. The main metabolite of the drug, carbamazepine-10, 11-epoxide, is also pharmacologically active.

Recently, there has been considerable interest in monitoring free carbamazepine serum levels and correlating these to seizure control (Agbato, et al., 1986). To measure free levels, an ultrafiltrate of the serum is obtained before analysis by EMIT, FPIA, or high performance liquid chromatography (HPLC). Therapeutic free serum levels for carbamazepine have been reported to be in the range 3.4 to 7.6 μmol/L (0.8 to 1.8 μg.mL) for the parent drug and 0.8 to 3.4 μmol/L (0.2 to 0.8 μg/mL) for the main active metabolite (Agbato, et al., 1986).

Ethosuximide (Zarontin).   Ethosuximide is a succinimide which is widely used in pe-tit-mal epilepsy because of its anticonvulsive properties. The trough specimen yields the most useful information concerning the therapeutic efficacy. It is usual to moni-tor the drug by immunoassay, especially FPIA or EIA on a regular basis, and occa-sionally to perform liver function and complete blood counts, as the use of ethosuximide has been associated with blood dyscrasias.

Phenobarbital.   Phenobarbital is a weak acid with a pK_a of 7.4 and is indicated for use in the management of generalized tonic-clonic seizures and complex partial seizures. It may also be used in patients with status epilepticus who do not respond to phenytoin therapy and also in the treatment of febrile seizures in children. Blood concentrations do not change rapidly because of the long elimination half-life and a serum specimen collected at trough is representative of the drug effect (Moyer, et al., 1987). Alcohol and central nervous system depressants increase the sedative effects of barbiturates, and warfarin, oral contraceptives, digoxin, and antiarrhythmics may have reduced potency due to their increased clearance when phenobarbital is taken.

Phenytoin (Dilantin).   Phenytoin is used in the treatment of generalized tonic-clonic seizures, status epilepticus and elementary-partial or complex-partial seizures, al-though it is not as effective for absence seizures. Unlike phenobarbital, phenytoin does not act by suppression of a seizure focus but prevents the spread to a general-ized seizure (Louis, et al., 1968). The drug is highly protein bound and its major metabolites do not exhibit anticonvulsant activity (Eadie, 1974). The degree of pro-tein binding can be reduced by other drugs (e.g., valproic acid), anemia and hypoal-buminemia, particularly in the geriatric population.

The sedation caused by phenytoin is further enhanced by coadministration of barbiturates, alcohol, and other central nervous system depressants (e.g., primidone). Metabolism of the drug is decreased with chloramphenicol, disulfiram, isoniazid, benzodiazepines, warfarin, estrogens, ethosuximide, and propoxyphene. Salicylate, valproic acid, phenylbutazone, and sulfonylureas compete with phenytoin for serum protein-binding sites. In situations of hypoalbuminemia, renal insufficiency, toxicity, and pregnancy, it is useful to measure free phenytoin levels to ensure adequate con-trol. The therapeutic range for free phenytoin is 5.9 to 11.9 μmol/L (1.5 to 3 μg/mL) (Levy and Schmidt, 1985).

Primidone (Mysoline).   Primidone and its main metabolite, phenobarbital are both active anticonvulsants. Primidone is used to treat tonic-clonic and complex-partial seizures and disposition of the drug is not known to be greatly influenced by other drugs or diseases. Toxicity is usually seen when levels are greater than 68.7 μmol/L (15 μg/mL), and symptoms include sedation, nausea, vomiting, diplopia, and ataxia.

When acetazolamide is simultaneously administered there is decreased gastrointestinal absorption of primidone and hence decreased plasma concentrations.

Valproic Acid (Depakene).   Valproic acid increases γ-aminobutyric acid (GABA) concentrations in the brain by inhibiting GABA transaminase and succinic semialdehyde dehydrogenase activity. It is used for treatment of absence seizures and is useful against tonic-clonic and partial seizures when given with other anticonvulsants. Valproic acid is highly protein bound and clearance is rapid, which can present a dosing dilemma. The drug is capable of displacing aspirin, warfarin, phenobarbital, primidone, and phenytoin while alcohol, tricyclic antidepressants, and monoamine oxidase inhibitors add to the sedative effects of the drug. Like other anticonvulsants, measurement of free valproic acid levels in serum has been proposed as a more rational approach in patient management (Cramer, et al., 1986). Free valproic acid levels measured by FPIA are usually in the range 49 to 160 μmol/L (7 to 23 μg/mL).

Antiarrhythmics

Disopyramide (Norpace).   Disopyramide is a quinidine-like Class 1a agent which reduces the incidence of ventricular and, to a lesser extent, atrial arrhythmias and has been used in the prevention of potentially serious arrhythmias following myocardial infarction. Basically, its mechanism of action involves shortening the sinus node recovery time, lengthening the effective refractory period, and increasing the duration of P waves, the QRS complex, and especially the QT interval (Howanitz and Howanitz, 1981). The *N*-dealkylated metabolite of the drug possesses anticholinergic activity and causes most of the reported side effects including the negative isotropic effect and congestive heart failure in patients with renal failure (Siddoway and Woosely, 1986).

Considerable drug-drug interaction has been observed with lidocaine, procainamide, propranolol, quinidine, and verapamil. Metabolism of disopyramide is increased with coadministration of phenytoin, phenobarbital, and rifampin and it enhances the effects of warfarin and various oral antihyperglycemic agents.

Flecainide (Tambocor).   Flecainide is a Class 1c drug producing slowing of cardiac impulse conduction with less effect on refractoriness, repolarization time, and action potential duration. It has the ability to prolong the PR interval, QRS complex, and QT interval. As it exhibits mild negative isotropic effects, it should be used with caution in patients with coronary artery disease, recent myocardial infarction, and congestive heart failure (Anderson, et al., 1981). Peak serum concentration occurs within 3 hours of an oral dose, the drug is bound primarily to α_1-acid glycoprotein, and the half-life ranges from 7 to 25 hours in adults. Changes in PR, QRS, and QT intervals do not correlate with increasing serum concentrations. Also flecainide interferes with the disposition of digoxin, increasing serum concentrations by approximately 20%.

Lidocaine (Xylocaine).   Lidocaine is a Class 1b drug of choice for the initial therapy of premature ventricular contractions and the prevention of ventricular arrhythmias.

Its half-life is usually 1 to 2 hours and it is principally metabolized by *N*-dealkylation to monethylglycinexylidide and glycinexylidide, which are not measured by the various immunoassays in use. Propranolol and other β-blockers decrease hepatic fusion thus affecting the clearance of the drug. Phenytoin and phenobarbital induce cytochrome P_{450} thus increasing hepatic biotransformation of lidocaine.

Procainamide (Pronestyl).   Procainamide, a *p*-aminobenzamide is used in the treatment of both atrial and ventricular cardiac arrhythmias. Its action on cardiac conduction tissues includes suppression of automaticity, delay in conduction, and increased refractoriness (Anderson, et al., 1978). Its biologic half-life is 3.5 hours and 15% is metabolized to *N*-acetylprocainamide (NAPA) in the liver by the enzyme *N*-acetyltransferase. NAPA, with a half-life approximately twice that of procainamide, has antiarrhythmic activity similar to that of the parent drug. Symptoms of toxicity include bradycardia, prolongation of the QRS interval, AV block, and induced arrhythmias. Procainamide induces heart block at serum concentrations greater than 85 μmol/L (20 μg/mL) or at NAPA plus procainamide sums in excess of 128 μmol/L (30 μg/mL). Treatment with procainamide can lead to development of systemic lupus erythematosus in patients who are slow acetylators of the drug and when used with other antiarrhythmic agents may aggravate cardiac problems.

Quinidine (Duraquin).   Quinidine is a cinchona alkaloid used in the treatment of both ventricular and supraventricular arrhythmias including ventricular premature contractions and atrial fibrillation. It has anticholinergic actions as well as a direct effect on the myocardium in that it depresses excitability and contractility and slows conduction. These effects result in the prolongation of the effective refractory period and widening of the QRS complex. Peak plasma concentrations are reached 4 to 5 hours after quinidine gluconate administration and the trough concentration occurs 1 to 2 hours before the next administration. When used in combination with other antiarrhythmics, quinidine can cause serious cardiac problems. Also, quinidine competes with digoxin for uptake into cardiac and muscle tissue, resulting in greater central nervous system digoxin toxicity.

Cardiac Glycosides

Digoxin (Lanoxin).   Digoxin is used to restore the force of cardiac contraction in congestive heart failure and in the management of supraventricular tachycardias. Chemically it has a characteristic ring structure (aglycone or genin) to which are coupled three sugars. The aglycone portion of the glycoside consists of a steroid nucleus with a lactone ring at the carbon-17 position. Absorption of digoxin is variable with a half-life of 26 days and it can take 24 weeks for patients receiving the drug to reach steady-state. Toxicity with digoxin use correlates with tissue concentration rather than plasma concentration and so samples should be taken when peak tissue concentration has been achieved, that is, 8 hours or more after the dose.

In patients with serum concentrations greater than 7.7 nmol/L (6 ng/mL) serious toxicity with resulting bradycardia and atrioventricular nodal block is often encountered. In cases of extreme toxicity an antibody product (digibind, Fab fragment [Burroughs Welcome]) may be administered and the drug carefully monitored by a rapid immunoassay procedure such as FPIA or EMIT. Verapamil reduces the hepatic clearance of digoxin, while anticonvulsants increase hepatic clearance. Coadministration with quinidine leads to increased digoxin concentration mainly due to decreased renal tubular secretion. The presence of interfering substances in serum samples can lead to problems with immunoassays (see Endogenous Interference in Immunoassays for Therapeutic Drug Monitoring above).

Digitoxin (Lanatoxin). Digitoxin is used less frequently than digoxin in cardiac disease states. It has a longer half-life and is greater than 90% protein bound resulting in a smaller volume of distribution. Toxicity begins to occur at 45 nmol/L (35 ng/mL) and immunoassays, mainly RIA, are available for the specific assay of digitoxin. It should be measured in all cases of suspected digitalis intoxication when digoxin cannot be detected. Digitoxin serum concentrations are reduced when barbiturates and anticonvulsants are coadministered.

New Antiarrhythmics and Antianginal Agents

Some newer antiarrhythmic drugs in use include *amiodarone* (Cordarone), *encainide* (Enkaid), *mexiletine* (Mexitil), and *tocainide* (Tonocard), while *verapamil* (Calan), *nifedipine* (Procardia), and *Diltiazem* (Cardizem) represent some of the newer antianginal medications. Immunoassays for their determination are not yet generally available, but they may be determined by HPLC and by gas chromatography with electron-capture detection.

Antibiotics

Aminoglycosides. Aminoglycoside antibiotics include streptomycin, neomycin, netilmicin, gentamicin, tobramycin, kanamycin, amikacin, and sisomicin and their mode of action is by inhibiting bacterial protein synthesis, particularly in aerobic and anaerobic gram-negative bacilli. Chemically, the aminoglycosides are carbohydrates composed of an aminocyclitol ring with one or more amino sugars attached to it by glycosidic linkage. Being very polar, they are poorly absorbed from the intestinal tract and are routinely administered intramuscularly or intravenously. Some recommend obtaining serum levels after the initial dose to provide data that can permit forecasting of maintenance doses (Lesar, et al., 1982). Trough and peak levels should be drawn when serum levels reach a steady-state condition, usually after 6 to 12 hours of therapy in patients with normal renal function. The toxic effect of aminoglycosides are usually delayed-onset vestibular and cochlear sensory-cell destruction and acute renal tubular necrosis. See Table 18-1 for therapeutic ranges (trough and peak).

Amikacin is the most stable and tobramycin the least stable drug in the presence of such drugs as carbenicillin, ticarcillin, ampicillin, and piperacillin. The chemical inactivation of the aminoglycosides is dependent on the concentration of the penicillin, contact time, and temperature (O'Bey, et al., 1982).

Chloramphenicol (Chloromycetin).   Chloramphenicol is a broad spectrum antibiotic used to treat many infections including those caused by ampicillin-resistant *Haemophilus influenzae*. It acts by binding to the 50 S ribosomal unit of bacteria and inhibiting protein synthesis. The drug is rapidly absorbed from the intestine and peak serum concentrations occur 1 to 2 hours after an oral dose with the free base form of the drug and 2 to 3 hours after a dose with the palmitate salt. Toxic effects include blood dyscrasias and cardiovascular collapse, both of which show a modest relationship to blood concentration.

Vancomycin (Vancocin).   Vancomycin is a glycopeptide antibiotic useful in the treatment of gram-positive infections. In fact, the use of vancomycin has increased over the last 10 years because of the emergence of methicillin-resistant *Staphylococcus aureus* and coagulase-negative staphylococcal species. Timing of the serum specimen is important for proper interpretation of the results. Usually two specimens are drawn: one just before a dose and the other 2 hours after infusion ends. Generally levels are measured on the second or third day of therapy when the steady-state is achieved.

Antidepressants

The tricyclic antidepressants include *amitriptyline* (Elavil), *desipramine* (Pertofran), *doxepin* (Sinequan), *imipramine* (Tofranil), *nortriptyline* (Aventyl), while the principal tetracyclic antidepressants include *maprotiline* (Ludiomil), and *oxaprotiline.* The tricyclic compounds consist chemically of two benzene rings connected by a central seven-member ring and an aliphatic side chain, that is, dibenzazepines or analogs such as dibenzocycloheptadienes and dibenzoxepines. The principal desired effect on the central nervous system appears to be related to the inhibition of the uptake of endogenous sympathomimetic amines.

The antidepressants are used to treat depression characterized by depressed mood, guilt, insomnia, appetite suppression, and weight change. They are also useful in the treatment of more severe cases, depersonalized behavior, suicidal tendencies, and paranoid behavior. With the exception of nortriptyline, which has a specific therapeutic window, 190 to 570 nmol/L (50 to 150 ng/mL), there is usually a reasonable linear relationship between serum concentrations of the tricyclic antidepressants and patient improvement. Toxicity is usually displayed as dry mouth and excessive perspiration and it should be stressed that for all of these antidepressants, serum concentrations in excess of 1700 ng/mL are associated with a high incidence of cardiac arrhythmias and permanent cardiac damage.

In terms of drug-drug interactions, barbiturates, smoking, and chloral hydrate all induce the metabolism of nortriptyline via increased cytochrome P_{450} enzyme complex induction. Trihexyphenidyl reduces absorption of nortriptyline thus decreasing serum concentrations, while cimetidine, chloramphenicol, and phenothiazines increase serum concentrations as a result of competition for biotransforming enzymes. A general rule is that there is a relative contraindication for the coadministration of monoamine oxidase inhibitors and tricyclic antidepressants.

Bronchodilators

Theophylline (Bronkodyl). Theophylline, which has been used to treat asthma for over 50 years, is also used clinically for apnea and bradycardia syndrome in neonates. It appears that the drug may affect prostaglandins and calcium metabolism in smooth muscle cells to relieve or prevent asthma (Ackerman and Pappas, 1991). Theophylline is eliminated from the blood by metabolism through hepatic biotransformation to inactive xanthine metabolites (Hendeles and Weinberger, 1983), and changes in renal function do not significantly affect the clearance of the drug. A variety of immunoassays, especially FPIA and EIA, are available for the determination of theophylline and are especially useful in the assessment of toxic symptoms, which include nausea, vomiting, diarrhea, and insomnia. Serum concentrations greater than 167 μmol/L (30 mg/L) can result in cardiac arrhythmias and seizures.

In terms of drug-drug interaction, cimetidine will reduce hepatic metabolism of theophylline resulting in significant serum concentrations, and coadministration of erythromycin reduces the clearance of the bronchodilator.

Caffeine. The therapeutic use of caffeine is limited to the treatment of neonates and infants with apnea and bradycardia syndrome. The half-life can exceed 100 to 150 hours in neonates, but can decrease over the first months of life to 2 to 4 hours (normal adult). Overdoses can be fatal and are characterized by cardiac arrest or arrhythmias.

Antineoplastics

Methotrexate is a folic acid antagonist which inhibits DNA synthesis by competitively inhibiting the enzyme dihydrofolate reductase thereby decreasing pyrimidine nucleotide synthesis. It has been used extensively in the treatment of various solid tumors (breast, tongue, pharynx, testes) and trophoblastic disease in women, as well as in the management of acute lymphoblastic leukemia in children. Common toxicities with high dose therapy include myelosuppression, renal toxicity, and hepatitis progressing to cirrhosis. Monitoring of the drug by RIA, EIA, or FPIA has substantially reduced patient mortality. Serum concentrations obtained 24 to 48 hours after administration reflect the extent of drug clearance and serum concentration. This is necessary in cases of rescue therapy to assess how much leucovorin (a folate analog) should be given. Criteria for methotrexate blood concentration indicative of a potential for toxicity after a single bolus, high dose therapy (>50 mg/m^2) are: (1) 10 μmol/L, 24 hours after dose; (2) greater than 1 μmol/L at 48 hours; and (3) greater than 0.1 μmol/L, 72 hours after dose.

Immunosuppressants

Cyclosporine (Cyclosporin A, Sandimmune). Cyclosporine is a cyclic peptide with 11 amino acid residues, isolated from the fungus *Tolypocladium inflatum*. The drug has been demonstrated to be effective in suppressing host-versus-graft rejection in organ transplants mainly by inhibiting the proliferation of lymphocytes due to the suppression of interleukin-2 production. Cyclosporine is 90% bound to blood cells or protein and has a low bioavailability with only about 36% of an oral dose being absorbed (Cohen, et al., 1984). There is a poor relationship between dose and whole blood concentration, and careful monitoring is required because the drug has inherent nephrotoxicity and hepatotoxicity. Cyclosporine blood concentrations have been reported to rise with concomitant treatment with amphotericin B and ketoconazole.

The methodology for cyclosporine determination and for the determination of the parent drug plus metabolites (of which there are more than 20) involves RIA with monoclonal antibodies supplied by Sandoz (East Hanover, NJ) and tritiated drug used as label. Also, an RIA is available with an iodinated label for measurement of the parent drug as well as various HPLC methods. As well as RIA, cyclosporine determinations by EMIT and FPIA are now available as alternatives to time-consuming HPLC procedures (McBride, et al., 1992).

Cyclosporine G.   Cyclosporine G (CsG) is a derivative of cyclosporine with the valine at position 2 on the molecule replaced by isoleucine. CsG has been demonstrated to be less nephrotoxic than cyclosporine and is now in clinical trials for use after renal transplantation. CsG levels are easily measured by RIA and FPIA for cyclosporine as the monoclonal antibody used in these assays cross-reacts strongly with CsG (Yatscoff, et al., 1993).

FK506 (Prograf).   FK506 isolated from the fungal strain *Streptomyces tsukubaensis*, has been shown to be a macrolide lactone with a hemiketal-masked-α, β-diketoamide incorporated into a 23 member ring (Kino, et al., 1987). The drug displays less nephrotoxicity, hepatoxicity and hypertensive episodes than cyclosporine, and its mode of action is thought to be as a potent inhibitor of peptidyl-prolyl *cis-trans* isomerase, an enzyme involved in accelerating the folding of intracellular proteins into their biologically active conformations in lymphocytes (Takahashi, et al., 1989). As FK506 is extensively metabolized by the liver and has limited and erratic bioavailability because of its hydrophobic nature and large "first-pass effect," it requires extensive therapeutic monitoring when in use. The time to peak concentration is usually 0.5 to 4 hours with a mean absorption of 27%. A rapid whole blood assay for FK506 with the IMx analyzer has also been developed (Abbott Laboratories, Chicago, ILL) (Grenier, et al., 1991). FK506 may also be measured by EIA (Wallemacq, et al., 1993).

DRUGS OF ABUSE

Acetaminophen

Acetaminophen (Tylenol) is widely used as a nonprescription analgesic, which is rapidly absorbed orally with a peak concentration observed 2 hours after ingestion. It is metabolized primarily by glucuronic acid conjugation and when taken in overdosage may produce liver toxicity due to the accumulation of the oxidative metabolite, *N*-acetyl-imidoquinone. *N*-Acetylcysteine provides an analog of glutathione and can be used a direct sequestering agent. When the serum level is greater than 930 mmol/L (150 μg/mL) at 4 hours, antidotal treatment is highly recommended.

Benzodiazepines

This class of compounds includes *diazepam* (Valium), *flurazepam* (Dalmane), *halazepam* (Paxipam), *alprazolam* (Xanax), *chlordiazepoxide* (Librium), and *lorazepam* (Ativan), which are administered for the relief of anxiety, insomnia, and for the control of epilepsy. The therapeutic effects of these drugs involve modulation of γ-aminobutyric acid. They are prescribed because of their low incidence of addiction and toxicity and as such, routine monitoring is not performed; however their levels are determined in assessing abuse. Toxicity is usually associated with serum levels of 18 to 70 μmol/L (5 to 20 μg/mL).

Barbiturates

Barbiturates are high on the list of leading offenders among overdose cases admitted to the emergency room. Since barbiturates are chemically similar to drugs with hypnotic, anticonvulsant and sedative properties, they are frequently used in suicide attempts. Structurally, they are substituted pyrimidine-ring compounds and may be classified as long acting (>6 hours, phenobarbital and mephobarbital), intermediate (3 to 6 hours, amobarbital and butabarbital), short acting <3 hours, pentobarbital, secobarbital) and ultrashort acting (10 minutes, thiopental).

Immunoassays may be used to determine levels of phenobarbital or total barbiturates. Immunoassays for total barbiturates are characterized by a list of drugs and the concentration of each giving a positive result; many are very sensitive to secobarbital. Barbiturates may be measured individually by differential ultraviolet spectrophotometric methods, gas-liquid chromatography (GLC), or HPLC.

Lethal blood levels are 16.3 to 21.7 μmol/L (30 to 40 μg/mL) for short-acting types, greater than 16.5 μmol/L (30 μg/mL) for intermediate-acting types and 35 to 64 μmol/L (80 to 150 μg/mL) for long-acting barbiturates (Pappas, et al., 1991).

Amphetamines

Amphetamine and its homolog methamphetamine are both phenylethylamine derivatives capable of central nervous system stimulation, and they have few legitimate uses. Other phenylethylamines are frequently used as decongestants, appetite suppressants, and antidepressants and may be abused for their hallucinogenic properties. Amphetamine and methamphetamine may be measured by GLC; however, the availability of rapid immunoassays enables the clinical laboratory to screen for these drugs by FPIA and EMIT techniques, which have a cutoff detection level of 2.22 μmol/L (300 ng/mL).

Cannabinoids

The primary active ingredient in marijuana is Δ^9-tetrahydrocannabinol (THC). THC is extremely lipophilic and is readily sequestered into the adipose tissue where it is slowly released into the circulation. The primary urinary metabolite measured in drug screening is 11-nor-Δ^9-THC-9 carboxylic acid. The peak effect of smoking THC occurs after 20 to 30 minutes and the effect may last up to 120 minutes after one cigarette. Urinary metabolites may be detected by immunoassay up to 310 days after smoking, and factors such as frequency and the amount smoked have an effect. Currently the sensitivity of FPIA using the Abbott AD_x is 0.07 μmol/L (25 ng/mL) and the sensitivity of EMIT using the Syva ETS is 0.28 μmol/L (100 ng/mL) for cannabinoid detection.

Cocaine

Cocaine is currently one of the most widely abused members of the Class I drugs and it has been established that over 20 million individuals in the United States have used the drug, with an addiction rate of 10%. The most common form of administration is by insufflation but the free base form of cocaine may be inhaled after heating and smoking. Urine may be screened for the presence of the principal urinary metabolite benzoylecgonine. Current immunoassays, both FPIA and EMIT, can detect the metabolite with an assay sensitivity of 1.39 μmol/L (200 ng/mL).

Opiates and Opioids

This class of drugs includes opiates (codeine and morphine), opioids derived from morphine (heroin, hydromorphone, and oxycodone) and the synthetic narcotics (fentanyl, meperidine, methadone, and propoxyphene). They are all well absorbed from the gastrointestinal tract and are metabolized in the liver where conjugation occurs with glucuronide or sulfate. In situations of opiate overdose, administration of naloxone will reverse coma, respiratory depression, and hypotensive episodes. Opiates and opioids are readily detected in the urine by FPIA or EMIT, although for toxicologic and forensic purposes, techniques such as gas chromatography (GC), HPLC, and GC/mass spectrometry are used. Therapeutic concentrations of morphine range from 0.18 to 0.23 mmol/L (0.07 to 0.08 μg/L) in serum and from 1.42 to 28.4 mmol/L (0.5 to 10 mg/L) in urine.

Phencyclidine

Phencyclidine (PCP, Sernyl) is structurally related to ketamine and is a highly popular drug of abuse taken in 1 to 3 mg amounts, usually by smoking. These doses typically result in lethargy, disorientation, loss of coordination, and hallucinations. PCP undergoes oxidative metabolism to inactive metabolites and by 72 hours 30% to

50% of a labeled intravenous dose is eliminated in the urine as unchanged drug (4% to 19%) and conjugated metabolites (25% to 30%). Only 2% of a dose is excreted in feces (Baselt and Cravey, 1989). In severe cases of overdose, acidification of blood and urine, usually by administration of ascorbic acid, causes a shift of PCP out of the brain and enhances renal excretion. The drug may be detected in urine by immunoassay and the usual cutoff value for detection is 308 nmol/L (75 µg/L) by both FPIA and EMIT.

Salicylate (Aspirin)

Aspirin is responsible for more cases of accidental poisoning in children than any other drug. Toxic doses produce a stimulation of the central nervous system, usually reflected by hyperventilation, flushing, and fever. Clinically, these symptoms may be thought to be due to infection and further aspirin administered may complicate the status of the patient.

Salicylate is also monitored in rheumatoid arthritis and other inflammatory diseases to achieve effective blood concentrations. Those patients with excessive salicylate ingestion and tinnitus usually have serum levels of 2.9 to 3.6 mmol/L (400 to 500 mg/L) and require hospitalization; levels of greater than 36 mmol/L (5 g/L) are associated with significant mortality. Classic methods for salicylate determinations include spectrophotometry and HPLC, although the drug may now be rapidly measured by FPIA using the Abbott TD$_x$ analyzer.

REFERENCES

Ackerman B, Pappas, AA. Therapeutic drug monitoring. In: Howanitz JH, Howanitz PJ, eds. Laboratory Medicine Test Selection and Interpretation. New York: Churchill Livingstone, 1991;13:333–368.

Agbato OA, Elyas AA, Patsalos PN, Brett EM, Lascelles PT. Total and free serum concentrations of carbamazepine and carbamazepine 10,11-epoxide in children with epilepsy. Arch Neurol 1986;43:1111–1116.

Anderson JL, Harrison DC, Meffin PJ, Winkle RA. Antiarrhythmic drugs: clinical pharmacology and therapeutic uses. Drugs 1978;15:271–276.

Anderson JL, Stewart JR, Perry BA, et al. Oral fecainide acetate for the treatment of ventricular arrhythmias. N Engl J Med 1981;305:473–477.

Baselt RC, Cravey RH. Phencyclidine. In: Baselt RC, Cravey RH, eds. Disposition of toxic drugs and chemicals in man. Chicago: Year Book Medical Publishers, 1989;661–663.

Berk LS, Imperio N, Eby WC. Evaluation of the powder-formulated enzyme multiplied immunoassay technique: quantitative single test for gentamicin. Ther Drug Monit 1986;8:111–114.

Blecka LJ, Shaffer M, Dworschack R. Inhibition enzyme immunoassays for the quantitation of various haptens: a review. In: Avramas S, ed. Immunoenzymatic Techniques. New York: Elsevier Science Publishers, 1983;207–214.

Blecka LJ, Jackson GJ. Immunoassays in therapeutic drug monitoring. In: Gerson B, ed. Clinics in Laboratory Medicine. Philadelphia: WB Saunders, 1987;7:357–370.

Boscato LM, Stuart MC. Heterophilic antibodies: a problem for all immunoassays. Clin Chem 1988;34:27–33.

Cohen DT, Loertscher R, Rubin MF, Tilney NL, Carpenter CB, Strom TB. Cyclosporine: a new immunosuppressive agent for organ transplantation. Ann Intern Med 1984;101: 667–682.

Cramer JA, Mattson RH, Bennett DM, Swick CT. Variable free and total valproic acid concentrations in sole- and multi-drug therapy. Ther Drug Monit 1986;8:411–415.

Eadie MJ. Laboratory control of anticonvulsant drugs. Drugs 1974;8:386–397.

Giegel JL, Brotherton MM. Solid phase system for ligand assay. U.S. Patent 4, 1985;517:288.

Gosling JP. A decade of development in immunoassay methodology (review). Clin Chem 1990;36:1408–1427.

Graves SW. Endogenous digitalis-like factors. Crit Rev Clin Lab Sci 1986;23:177–200.

Grenier FC, Luizkiw J, Bergmann M, et al. A whole blood FK506 assay for the IM_x® analyzer. Transplant Proc 1991;23:2748–2749.

Hendeles L, Weinberger M. Theophylline: a "state of the art" review. Pharmacotherapy 1983;3:2–44.

Howanitz JH, Howanitz PJ. Antiarrhythmic drug monitoring. In: Henry JB, ed. Clinics in Laboratory Medicine. Philadelphia: WB Saunders, 1981;501–522.

Jolley ME, Stroupe SD, Wang CHJ, et al. Fluorescence polarization immunoassay. I. Monitoring aminoglycoside antibiotics in serum and plasma. Clin Chem 1981;27:1190–1197.

Khanna PL, Dworschack RT, Manning WB, Harris JD. A new homogenous enzyme immunoassay using recombinant enzyme fragments. Clin Chem Acta 1989;185:231–240.

Kino T, Hatanaka H, Hashimoto M, et al. FK506, a novel immunosuppressant isolated from Streptomyces. I. Fermentation, isolation and physiochemical and biological characteristics. J Antibiot (Tokyo) 1987;40:1249–1255.

Lesar TS, Rotchafer JC, Strand LM, Solem L, Zaske D. Gentamicin dosing errors with four commonly used nomograms. JAMA 1982;248:1190–1193.

Levy RH, Schmidt D. Utility of free level monitoring of antiepileptic drugs. Epilepsia 1985;26:199–205.

Longerich L, Vasder S, Johnson E, Gault MH. Disposable-column radioimmunoassay for serum digoxin with less interference from metabolites and endogenous digitalis-like factors. Clin Chem 1988;34:2211–2216.

Louis S, Kutt H, McDowell F. Intravenous diphenylhydantoin in experimental seizures. II. Effect on penicillin induced seizures in the cat. Arch Neurol 1968;18:472–477.

McBride JH, Kim SS, Rodgerson DO, Reyes AF, Ota MK. Measurement of cyclosporine by liquid chromatography and three immunoassays in blood from liver, cardiac and renal transplant recipients. Clin Chem 1992;38:2300–2306.

Moyer TP, Pippenger CE, Blanke RV, Blouin RA. Therapeutic drug monitoring. In: Tietz NW, ed. Fundamentals of Clinical Chemistry. Philadelphia: WB Saunders, 1987;26: 842–868.

O'Bey KA, Jim LK, Gee JP, Johnson R. Temperature dependence of the stability of tobramycin mixed with penicillins in human serum. Am J Hosp Pharm 1982;39:1005–1008.

Pappas AA, Taylor EH, Ackerman B. Toxicology and drugs of abuse. In: Howanitz JH, Howanitz PJ, eds. Laboratory Medicine Test Selection and Interpretation. New York: Churchill Livingstone, 1991;14:369–398.

Price CP. Analytical techniques for therapeutic drug monitoring. Clin Biochem 1984;17: 52–56.

Sandrzadeh SMH, Vincenzi FF, Dasgupta A, Amhad S, Kenny M. Biochemical characterization of digoxin-like immunoreactive substances. Clin Chem 1988;34:1222–1223.

Schultz SG, Hollen JT, Donohue JP, Francoeur TA. Two-dimensional centrifugation for desktop clinical chemistry. Clin Chem 1985;31:1457–1463.

Shaykh M, Bazilinski N, McCaul DS, Ahmed S. Fluorescent substances in uremic and normal serum. Clin Chem 1985;31:1988–1992.

Siddoway LA, Woosely RL. Clinical pharmacokinetics of disopyramide. Clin Pharmacokinet 1986;11:214–222.

Takahashi N, Hagano T, Suzuki M. Peptidyl-prolyl cis-trans isomerase is the cyclosporine A binding protein cyclophilin. Nature 1989;337:473–475.

Valdes R. Endogenous digoxin-like immunoreactive factors: impact on digoxin measurements and potential physiological implications. Clin Chem 1985;31:1525–1532.

Wallemacq PE, Firdaous I, Hassoun A. Improvement and assessment of enzyme-linked immunosorbent assay to detect low FK506 concentration in plasma or whole blood within 6 hours. Clin Chem 1993;39:1045–1049.

Weber TH, Käpyaho KI, Tanner P. Endogenous interference in immunoassays in clinical chemistry: a review. Scand J Clin Lab Invest 1990; 50 (suppl 201):77–82.

Yatscoff RW, Langman LJ, LeGatt DF. Cross-reactivities of cyclosporin G (NVa^2 cyclosporin) and metabolites in cyclosporin A immunoassays. Clin Chem 1993;39:1089–1092.

Zuk RF, Ginsberg VK, Houts T, et al. Enzyme immunochromatography—a quantitative immunoassay requiring no instrumentation. Clin Chem 1985;31:1144–1150.

Appendix 1

Endocrine S.I. Unit Conversion Table
Part 1: To S.I. Units

Hormone	When You Know	Multiply By	To Find
ACTH (Corticotropin)	pg/mL	0.2222	pmol/L
Antidiuretic hormone (ADH)	pg/mL	0.9225	pmol/L
Albumin	g/dL	10.0000	g/L
Aldosterone, serum	ng/dL	27.7469	pmol/L
Aldosterone, urine	μg/24 h	2.7747	nmol/day
Aldosterone/creatinine	μg/g	0.3139	nmol/mmol
Androstanediol	ng/dL	34.1997	pmol/L
Androstanediol glucuronide	ng/dL	21.3447	pmol/L
Androstenedione	ng/dL	34.9162	pmol/L
Androsterone, urine	mg/24 h	3.4423	μmol/day
Androsterone/creatinine	mg/g	0.3894	μmol/mmol
Angiotensin-I	pg/mL	0.7716	pmol/L
Angiotensin-II	pg/mL	0.9560	pmol/L
Angiotensin-III	pg/mL	1.0741	pmol/L
Angiotensin I converting enzyme	mU/mL	1.0000	U/L
Atrial natriuretic peptide (ANP)	pg/mL	0.3247	pmol/L
C-Peptide	ng/mL	0.3310	nmol/L
C-Peptide, urine	ng/mL	0.3310	nmol/L
C-Peptide/creatinine	μg/g	0.0374	nmol/mmol
Calcitonin	pg/mL	0.2926	pmol/L
Calcium	mg/dL	0.2495	nmol/L
Calcium, urine	mg/24 h	0.0250	mmol/d
Catecholamines, urine	μg/24 h	5.6770	nmol/d
Catecholamines/creatinine	μg/g	0.6422	nmol/mmol
Corticosterone	ng/dL	28.8600	pmol/L
18-Hydroxycorticosterone	ng/dL	27.5938	pmol/L
Cortisol, serum	μg/dL	27.5862	nmol/L
Cortisol, urine	μg/24 h	2.7586	nmol/d
Cortisol/creatinine	μg/g	0.3121	nmol/mmol
Cortisone	ng/dL	27.7393	pmol/L
Creatinine, urine	mg/24 h	8.8420	μmol/d
Cyclic AMP, urine	nmol/mL	1.000	μmol/L

Endocrine S.I. Unit Conversion Table *(continued)*

Hormone	When You Know	Multiply By	To Find
Cyclic AMP/creatinine	μmol/g	113.1000	nmol/mmol
Dehydroepiandrosterone (DHEA)	ng/dL	34.6741	pmol/L
Dehydroepiandrosterone sulfate (DHEAS)	μg/dL	27.2109	nmol/L
Deoxycorticosterone (DOC)	ng/dL	30.2572	pmol/L
18-Hydroxydeoxycorticosterone (18-OH-DOC)	ng/dL	28.8600	pmol/L
11-Desoxycortisol (Compound S)	ng/dL	28.8684	pmol/L
Dexamethasone	ng/dL	25.4777	pmol/L
Dihydrotestosterone	ng/dL	34.4353	pmol/L
Dopamine, plasma	pg/mL	6.5359	pmol/L
Dopamine, urine	μg/24 h	6.5359	nmol/day
Dopamine/creatinine	μg/g	0.7392	nmol/mmol
Endorphin, BETA	pg/mL	0.2500	pmol/L
Epinephrine, plasma	pg/mL	5.4615	pmol/L
Epinephrine, urine	μg/24 h	˙5.4615	nmol/d
Epinephrine/creatinine	μg/g	0.6178	nmol/mmol
Estradiol	ng/dL	36.7107	pmol/L
Estriol	ng/dL	34.6741	pmol/L
Estrogens, serum	ng/dL	36.8450	pmol/L
Estrone	ng/dL	36.9822	pmol/L
Estrone sulfate	ng/dL	28.6123	pmol/L
Folic acid	ng/dL	22.6552	pmol/L
Follicle-stimulating hormone, (FSH)	mIU/mL	1.0000	IU/L
Follicle-stimulating hormone, urine	IU/24 h	1.0000	IU/d
FSH/creatinine	IU/g	0.1131	IU/mmol
Gastrin	pg/mL	1.0000	ng/L
Glucagon	pg/mL	1.0000	ng/L
Growth hormone	ng/mL	1.0000	μg/L
Human chorionic gonadotrophin (HCG)	mIU/mL	1.0000	IU/L
HCG, urine	IU/24 h	1.0000	IU/day
HCG/creatinine	IU/g	0.1131	IU/mmol
5-Hydroxyindole acetic acid (5-HIAA), urine	μg/24 h	5.2301	nmol/day
5-HIAA/creatinine	μg/g	0.5915	nmol/mmol
Homovanillic acid (HVA), urine	μg/24 h	5.4885	nmol/day
HVA/creatinine	μg/g	0.6207	nmol/mmol
17-Hydroxycorticosteroids, urine	μg24 h	2.7586	nmol/day
17-Hydroxycorticosteroids/ creatinine	μg/g	0.3121	nmol/mmol
IGF-I (Somatomedin-C)	ng/mL	0.1307	nmol/L

Endocrine S.I. Unit Conversion Table (*continued*)

Hormone	When You Know	Multiply By	To Find
IGF-II	ng/mL	0.1333	nmol/L
Inhibin	U/mL	1000	U/L
Insulin	μU/mL	7.1750	pmol/L
17-Ketosteroids, urine	mg/24 h	3.4674	μmol/day
17-Ketosteroids/creatinine	mg/g	0.3922	μmol/mmol
Luteinizing hormone (LH)	mIU/mL	1.0000	IU/L
Luteinizing hormone, urine	IU/24 h	1.0000	IU/day
LH/creatinine	IU/g	0.1131	IU/mmol
Metanephrine, urine	μg/24 h	5.0710	nmol/day
Metanephrine/creatinine	μg/g	0.5736	nmol/mmol
Metanephrines, total, urine	μg/24 h	5.2576	nmol/day
Metanephrines, total/creatinine	μg/g	0.5948	nmol/mmol
Methoxytyramine, urine	μg/24 h	5.9809	nmol/day
Methoxytyramine/creatinine	μg/g	0.6764	nmol/mmol
Norepinephrine, plasma	pg/mL	5.9100	pmol/L
Norepinephrine, urine	μg/24 h	5.9100	nmol/day
Norepinephrine/creatinine	μg/g	0.6685	nmol/mmol
Normetanephrine, urine	μg/24 h	5.4585	nmol/day
Normetanephrine/creatinine	μg/g	0.6175	nmol/mmol
Osteocalcin	ng/mL	0.1538	nmol/L
Parathyroid hormone	pg/mL	0.1053	pmol/L
Prednisolone	ng/dL	27.7393	pmol/L
Prednisone	ng/dL	27.9018	pmol/L
Pregnanediol, urine	mg/24 h	3.1201	μmol/d
Pregnanediol/creatinine	mg/g	0.3530	μmol/mmol
Pregnanetriol, urine	mg/24 h	2.9718	μmol/day
Pregnanetriol/creatinine	mg/g	0.3362	μmol/mmol
Pregnenolone	ng/dL	31.5956	pmol/L
17-Hydroxypregnenolone	ng/dL	30.0752	pmol/L
Progesterone	ng/dL	31.7965	pmol/L
17-Hydroxyprogesterone	ng/dL	30.2572	pmol/L
20-Hydroxyprogesterone	ng/dL	31.5956	pmol/L
Prolactin	ng/mL	1.0000	μg/L
Renin (plasma renin activity)	ng/mL/h	0.2778	ng/L/sec
Reverse T_3	ng/dL	15.3610	pmol/L
Secretin	pg/mL	0.3273	pmol/L
Somatostatin-14	pg/mL	0.6105	pmol/L
Somatostatin-28	pg/mL	0.3053	pmol/L
Testosterone-estrogen binding globulin (TeBG) (binding capacity)	μg/dL	34.6741	nmol/L
Testosterone	ng/dL	34.6741	pmol/L
Free testosterone	pg/mL	3.4674	pmol/L
Testosterone, urine	μg/24 h	3.4674	nmol/day

Endocrine S.I. Unit Conversion Table (*continued*)

Hormone	When You Know	Multiply By	To Find
Testosterone/creatinine	μg/g	0.3922	nmol/mmol
Thyroglobulin	ng/mL	1.0000	μg/L
Thyroid-stimulating hormone (TSH)	μU/mL	1.0000	mU/L
Thyroxine (T_4)	μg/dL	12.8717	nmol/L
Thyroxine-binding globulin	mg/dL	10.0000	mg/L
TSH releasing hormone (TRH)	pg/mL	2.7624	pmol/L
Triiodothyronine (T_3)	ng/dL	15.3610	pmol/L
Vanillylmandelic acid (VMA), urine	μg/24 h	5.0454	nmol/day
VMA/creatinine	μg/g	0.5706	nmol/mmol
Vitamin B_{12}	ng/dL	7.3779	pmol/L
25-Hydroxyvitamin D	ng/mL	2.4963	nmol/L
1,25-Dihydroxyvitamin D	pg/mL	2.4004	pmol/L

Endocrine S.I. Unit Conversion Table
Part 2: From S.I. Units

Hormone	When You Know	Multiply By	To Find
ACTH (Corticotropin)	pmol/L	4.5000	pg/mL
Antidiuretic hormone (ADH)	pmol/L	1.0840	pg/mL
Albumin	g/L	0.1000	g/dL
Aldosterone, serum	pmol/L	0.0360	ng/dL
Aldosterone, urine	nmol/day	0.3604	μg/24 h
Aldosterone/creatinine	nmol/mmol	3.1859	μg/g
Androstanediol	pmol/L	0.0292	ng/dL
Androstanediol glucuronide	pmol/L	0.0469	ng/dL
Androstenedione	pmol/L	0.0286	ng/dL
Androsterone, urine	μmol/day	0.2905	mg/24 h
Androsterone/creatinine	μmol/mmol	2.5680	mg/g
Angiotensin-I	pmol/L	1.2960	pg/mL
Angiotensin-II	pmol/L	1.0460	pg/mL
Angiotensin-III	pmol/L	0.9310	pg/mL
Angiotensin I converting enzyme	U/L	1.0000	mU/mL
Atrial natriuretic peptide (ANP)	pmol/L	3.0800	pg/mL
C-Peptide	nmol/L	3.0210	ng/mL
C-Peptide, urine	nmol/L	3.0210	ng/mL
C-Peptide/creatinine	nmol/mmol	26.7109	μg/g
Calcitonin	pmol/L	3.4180	pg/mL
Calcium	mmol	4.0080	mg/dL

Endocrine S.I. Unit Conversion Table (*continued*)

Hormone	When You Know	Multiply By	To Find
Calcium, urine	mmol/day	40.0800	mg/24 h
Catecholamines, urine	nmol/day	0.1762	μg/24 h
Catecholamines/creatinine	nmol/mmol	1.5572	μg/g
Corticosterone	pmol/L	0.0347	ng/dL
18-Hydroxycorticosterone	pmol/L	0.0362	ng/dL
Cortisol, serum	nmol/L	0.0363	μg/dL
Cortisol, urine	nmol/day	0.3625	μg/24 h
Cortisol/creatinine	nmol/mmol	3.2045	μg/g
Cortisone	pmol/L	0.0361	ng/dL
Creatinine, urine	μmol/d	0.1131	mg/24 h
Cyclic AMP, urine	μmol/L	1.0000	nmol/mL
Cyclic AMP/creatinine	nmol/mmol	0.0088	μmol/g
Dehydroepiandrosterone (DHEA)	pmol/L	0.0288	ng/dL
Dehydroepiandrosterone sulfate (DHEAS)	nmol/L	0.0368	μg/dL
Deoxycorticosterone (DOC)	pmol/L	0.0331	ng/dL
18-Hydroxydeoxycorticosterone (18-OH-DOC)	pmol/L	0.0347	ng/dL
11-Desoxycortisol (Compound S)	pmol/L	0.0346	ng/dL
Dexamethasone	pmol/L	0.0393	ng/dL
Dihydrotestosterone	pmol/L	0.0290	ng/dL
Dopamine, plasma	pmol/L	0.1530	pg/mL
Dopamine, urine	nmol/day	0.1530	μg/24 h
Dopamine/creatinine	nmol/mmol	1.3528	μg/g
Endorphin, BETA	pmol/L	4.0000	pg/mL
Epinephrine, plasma	pmol/L	0.1831	pg/mL
Epinephrine, urine	nmol/day	0.1831	μg/24 h
Epinephrine/creatinine	nmol/mmol	1.6186	μg/g
Estradiol	pmol/L	0.0272	ng/dL
Estriol	pmol/L	0.0288	ng/dL
Estrogens, serum	pmol/L	0.0271	ng/dL
Estrone	pmol/L	0.0270	ng/dL
Estrone sulfate	pmol/L	0.0350	ng/dL
Folic acid	pmol/L	0.0441	ng/dL
Follicle-stimulating hormone, (FSH)	IU/L	1.0000	mIU/mL
Follicle-stimulating hormone, urine	IU/day	1.0000	IU/24 h
FSH creatinine	IU/mmol	8.8420	IU/g
Gastrin	ng/L	1.0000	pg/mL
Glucagon	ng/L	1.0000	pg/mL
Growth hormone	μg/L	1.0000	ng/mL
Human chorionic gonadotrophin (HCG)	IU/L	1.0000	mIU/mL

Endocrine S.I. Unit Conversion Table (*continued*)

Hormone	When You Know	Multiply By	To Find
HCG, urine	IU/day	1.0000	IU/24 h
HCG/creatinine	IU/mmol	8.8420	IU/g
5-Hydroxyindole acetic acid (5-HIAA), urine	nmol/day	0.1912	μg/24 h
5-HIAA/creatinine	nmol/mmol	1.6906	μg/g
Homovanillic acid (HVA), urine	nmol/day	0.1822	μg/24 h
HVA/creatinine	nmol/mmol	1.6110	μg/g
17-Hydroxycorticosteroids, urine	nmol/day	0.3625	μg/24 h
17-Hydroxycorticosteroids/ creatinine	nmol/mmol	3.2045	μg/g
IGF-I (Somatomedin-C)	nmol/L	7.6490	ng/mL
IGF-II	nmol/L	7.5000	ng/mL
Inhibin	U/L	0.0010	U/mL
Insulin	pmol/L	0.1394	μU/mL
17-Ketosteroids, urine	μmol/day	0.2884	mg/24 h
17-Ketosteroids/creatinine	μmol/mmol	2.5495	mg/g
Luteinizing hormone (LH)	IU/L	1.0000	mIU/mL
Luteinizing hormone, urine	IU/day	1.0000	IU/24 h
LH/creatinine	IU/mmol	8.8420	IU/g
Metanephrine, urine	nmol/day	0.1972	μg/24 h
Metanephrine/creatinine	nmol/mmol	1.7432	μg/g
Metanephrines, total, urine	nmol/day	0.1902	μg/24 h
Metanephrines, total/creatinine	nmol/mmol	1.6814	μg/g
Methoxytramine, urine	nmol/day	0.1672	μg/24 h
Methoxytramine/creatinine	nmol/mmol	1.4786	μg/g
Norepinephrine, plasma	pmol/L	0.1692	pg/mL
Norepinephrine, urine	nmol/day	0.1692	μg/24 h
Norepinephrine/creatinine	nmol/mmol	1.4957	μg/g
Normetanephrine, urine	nmol/day	0.1832	μg/24 h
Normetanephrine/creatinine	nmol/mmol	1.6195	μg/g
Osteocalcin	nmol/L	6.5000	ng/mL
Parathyroid hormone	pmol/L	9.5000	pg/mL
Prednisolone	pmol/L	0.0361	ng/dL
Prednisone	pmol/L	0.0358	ng/dL
Pregnanediol, urine	μmol/d	0.3205	mg/24 h
Pregnanediol/creatinine	μmol/mmol	2.8332	mg/g
Pregnanetriol, urine	μmol/day	0.3365	mg/24 h
Pregnanetriol/creatinine	μmol/mmol	2.9747	mg/g
Pregnenolone	pmol/L	0.0317	ng/dL
17-Hydroxypregnenolone	pmol/L	0.0333	ng/dL
Progesterone	pmol/L	0.0315	ng/dL
17-Hydroxyprogesterone	pmol/L	0.0331	ng/dL
20-Hydroxyprogesterone	pmol/L	0.0317	ng/dL
Prolactin	μg/L	1.0000	ng/mL

Endocrine S.I. Unit Conversion Table (*continued*)

Hormone	When You Know	Multiply By	To Find
Renin (plasma renin activity)	ng/L/sec	3.6000	ng/mL/h
Reverse T_3	pmol/L	0.0651	ng/dL
Secretin	pmol/L	3.0550	pg/mL
Somatostatin-14	pmol/L	1.6380	pg/mL
Somatostatin-28	pmol/L	3.2760	pg/mL
Testosterone-estrogen binding globulin (TeBG) (binding capacity)	nmol/L	0.0288	µg/dL
Testosterone	pmol/L	0.0288	ng/dL
Free testosterone	pmol/L	0.2884	pg/mL
Testosterone, urine	nmol/day	0.2884	µg/24 h
Testosterone/creatinine	nmol/mmol	2.5496	µg/g
Thyroglobulin	µg/L	1.0000	ng/mL
Thyroid-stimulating hormone (TSH)	mU/L	1.0000	µU/mL
Thyroxine (T_4)	nmol/L	0.0777	µg/dL
Thyroxine-binding globulin	mg/L	0.1000	mg/dL
TSH releasing hormone (TRH)	pmol/L	0.3620	pg/mL
Triiodothyronine (T_3)	pmol/L	0.0651	ng/dL
Vanillylmandelic acid (VMA), urine	nmol/day	0.1982	µg/24 h
VMA/creatinine	nmol/mmol	1.7525	µg/g
Vitamin B_{12}	pmol/L	0.1355	ng/dL
25-Hydroxyvitamin D	nmol/L	0.4006	ng/mL
1,25-Dihydroxyvitamin D	pmol/L	0.4166	pg/mL

Index